Community Mental Health in Texas: Four Case Studies

by the

Policy Research Project

on

Financing Care

for the

Chronically Mentally Ill

Sponsored by

Hogg Foundation for Mental Health

and

Commission on the Community

Care of the Mentally Ill

Special Project Report

Lyndon B. Johnson School of Public Affairs

The University of Texas at Austin

ISBN: 0-89940-869-9
Library of Congress Catalog Card No.: 90-61734

Printed in the U.S.A.

Cover design by María de la Luz Martínez
and Carol Sjollema

Project Participants

Students

Jana Biasi, B.A. (Political Science), North Texas State University

Charles Blissett, Ph.D. (Pharmacy/Microbiology), University of Florida at Gainsville

Hugh F. Crean, B.A. (Psychology), St. Michaels College

Pamela Diamond, M.A. (Psychology), Texas Women's University

Kathleen A. Fahey, A.B. (Psychology), Occidental College

Minh Ly Griffin, B.A. (Plan II), University of Texas

Joellen Harper, B.A. (Economics and Government), Skidmore College

Nicholas C. Hoover, B.A. (Sociology), Trinity University

Ronnie Jung, B.B.A. (Accounting), University of Texas at Austin

Carolina Martinez, B.A. (Political Science, Psychology), Pan American University

Lynn Parrish, B.A., University of Pennsylvania

Jan Rienstra, B.A., (Chemistry), University of Texas at Austin

Norma Rodriguez, B.A. (Psychology), University of Texas at Austin

Timothy J. Tompkins, B.A. (Spanish, Business), Appalachian State University and The University of Madrid, Spain

Rudolfo R. Vega, B.A. (Psychology), San Jose State University

Project Directors

David Warner, Ph.D., Professor, Lyndon B. Johnson School of Public Affairs

L. Connie Harris, Ph.D., Participating Faculty, Hogg Foundation for Mental Health (Fall 1988)

Scott Kier, Ph.D., Participating Faculty, Hogg Foundation for Mental Health (Spring 1989)

Reymundo Rodriguez, M.Ed., M.P.A., Participating Faculty, Hogg Foundation for Mental Health

Contents

List of Tables

List of Figures

Preface

This volume of case studies of three community mental health and mental retardation centers and one state hospital outreach center in Texas is part of a larger study on financing care for the chronically mentally ill in Texas, which was conducted as a Policy Research Project during 1988 and 1989 at the LBJ School of Public Affairs at the University of Texas at Austin. The longer study, entitled Financing Community Care for the Chronically Mentally Ill in Texas, analyzes the clients, services, and financing of care in the state as a whole. This volume is an offshoot of that. As we began to study the broader topic, we came to the conclusion that we needed to go into the field to understand how these services were arranged at the community level.

In Texas the community-level entity is the community mental health and mental retardation center (CMHMRC). We decided to study three fairly diverse community centers and one state hospital outreach center. In the fall and winter of 1988-89, groups of students visited each of the three community centers (San Angelo, Dallas, and Tri-County in Conroe) and the San Antonio State Hospital Outreach Center several times. These visits and the help provided by persons at all levels of the system helped us immeasurably and made the issues far less "theoretical" than they had been before. We hope this volume will provide the reader with some of this same specificity and understanding.

The genesis of the larger project was in the fall of 1987, when Reymundo Rodriguez, who was also one of the participating faculty for the project, and Wayne Holtzman encouraged me to develop this project to be a parallel activity to the Commission on the Chronically Mentally Ill in Texas, which the Hogg Foundation had formed earlier in the year. The primary sources of funding for the entire project were the Hogg Foundation and the University of Texas. Other funding has been provided by the John Sharpe Fellowship, the Mike Hogg Endowment, and the Wilbur Cohen Professorship at the LBJ School of Public Affairs.

The process of doing the research and writing up our findings has been an educational process for everyone involved. We hope that the results will help others to understand the issues and institutions involved and lead to more services at the community level for the chronically mentally ill.

David C. Warner
December 1989

Acknowledgments

The work of the students who wrote this volume was enhanced and made possible by a large number of persons at the community centers, in state government, and elsewhere who graciously answered questions and provided guidance at each point of the project.

Although many of the students worked hard throughout the project, several should be mentioned for their continuing and outstanding contributions. Jan Rienstra was in many ways the de facto director of this project. She contributed her experience, her insights, and her hard work to making sure that we treated this project seriously and completely. Pam Diamond, Nicholas Hoover, and Hugh Crean also continued to work on the project over the summer and were crucial in making sure that it got to the publication stage. None of them should be held unduly accountable for errors or omissions, for all of us involved in the project stand jointly responsible. Melanie Padgett selflessly produced many drafts of this text and has contributed in many ways to the final product.

During the spring of 1988, Gary Watts, M.D., worked with Connie Harris, Ph.D., Reymundo Rodriguez, and me to develop bibliographic material as well as a taxonomy of issues that provided resources and structure to the project. Laurie Crumpton worked during the summer of 1988 to further refine this information, and participated in the class during the fall semester. Scott Kier, Ph.D, joined the project in March 1989, replacing Connie Harris as a co-director of the project, and as the research director for the three Hogg Foundation commissions.

Persons at the Texas Department of Mental Health and Mental Retardation who have helped in this project include Dennis Jones, Commissioner; Tom Suehs, former Deputy Commissioner for Management and Support; Sally Anderson and Julie Bonner of Information Services; Leilani Rose, Clyde Allen, Debra Watson, and Virgina Leininger of Budget and Fiscal Services; Tom Martinec of Internal Audit; Jim Dalton and Dan Kern of Claims; Mike Laritz of Contracts; Don Vaughn, Assistant Deputy Commissioner; and Bruce Nunn and Gary Anderson, Management Analysis and Reporting Unit (MARU); Cathy Collier, Carolee Moore, and Phyllis Gipson, Assistant Deputy Commissioners for Mental Health Services; Nancy Ditmar, Ph.D., Director of Special Programs, Mental Health Services; Ann Denton, Coordinator, Adult Residential Services; Linda Logan, SQA; Rush Russell, Revenue Officer; and Vijay Ganju, Ph.D., and Carol Bouchard of the Office of Strategic Planning.

Persons who addressed the class in the course of the year and shared their expertise and insights included Karen Hale, Mental Health Association of Texas; David Pharis, special monitor for the R. A. J. v. Jones settlement agreement; Spencer McClure, Executive Director of the Texas Council of Community Mental Health and Mental Retardation Centers; John Brubaker, Executive Director, Mildred Vuris, Director, Mental Health Services, Scott Kier, Director of Evaluation, Alan McCoy, Executive Assistant, and Michael Figer, Director of Finance, all at Austin-Travis County MHMR; Genevieve Hearon, President of the Texas Alliance for the Mentally Ill; Don Green, Legislative Budget Board; George Fairweather, Ph.D., Michigan State University; Ira Iscoe, Ph.D., Professor of Psychology, Hogg Foundation, University of Texas; Robert Campbell, Touche Ross; Rush Russell, Revenue Officer, Linda Logan, SQA, and Cathy Collier, Assistant Deputy Commissioner of Mental Health Services, all of the Texas Department of Mental Health and Mental Retardation; and Charles Holzer and Fernando Trevino of the University of Texas Medical Branch at Galveston.

With regard to this volume, the staff members of each of the community centers and outreach center unselfishly provided us with information, reviewed drafts of case studies, and provided feedback to endless queries. Under no circumstances should anyone but the authors be held responsible for any errors of commission or omission.

At Dallas County MHMR, many staff members provided their support, cooperation, and information. These staff members include John Gill, Ph.D., Marilyn Charlesworth, Florence Gonzales, Cynthia Bursey, Larry Cotten, Dan Schafer, Dwight Walker, Jon Baughman, Jonathan Beard, Mary Blegen-Sola, Diane Boardman, Carolyn Long, Alan Tanowitz, and Marvin Williams. The many other staff members interviewed were also very helpful. In addition, Douglas Puryear, M.D., offered many helpful comments on a draft of the report, as did Phyllis Gipson, Assistant Deputy Commissioner for Mental Health Services, Texas Department of Mental Health and Mental Retardation. The department's other Central Office sections which provided information and assistance in the Dallas case study include Information Services, Internal Audit, and Budget and Fiscal Services.

The staff and clients of the Concho Valley Center for Human Advancement were very helpful, especially Shelby Blaydes, Program Director, Mental Health Services; James Young, Executive Director; and Carol Jeffers, Director of Community Support Programs. They were generous with their time and resources during two visits and also graciously responded to many subsequent questions. We would also like to thank Charles Shannon, a member of the San Angelo Alliance for the Mentally Ill, for taking time out of his day to meet with us.

At the San Antonio State Hospital Outreach, we would first of all like to express our appreciation to the staff at San Antonio State Hospital for their cooperation, especially Steven B. Schnee, Ph.D., Superintendent; Calvin Bayne, Business Manager; and Porfirio Esparza, Director of Outreach Services. A special note of thanks also goes to Allen Rossett and the rest of the staff of the Karnes County Mental Health Clinic in Kenedy for graciously answering all of our questions during our unannounced visit to their facility. We would also like to thank all of those who responded to our phone interviews: Susie Battle-Ledford, Director of the Comal County Mental Health Clinic; Vivian Bruce, Director of the Atascosa County Mental Health Clinic; Frances Burk, LVN and Acting Director, San Patricio County Mental Health Clinic; Shirley Crabtree, Director, Gonzales County Mental Health Clinic; Raymond Flores, Director, Dimmit County Mental Health Clinic; Ann Parsons, Director, Multi-County Mental Health Clinic; Allen Rossett, LVN and Director, Karnes County Mental Health Clinic; and John Stockley, Director, Maverick County Mental Health Clinic.

We would also like to extend thanks to several staff members at the Texas Department of Mental Health and Mental Retardation who helped on this project. James Smith, Budget Analyst, was central to figuring out some of the budget processes for outreach services. Cathy Collier, Assistant Deputy Commissioner, Mental Health Services, provided invaluable information on the reality of administering rural mental health care delivery.

Finally, at Tri County MHMR in Conroe, Leon Evans, Executive Director, and Dot Young, Associate Executive Director, were extraordinarily hospitable, encouraging, and helpful. We also received a great deal of help from Carol Audis, Larry George, Rosa de Luna Gonzales, Tom Mitchell, Johnny Phillips, Faith Ray, Rona Riolo, Adelle Taylor, Mary Ellen Thompson, and Mike Thompson. Tri County staff agreed to brief us on a wide assortment of issues and problems with regard to the mental health system and gave us enormous support throughout. They patiently corrected a number of errors of commission and omission promptly and conscientiously.

We hope that these cases will give readers a greater understanding of the complexity of providing care for the chronically mentally ill at the community level in Texas and that through a better understanding of the configuration and organization of local community centers, as citizens we will all be more effective at facilitating their mission.

Chapter 1. Introduction

In order to place these four case studies of community mental health in context, it may be useful to the reader to have a brief history of the community center as well as an account of some of the developments nationally and in Texas in treating the chronically mentally ill.

COMMUNITY-BASED MENTAL HEALTH SERVICES

The community mental health center movement was a creation of the Kennedy administration. The 1963 Community Mental Health Center Act (PL 88-164) was oriented to promoting community mental health. The act provided federal funds for the creation of community centers for mental health services that were far more broadly conceived than the community clinics which had been proposed by earlier blue ribbon task forces (Connery et al., 1968, p. 48).

Indeed these local community centers were mandated to take a public health approach to mental health services, including performing a needs assessment for the specific geographic service area served, identifying and attacking environmental factors underlying mental health problems, providing early detection and early treatment, injecting mental health precepts into the work of human service agencies, and providing mental health education and information to the public. (Wagenfield, Lemkau, and Justice, 1982, p. 50).

The act bypassed the states by allocating the funds directly to the local community centers and their boards. Because this new federal money was far more than the states had been spending on community-based care of the mentally ill, the community mental health center (CMHC) became the local component of the mental health system. Yet there was no effort to define the basic functions of the CMHCs or to develop mechanisms for some integration with state hospitals (Grob, 1987). Over the next decade, $1.2 billion in direct federal grants was awarded to 603 CMHCs throughout the country (Comptroller General of the United States, 1976).

The Community Mental Health Center Act was passed after it was discovered that psychotropic drugs significantly increased the ability of persons with severe mental illness to function in the community. Of even greater significance, the implementation of Medicare and Medicaid (Titles 18 and 19 of the Social Security Act) in 1966 provided federal payment for care in nursing homes of many of the chronically mentally ill, which led many states to shift patients from the state hospitals where the patients were the sole responsibility of the state. In 1955 there were 560,000 patients in U.S. mental hospitals on an average day; by 1985 the average daily census had declined to roughly 125,000 (Mechanic, 1985, pp. 76-77).

The Mental Health Systems Act replaced the CMHC Act in 1980; however, the Reagan administration repealed the Mental Health Systems Act in 1981 and consolidated its appropriated funds with those of 25 other categorical health programs into block grants made directly to the states under the Omnibus Reconciliation Act of 1981. Though states continue to receive mental health block grant funds, the amounts of money have declined relative to costs over the past decade. The block grant appropriations increased only 16 percent from FY 1982 to FY 1987, which is still 9 percent below what CMHC programs received in FY 1981 (Rochefort, 1987).

As mental health centers came more directly under the control of the states and as federal funding was reduced, the orientation of the centers has become increasingly sensitive to state priorities. With the mentally ill this has been translated into providing care at the community level to persons who in the past would have to be in a state hospital. Exactly how this mandate has developed and the level of its articulation varies of course around the country. In some states where the county is the locus of most social welfare authority, the coordination is quite explicit and centered at the local level. In Wisconsin, for instance, which is often cited as a model state for community-based care, the state grants a great deal of authority to the individual counties. State funds go directly to the county, which must provide basic services and pay for care provided at state hospitals to clients.

With deinstitutionalization and the development of far more vocal advocacy groups for the mentally ill, there has come an increased realization that adequate community-level services and treatments are needed. This population is generally in need of an array of support services, including housing, supported employment, medication, and various core services such as crisis intervention, family support, and case management. For this population of severely and chronically mentally ill persons, the community center must be far more than a local outpost of public health principles applied to mental health. It must be the locally responsible entity for arranging for the care, treatment, and in many cases the living arrangements for persons entrusted to them by the community.

As perspectives have changed, the federal government has changed its initiatives as well. Public Law 99-660, which was implemented on October 1, 1987, requires that states prepare a three-year plan for comprehensive community mental health services for adults and children with serious mental illness. State plans must also address the needs of special populations such as minorities, the elderly, and homeless persons with serious mental illness. These plans are required to contain quantitative targets for the implementation of the plan, a description of how access to services will be provided and how these services will reduce the rate of hospitalization, and a design for case management services for all persons with severe mental illness who receive substantial amounts of public funds or services. This mandated planning system is of course being grafted on 50 different state mental health systems and their respective community mental health agencies.

COMMUNITY MENTAL HEALTH IN TEXAS

Before the 1963 Community Mental Health Center Act, virtually all public mental health care in Texas was provided by the state mental hospitals. The Texas Department of Health, then the state mental health authority, was funded by the National Institute of Mental Health in 1963 to develop a state mental health plan. The planning committee proposed legislation which would reorganize the administration of mental health and mental retardation services in Texas and permit the creation of CMHCs (McKlesky, 1968).

The legislation which was passed (House Bill 3) created the Texas Department of Mental Health and Mental Retardation (TDMHMR) and established it as the state mental health authority for state institutions. The Board of Hospitals and Schools was abolished and administrative oversight of the state tuberculosis hospitals was transferred to the state health department. The bill also authorized the creation of nonprofit CMHCs by local sponsoring agencies. The statutory authority for the creation of CMHCs is found in Article 5547-203 of Vernon's Texas Civil Statutes, which authorizes certain local agencies to establish and operate community centers. The local agencies are limited to counties, cities, hospital districts, school districts, or organizational combinations of two or more of these.

In effect the CMHCs are public nonprofit entities whose boards are wholly designated by their governmental sponsors; but they do not have taxing authority themselves. It was thought that by making their sponsors local taxing authorities there would be some possibility that local effort could be required to qualify for state matching funds. In 1965, these CMHCs were able to apply for federal funds which were available under the federal CMHC act. The state also provided some grant-in-aid funds which had to be matched by local funds. Centers were also required by both federal and state legislation to provide free services to indigent persons. For the 1966-67 biennium, the total state appropriation for new Texas CMHCs was $600,000 (Frazier, 1978, p. 79).

The new TDMHMR inherited three entities and three methods of state support for community services: (1) state-operated outpatient clinics; (2) contracts with local agencies for services to indigent persons; and (3) new grants-in-aid to CMHCs. In 1966-67, state funds for all these community services were budgeted in one line item, a total of $1,350,000 for the biennium. The TDMHMR board had to decide how to allocate the funds among the competing entities. Each method had different consequences and implications (McCleskey, 1968, p. 157).

Within 18 months of the passage of HB 3, 24 community centers had been established in Texas (DeMoll, 1978, p. 62). The federal grant funds that most of these centers received came with the attendant regulations, including minimum limits on the jurisdictional size or catchment area of a community center. Thus, although community centers were established in virtually all urban areas of the state, very few were created in the large, sparsely populated areas of west and south Texas.

PL 88-164, as echoed in HB 3, established the CMHC as a new entity, separate and distinct from the state mental health authority and the state institutions. In the late 1960s and early 1970s, most Texas community mental health centers operated almost wholly independent of the state and of each other. Those with federal grants received their federal funds directly. The amount of state grant-in-aid available through the department was only $4 million in 1969 (Rienstra, 1990). During this time the CMHCs were often criticized for lack of fiscal accountability, failure to lower admissions to the state hospitals, failure to serve chronic and severely disabled clients, and an attempt to be "all things to all people" (Burke, 1978, p. 63).

During the period of rapid growth of the community mental health centers, TDMHMR was undergoing some substantial changes. The state hospital census dropped from 16,000 in 1966 to below 8,000 by 1975. TDMHMR established five state centers to provide services in areas of the state not served by community centers. The state hospitals opened community outreach programs to serve nearby rural areas.

The first patients to leave the state hospitals were the elderly; usually they were placed in nursing homes. In most instances, the new CMHCs were ill equipped to take care of the persons who were discharged. The result was that Texas went through a period of "transinstitutionalization" rather than deinstitutionalization (Farabee, 1978, p. 72).

In the late 1970s and early 1980s, a series of significant events occurred which moved TDMHMR and the CMHCs closer together, both operationally and in statute. The federal staffing grants to CMHCs began to expire, so the centers looked increasingly to the state for continuation funds. A cluster of legislative oversight committee reports on mental health services resulted in a new state law that mandated a role for CMHCs in the state's public mental health system. The respective responsibilities of the state institutions and community centers in providing a continuum of care were defined in state law for the first time in 1981 as Senate Bill 791.

A major federal class-action lawsuit, Jenkins v. Cowley, originally filed in 1974 against all Texas state hospitals on behalf of all past, current, and future patients of the hospitals, was settled in 1981. Now known as R. A. J. v. Jones, the suit alleged that the hospitals failed to provide adequate treatment in the least restrictive environment, the facilities were understaffed, patients were overmedicated, and living conditions were oppressive and unhealthy (TDMHMR, 1989, p. 30). The settlement agreement signed March 2, 1981, mandated many improvements in the hospitals, including stringent staff-to-patient ratios (Harper, 1989, pp. 36-37). Funds had to be moved to the CMHCs from the hospitals in order to comply with this requirement.

The TDMHMR appropriations structure at the time was fairly restrictive. Line-item appropriations were made to individual hospitals; another line item was for all CMHC grants-in-aid. The board had only limited authority to transfer funds from one line item to another. In 1983, TDMHMR requested and received legislative approval for unprecedented authority to transfer funds between line items. Under the agreement reached, a new appropriation line item, Staff-to-Patient Ratios, was created. TDMHMR could then allocate funds to either the CMHCs to help fund services for hospital patients discharged to them or directly to state hospitals for additional staff to meet the required staffing ratios. Initially called the "$35.50 program," this is now called the Mental Health Incentive Diversion Program.

In 1983, the legislature enacted substantive revisions to the 1957 Mental Health Code. As a result of many of the federal court decisions on the civil rights of mentally ill persons in the 1970s and early 1980s, many provisions of the code had to be changed. In 1979, the U.S. Supreme Court decided in Addington v. Texas that the substantive due-process standard used in civil commitments, preponderance of the evidence, was not sufficient. The next higher standard, clear and convincing evidence, was to be used. Other changes included stricter definitions of mental illness required for commitment; replacement of indefinite commitments with extended (up to one year) commitments; and authorization for peace officers to take a person to an inpatient unit for emergency evaluation without a warrant. In 1987, provisions for single portal authorities were added to the code (Churgin, 1988, p. 5).

In response to growing economic pressure from the R.A.J. settlement agreement, Lieutenant Governor Bill Hobby and Speaker Gib Lewis established a Legislative Oversight Committee in June 1984 to study TDMHMR and present recommendations to the 69th Legislature for allocating the resources available to meet the mandate of the settlement agreement and for the future directions of public mental health services in Texas. The committee's three-volume report contained 93 recommendations for TDMHMR; most of these were enacted in Senate Bill 633 by the 69th Legislature in 1985 (LOC, 1985). The major requirements of SB 633 included more citizen involvement in planning, the development of a long-range strategic plan, the definition of priority client populations for mental health services, replacement of the grant-in-aid mechanism with performance contracts for the community centers, and requirements for certain core services in all local service areas.

The most recent legislative initiative was the first formal review of TDMHMR in 1985 by the Sunset Advisory Commission. The resulting TDMHMR sunset legislation, Senate Bill 257, enacted by the 70th Legislature, is replete with privatization initiatives for current state hospital services, with strong emphasis on community services. SB 257 also mandated that two more core services be provided in local areas and removed the requirement that the TDMHMR commissioner be a psychiatrist.

Concurrently with these reforms and developments the TDMHMR has divided the state into 63 Local Service Areas (see Appendix 1.A). The department has designated a local Mental Health Authority (MHA) responsible for providing services to children and adults with serious mental illness for each Local Service Area. Each CMHMRC is the MHA for its respective service area. When a local service area does not have a CMHMRC, then the state facility in the region serves as the local MHA. A list of the MHAs by service area is in Appendix 1.B. (TDMHMR, 1989, p. 13).

The legislature has mandated seven essential or core services which every local mental health authority must provide to eligible persons in the local service areas for which they are responsible. These core services are (1) crisis stabilization; (2) 24-hour emergency screening and referral; (3) multidisciplinary assessments; (4) family support services, including respite care; (5) case management; (6) medication-related services; and (7) psychosocial rehabilitation.

These mandated core services are used as a primary mechanism to improve community-based services for persons with serious mental illness. The seven core services must be provided by all CMHMRCs. In fact, if a CMHMRC fails to provide the core services, Senate Bill 633 requires the department to contract for these services from another provider. The state-operated community programs are also, in principle, responsible for providing all of the core services in the areas that they serve. But the low level of funding of the state-run programs and the geographic distance faced by these providers seem to mandate against provision of all the services in each area.

No one would claim that these seven core services are the only ones needed by this population in order to minimize risk of readmission to state hospitals. In fact, most would agree that adequate housing and income support are probably the key missing ingredients for most chronically mentally ill persons in Texas, since lack of these support services causes many chronically mentally ill persons to fall through the cracks. Lack of housing also may explain why so many persons seem to migrate away from rural or suburban locations to the larger cities. This migration makes it increasingly difficult to delineate just which patients should be allocated to a particular mental health authority.

These core services are not available to all who need them. Rather, the state has established priority service groups who are to be served first by the public mental health system. These groups are defined as follows:

SERVICE GROUP I
Chronically dysfunctional mental disorder with present dangerousness and/or dependency: a person with mental disorder of at least two years' duration (or six months' duration, if a disorder of infancy, childhood, or adolescence) with present dangerousness* and/or dependency.**

SERVICE GROUP II
Historically dysfunctional mental disorder with present dangerousness and/or dependency: a person with mental disorder of less than two years' duration (or less than six months' duration, if a disorder of infancy, childhood, or adolescence) with presence of dangerousness and/or dependency, and at least one previous psychiatric hospitalization or at least one involuntary commitment to psychiatric services.

---

*Present dangerousness involves a condition of substantial likelihood for inflicting injury on self or others, including such recent acts as combative aggressive behaviors or convincing verbalizations or menacing overtures toward others; or convincing self-injurious verbalizations, self-injury, or actions conveying self-injurious intent.

**Present dependency involves a condition of inability, because of mental disorder, to meet basic life support needs (e.g. food, shelter, medical care) without extensive support from others outside the natural support system. Criteria for dependency include: unemployment due to mental disorder; or education disruption in the case of children and adolescents; or strong reliance on financial entitlements; or marked social dysfunction such as failure to meet household health standards or disorderly conduct.

SERVICE GROUP III

Chronically dysfunctional mental disorder with threat of deterioration to dangerousness and/or dependency: a person with mental disorder of at least two years' duration (or six months' duration, if a disorder of infancy, childhood, or adolescence) who exhibits a threat of deterioration to dangerousness and/or dependency, i.e., it is probable that without external intervention a worsening of the condition will occur so that the person will require further intervention for acute dangerousness and/or dependency.

SERVICE GROUP IV

Dysfunctional mental disorder with threat of deterioration to dangerousness and/or dependency: a person who exhibits a threat of deterioration to dangerousness and/or dependency, i.e., it is probable that a worsening of the condition will progress to a level requiring a primary commitment for reason of dangerousness and/or dependency, without external intervention.

SERVICE GROUP V (Nonpriority Population)

All other persons receiving mental health services: this category includes *(a) dysfunctional mental disorder*, without threat of deterioration to dangerousness and/or dependency: a person with a history of either short- or long-term mental dysfunction, i.e., of either less than or more than two years' duration, who exhibits no evidence of deterioration to a condition of dangerousness or dependency. This person, despite mental disorder, remains capable of satisfying basic life support needs without the natural support system, and exhibits no overt or implicit behaviors which convey dangerousness to self or others; *(b) at risk of dysfunctional mental disorder:* a person with increased likelihood of dysfunctional mental disorder who remains capable of satisfying basic life support needs in the natural support system, and who is not indicating deterioration toward dangerousness. Failure to receive psychiatric service may result in subsequent dysfunctional mental disorder; *(c) all other persons receiving services*, or screened and referred to other community resources.

Both the state and the federal governments are increasingly defining their roles in community mental health as that of arranging for the funding of core services to priority chronically mentally ill clients. Currently the CMHMRCs must provide all of the core services and set priorities for clients served. They cannot provide these services to all of the priority service groups who need them since they lack the funds to do this. In fact, at one center in our study, there is just one contracted bed for crisis stabilization; when the funds to pay for that bed run out partway through the fiscal year, persons needing crisis stabilization are referred to the state hospital serving that CMHMRC's area.

In its biennial performance report to the legislature, the Legislative Budget Board (LBB) called for increased contract accountability between the community centers and TDMHMR. The report stated that the latitude given to community centers in determining level of services hinders the department's ability to provide systematic and uniform community services. The LBB recommended TDMHMR convert all contracts for mental health and mental retardation client services to a purchase-of-service contract by fiscal year 1991. The LBB also called for developing a unit cost per service for all services contracted with outside entities. And it further recommended that TDMHMR target community centers with below-average service availability for service expansion under a purchase-of-service contract system (LBB, 1989).

Although Texas still spends far less on its chronically mentally ill per capita than most states, the aggregate levels of expenditure are far from trivial. We estimate that in 1984 total state and federal spending through TDMHMR for mental health services was $307.6 million, of which $45.7 million was contracted to community centers. By fiscal year 1988 this amount had increased to $353.8 million, of which $70.9 million was channeled to through direct contracted services as well as the staff-to-patient funding program or the so-called $35.50 program.*

For the 1990-91 fiscal year, the budgeted funds for mental health services in the department as a whole will be $356,148,639, of which the community centers will receive $123,928,475. It must be remembered that in addition to the funds received from TDMHMR, the community centers may receive funds from a variety of local sources and state contracts. Some of these funds go to care for the chronically mentally ill and some of them may be spent on other activities.

COMMUNITY MENTAL HEALTH CENTERS IN TEXAS

By August 31, 1988, there were 35 CMHMRCs in Texas; their service areas contained a total population of 14.8 million persons---roughly 88 percent of the state's population. Table 1.1 shows the 1988 revenues for each of these centers by source. It should be noted that local revenues include funds from a variety of state contracts as well as patient fees and local tax revenues and contracts.

Since the passage of HB 3, financial support for CMHMRCs by local governments has been extremely uneven across the state and varies from year to year. Many cities and counties which are served by a CMHMRC contribute no financial support. A few others, Harris County being the most notable, have provided consistent and occasionally significant financial support. Today, local tax funds average 10 percent of the total CMHMRC's annual budgets. Figure 1.1 illustrates recent trends in local tax funding for Texas CMHMRCs. Financial support from Harris and Dallas counties for their respective CMHMRCs alone represents more than two-thirds of the total local tax dollars for all 35 CMHMRCs in the state.

In a recent survey on Texas mental health services, local community leaders were about equally divided on the question of who should have primary responsibility for meeting local mental health needs. State government, a coalition of different levels of government, and a coalition of various groups (i.e., private, public, family, consumer, and community) were all ranked approximately equally (League of Women Voters, 1985, p. 90).

Today, Texas CMHCs provide services to 141 of the state's 254 counties. These 141 counties contain 88 percent of the total state population. Local tax support for CMHC services in these counties ranges from a low of $0.00 per capita in Lubbock to a high of $4.62 per capita in Travis County. In the 113 counties for which the state provides community mental health services through hospital and state center outreach units, the local governments contribute virtually no financial support other than to bear the costs of court commitments and transportation of committed persons to the state hospital.

THE CASE STUDIES

The four case studies in this volume illustrate some of the diversity and complexity of the organization of community care for the seriously mentally ill. They were chosen so as to include an urban center (Dallas County MHMR), a suburban center with a number of innovative programs (Tri County in Conroe), a relatively isolated center which serves an extensive rural area (Concho Valley in San Angelo), and a state outreach center (San Antonio State Hospital Outreach). These centers were chosen because of reasonable accessibility to Austin and the willingness of the staff to work with the class. As with all case studies there is no guarantee that what was found can necessarily be generalized to

---

*This is discussed in more detail in Section 4 of the companion volume, Financing Care for the Chronically Mentally Ill in Texas, to be published by the LBJ School of Public Affairs.

Table 1.1. Community MHMR Centers Revenue of 1988

Center	Local	State	Federal	Total
Abilene	1,228,884	3,942,183	222,533	5,393,600
Austin-Travis MHMR	4,670,866	6,981,873	873,047	12,525,786
Bexar County	2,997,979	11,709,245	352,300	15,059,524
Brazos Valley	691,713	2,780,164	326,016	3,797,893
Central Counties Ctr.	1,147,784	4,028,839	736,514	5,913,137
Central Plains MHMR	807,846	2,411,087	175,102	3,394,035
Central Texas MHMR Ctr.	1,242,812	1,597,296	481,077	3,321,185
Collin County MHMR Ctr.	420,605	1,701,447	443,478	2,565,530
Concho Valley Ctr.	705,883	1,908,429	148,694	2,763,006
Dallas County MHMR Ctr.	6,944,247	16,100,815	1,111,413	24,156,475
Deep East Texas MHMR	4,756,704	5,020,421	679,845	10,456,970
Denton County MHMR Ctr.	1,073,739	1,639,506	322,478	3,035,723
MHMR Ctr. of East Texas	2,781,812	4,968,043	441,260	8,191,115
Gulf Bend MHMR Center	1,045,913	1,955,185	175,165	3,176,263
Gulf Coast Regional MHMR	2,585,894	4,574,787	520,313	7,680,994
MHMR Authority of Harris	17,783,511	20,682,907	2,718,183	41,184,601
Heart of Texas MHMR Ctr.	1,488,982	3,370,034	727,915	5,586,931
Hunt County Family Service	750,508	992,483	346,026	2,089,017
Johnson County MHMR Ctr.	403,456	1,078,903	199,831	1,682,190
Life Management Ctr.	2,472,195	161,935	505,132	3,139,262
Lubbock Management Ctr.	2,596,692	4,160,755	378,245	7,135,692
Navarro County MHMR Ctr.	81,296	447,330	7,520	536,146
Northeast Texas MHMR Ctr.	318,389	1,351,181	66,915	1,736,485
Nueces County MHMR Ctr.	1,554,216	3,960,847	416,739	5,931,802
Pecan Valley MHMR Region	445,863	2,021,894	738,657	3,206,414
Permian Basin MHMR Ctr.	958,144	2,941,403	678,434	4,577,981
Sabine Valley MHMR	3,686,446	4,018,518	801,347	8,506,311
MHMR of Southeast Texas	1,349,791	4,363,286	120,829	5,833,906
Tarrant County MHMR	6,462,498	9,610,623	1,149,773	17,222,894
Texas Panhandle MH	431,941	3,028,967	89,695	3,550,603
MHMR Services of Texoma	1,094,229	1,900,574	790,898	3,785,701
Tri-County MHMR Services	5,215,737	3,759,087	329,781	9,304,605
Tropical Texas MHMR Ctr.	2,730,711	5,022,035	1,318,288	9,071,034
Wichita Falls MHMR Ctr.	1,582,841	2,113,230	110,623	3,806,694
Total	**84,510,127**	**146,305,312**	**18,504,066**	**249,319,505**
Percentage	**34**	**59**	**7**	**100**

Source: Financing Care for the Chronically Mentally Ill in Texas, LBJ School of Public Affairs, Policy Research Project, 1989, (Draft).

Figure 1.1. Trends in Local Tax Funds to Texas CMHCc

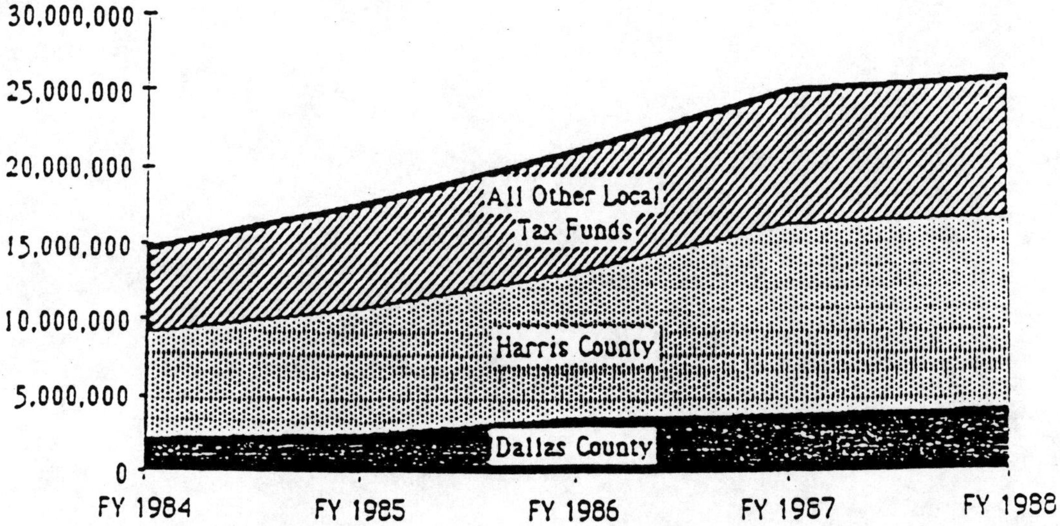

Source: Austin-Travis County MHMR, 1988.

apply to all community centers. Nonetheless, by trying to gather reasonably parallel data, we hope some comparisons will be possible. The main purpose of the exercise has been to provide case information that makes the community center less of a black box.

Each of the case studies begins with a discussion of the geographic area served by the center, a history of the center, and a description of its organizing entities. Then each case study examines the core services and noncore services delivered by the center and the populations to which these services are delivered. It is illuminating to see the variety of arrangements which have been developed to meet the requirements of TDMHMR and to see how short the state funds generally fall in financing the necessary core services to the priority populations.

Next each study examines the center's budget and financing to understand the sources and uses of funds which are available. Finally we examine issues in each of the centers which the staff or the analysis has identified as worthy of consideration.

The authors hope that these case studies will provide the reader with a more informed perspective regarding the strengths and weaknesses of community care of the chronically mentally ill. In any event we believe that the cases document the work of a number of committed professionals who have kept providing services to a variety of clients even as the higher authorities at the state and federal levels have changed the rules of the game with some regularity. In the end, the concern of this study is to improve the conditions of persons with serious mental illness.

Appendix 1.A. Map of Texas Showing the 63 Local Service Areas

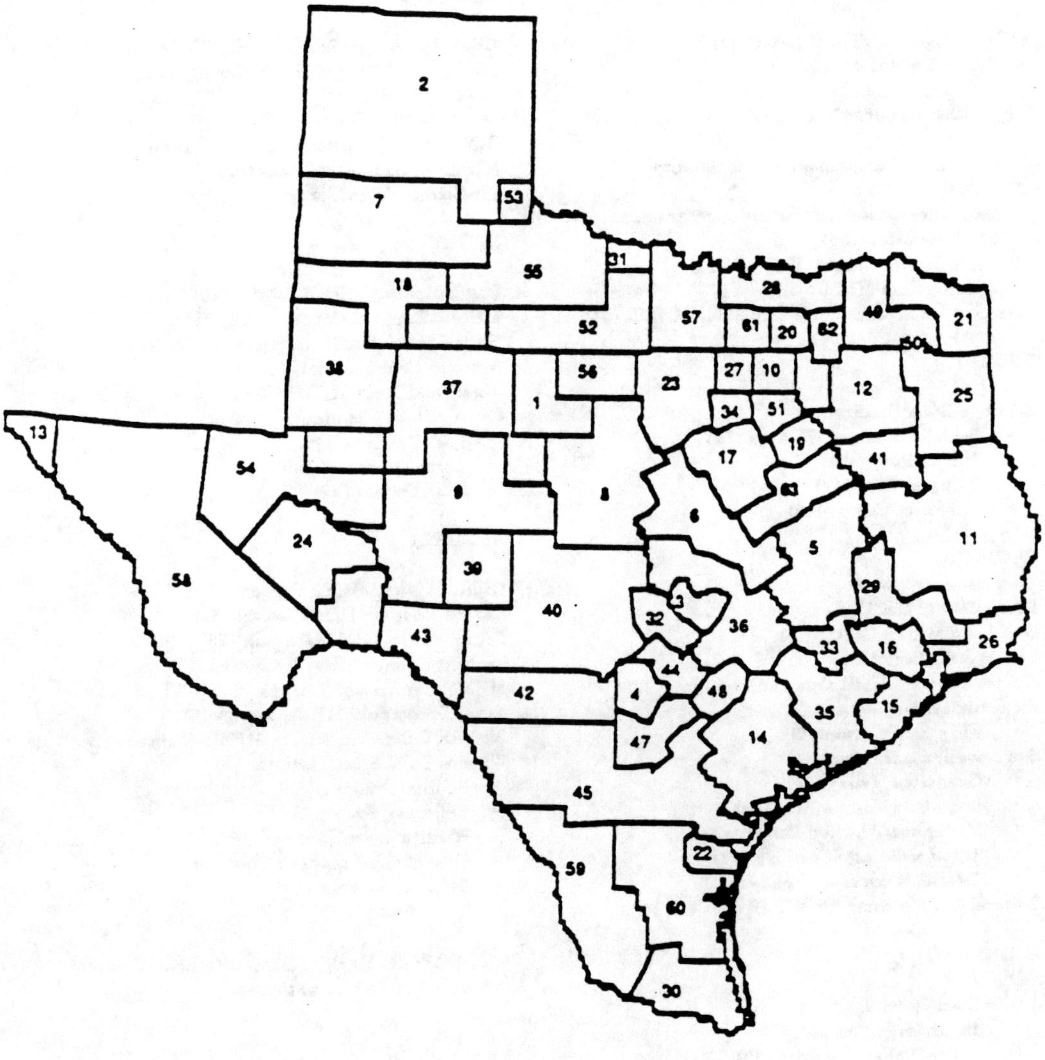

Source: TDMHMR, "Future Directions for Comprehensive Community-Based Mental Health Services in Texas" Austin, September 15, 1989. Working Draft.

Appendix 1.B. Mental Health Regional Councils and MHAs by Service Area

REGION 1

Abilene Regional MHMR Center (1)*
Big Spring State Hospital
- Great Plains (37)
- Staked Plains/Caprock (38)
- Pecos River (54)

Central Plains Comprehensive Community MHMR Center (7)
Concho Valley Center for Human Advancement (9)
El Paso State Center (58)
Life Management Center (El Paso) (13)
Lubbock Regional MHMR Center (18)
Permian Basin Community Center for MHMR (24)

REGION 2

Kerrville State Hospital
- Schleicher/Sutton Counties (39)
- Hill Country (40)
- Balcones Area (42)
- Val Verde County (43)

REGION 3

Bexar County MHMR Center (4)
Gulf Bend MHMR Center (14)
Laredo State Center (59)
Nueces County MHMR Community Center (22)
Rio Grande State Center
- King Ranch Area (60)

San Antonio State Hospital
- Guadalupe Valley (44)
- Brushland Coastal Area (45)
- Matagorda/Wharton Counties (46)
- Atascosa/Wilson Counties (47)
- Colorado/Gonzales Counties (48)

Tropical Texas Center for MHMR (30)

REGION 4

Austin State Hospital
- Blanco/Hays Counties (32)
- Austin/Waller Counties (33)
- Capital Area (36)

Austin-Travis County MHMR (3)
MHMR Authority of Brazos Valley (5)
Central Counties Center for MHMR (6)
Central Texas MHMR Center (8)
Gulf Coast Regional MHMR Center (15)
Heart of Texas Regional MHMR Center (17) (63)
Johnson County MHMR Center (34)
Riceland Regional MH Authority (35)

REGION 5

Deep East Texas Regional MHMR Center (11)
MHMR Authority of Harris County (16)
Rusk State Hospital
- Anderson/Cherokee Counties (41)

Sabine Valley Regional MHMR Center (25)
MHMR of Southeast Texas (26)
Tri-County MHMR Services (29)

REGION 6

Dallas County MHMR Center (10)
MHMR Regional Center of East Texas (12)
Hunt County Family Services Center (62)
Navarro County MHMR Center (19)
Northeast Texas MHMR Center (21)
Terrell State Hospital
- Post Oak Area (49)
- Camp County (50)
- Ellis County (51)

REGION 7

Collin County MHMR Center (20)
Denton County MHMR Center (61)
Pecan Valley MHMR Region (23)
Tarrant County MHMR Services (27)
MHMR Services of Texoma (28)
Texas Panhandle MH Authority (2)
Wichita Falls Community MHMR Center (31)
Wichita Falls State Hospital
- Rolling Prairies (52)
- Childress County (53)
- Wichita River (55)
- Shackelford/Stephens Counties (56)
- Grasslands Area (57)

* Each Mental Health Authority's Local Service Area is listed in parentheses.

Source: TDMHMR, "Future Directions for Comprehensive Community-Based Mental Health Services in Texas" Austin, September 15, 1989. Working Draft.

References

Austin-Travis County MHMR. 1988. "Summary Data Books, FY 1984-FY 1988." Austin, Texas.

Burke, W. 1978. "Community Centers in Transistion." In Mental Health for the People of Texas, ed. Louis E. DeMoll. Austin: Hogg Foundation for Mental Health, University of Texas.

Churgin, M. 1988. An Analysis of the Texas Mental Health Code. Austin, Texas: Hogg Foundation for Mental Health, University of Texas.

Comptroller General of the United States. 1976. "Returning the Mentally Disabled to the Community: Government Needs to Do More." HRD-76-152. Washington, DC.

Connery, Robert H., et al. 1968. The Politics of Mental Health: Organizing Community Mental Health in Urban Areas. New York: Columbia University Press.

Farabee, H. 1978. "Taking the Next Steps for Community Mental Health." In Mental Health for the People of Texas, ed. Louis E. DeMoll. Austin, Texas: Hogg Foundation for Mental Health, University of Texas.

Frazier, S. 1978. "From a Decade Ago to the Decades Ahead." In Mental Health for the People of Texas, ed. Louis E. DeMoll. Austin, Texas: Hogg Foundation for Mental Health, University of Texas.

Grob, Gerald N. 1987. "Mental Health Policy in Post World War II America." In Improving Mental Health Services: What the Social Sciences Can Tell Us, ed. David Mechanic. San Francisco: Jossey-Bass, Inc.

Harper, Joellen. 1989. "Financing Mental Health Care in Texas: Issues and Alternatives." Professional report, LBJ School of Public Affairs, The University of Texas at Austin.

League of Women Voters. 1985. "Perceptions of Community-Based Services for People with Serious Mental Illness in Texas: A Survey of Consumers and Community Leaders." Austin, Texas.

Legislative Budget Board (LBB). 1989. "Texas Department of Mental Health and Mental Retardation: Performance Report to the 71st Legislature." Austin. (January 10.)

Legislative Oversight Committee (LOC). 1985. Report to the Texas Legislature: Volume I Mental Health. Austin, Texas.

McCleskey, C. 1968. "The Metropolitan Milieu: Houston." In The Politics of Mental Health: Organizing Community Mental Health in Urban Areas, ed. Robert H. Connery, et al. New York: Columbia University Press.

Mechanic, David. 1985. "Mental Health and Social Policy: Initiatives for the 1980s." Health Affairs, vol. 4 (Spring), pp. 76-77.

Mechanic, David, ed. 1987. Improving Mental Health Services: What the Social Sciences Can Tell Us. San Francisco: Jossey-Bass, Inc.

Rienstra, Jan. 1990. "Public Mental Health Services in Texas 1856-Present." In Financing Care for the Chronically Mentally Ill in Texas. Austin: LBJ School of Public Affairs, Policy Research Project. (Draft)

Rochefort, David A. 1987. "The Political Context of Mental Health Care." In Improving Mental Health Services: What the Social Sciences Can Tell Us, ed. David Mechanic. San Francisco: Jossey-Bass, Inc.

Texas Department of Mental Health and Mental Retardation (TDMHMR). 1989. Future Directions for Texas Comprehensive Community Based Mental Health Services, (Second Working Draft, June 23.)

Wagenfield, M., P. Lemkau, and B. Justice. eds. 1982. "Public Mental Health: Perspectives and Prospects." In Sage Studies in Community Mental Health, Vol. 5. Beverly Hills, Calif.: Sage Publications.

Chapter 2. Dallas County MHMR Center

Jana Blasi, Lynn Parrish, Jan Rienstra, and Charles Blissett

INTRODUCTION

The Dallas County MHMR Center (DCMHMR) is the second largest center in Texas, and it is among the three or four largest centers in the country (DCMHMR, n.d., p. 9). DCMHMR was chosen as the subject of this case study because it is located within a large metropolitan area; its local social, economic, and political contexts have influenced its service philosophy and practices. Operationally, it faces problems which are very different from those of smaller urban or rural centers.

DALLAS COUNTY DEMOGRAPHICS

Dallas is the second largest city in Texas and the seventh largest in the country. Dallas County is also one of the state's most affluent; it ranks second, behind the Midland-Odessa SMSA, in per capita income. With 2,077 persons per square mile, Dallas County is the most densely populated county in the state. In addition to the city of Dallas, Dallas County contains a number of smaller but rapidly growing cities, including Garland, Irving, Mesquite, and Richardson.

The Dallas County population was estimated to be 1,864,238 in 1986. The projections in Table 2.1 show that, according to the median projections of the Texas Department of Commerce, the Anglo population is expected to decrease from 65 percent in 1986 to 56 percent in 2000. The black population should remain fairly stable, from 20 percent in 1986 to 22 percent in 2000. The Hispanic population is projected to increase from 14 percent in 1986 to 20 percent in 2000.

Table 2.2 lists the projected population changes in Dallas County by age group and ethnicity. According to these projections, the number of Hispanic children and adolescents is projected to nearly double between 1986 and 2000. The number of persons 65 years old or older is also projected to increase significantly for all groups.

Levels of average family incomes in Dallas County are listed in Table 2.3. In 1979, 14.5 percent of all households had annual incomes less than $10,000, compared with 19.3 percent for the state and 18.8 percent for the nation.

Dallas County is a major center for commerce, banking, insurance, transportation, retail and wholesale trade, manufacturing, data processing, conventions, trade shows, and tourism. More than 3,000 manufacturing plants make apparel, building materials, food products, oil field supplies, and electronic products. The city of Dallas has more home offices of insurance firms than any other major city in the United States (Texas Almanac, 1987, p. 269).

In addition to a number of colleges and universities, Dallas County has an abundance of hospitals and related medical facilities. The University of Texas Health Science Center, affiliated with many local hospitals, has three schools: Southwestern Medical School, the School of Allied Health Sciences, and the Graduate School of Bio-Medical Sciences. Parkland Memorial Hospital, operated by the Dallas County Hospital District, is the primary provider of indigent hospital care. The hospital district has taxing authority (up to 75 cents per $100 valuation) to raise funds to support Parkland. Table 2.4 lists the major revenues for Parkland in 1988.

Table 2.1. Projected Population Change in Dallas County by Ethnicity, 1986 to 2000

Year	Age	Total	Anglo	Black	Hispanic	Other
1986	All Ages	1,864,238	1,205,252	373,053	255,280	30,653
			65 percent	20 percent	14 percent	02 percent
1990	All Ages	1,961,485	1,221,980	397,873	310,046	31,586
			62 percent	20 percent	16 percent	02 percent
1995	All Ages	2,065,091	1,224,754	433,226	373,767	33,344
			59 percent	21 percent	18 percent	02 percent
2000	All Ages	2,151,455	1,209,960	467,583	439,172	34,740
			56 percent	22 percent	20 percent	02 percent

Source: Texas Department of Commerce.

Table 2.2. Projected Population Change in Dallas County by Age and Ethnicity, 1986 to 2000

Year	Age	Total	Anglo	Black	Hispanic	Other
1986	0 - 4	162,190	85,247	39,226	35,354	2,363
1990	0 - 4	159,257	70,995	41,357	44,829	2,076
1995	0 - 4	151,873	60,468	40,421	49,022	1,962
2000	0 - 4	140,722	49,537	38,094	51,250	1,841
1986	5 - 17	342,312	190,259	85,243	60,059	6,751
1990	5 - 17	348,524	182,572	87,098	72,501	6,353
1995	5 - 17	378,195	180,588	96,978	94,928	5,701
2000	5 - 17	392,612	164,621	104,612	118,286	5,093
1986	18-44	890,468	566,513	177,882	129,902	16,171
1990	18-44	945,250	583,893	190,414	154,521	16,422
1995	18-44	948,574	555,909	200,427	175,844	16,394
2000	18-44	901,602	497,344	201,671	187,607	14,980
1986	45-64	315,797	237,511	50,483	23,442	4,361
1990	45-64	335,368	243,775	56,561	29,537	5,495
1995	45-64	394,764	274,833	69,880	42,312	7,739
2000	45-64	504,726	333,714	93,311	66,938	10,763
1986	65+	153,471	125,722	20,219	6,523	1,007
1990	65+	173,086	140,745	22,443	8,658	1,240
1995	65+	191,685	152,956	25,520	11,661	1,548
2000	65+	211,793	164,744	29,895	15,091	2,063

Source: Texas Department of Commerce.

Table 2.3. Average Family Income Levels in Dallas County

Age of Head of Household	Average Annual Income	Number of Families	Average Annual Income
15-24 years	$14,738	23,672	< $5,000
25-34 years	$20,387	18,852	$5,000-$7,000
35-44 years	$25,500	22,840	$7,500-$9,999
45-54 years	$28,380	54,397	$10,000-$14,999
55-64 years	$25,117	58,188	$15,000-$19,999
65 + years	$13,852	57,065	$20,000-$24,999
		82,201	$25,000-$34,999
		51,726	$35,000-$49,999
		34,000	> $50,000

Source: U.S. Census Bureau, 1980; Bureau of Business Research, University of Texas at Austin, 1985.

Table 2.4. Parkland Memorial Hospital 1988 Budget

Revenues	(In millions)
Dallas County Hospital District	$111.10
Net Patient Service Receipts	$83.50
Other(parking, vending, etc.)	$2.40
Non-operating Revenues	$5.70
Total	$202.70
Expenditures (excluding capital bond issues)	$198.50

Source: William Hatton and John Moore, Office of the Comptroller, Parkland Memorial Hospital, Dallas, Texas, March 23, 1989.

Dallas County also has many private psychiatric facilities. The nearest state hospital is located in Terrell, a small town in Kaufman County about 40 miles east of Dallas.

THE DEVELOPMENT OF PUBLIC MENTAL HEALTH SERVICES IN DALLAS COUNTY

In 1958, TDMHMR opened a state-operated outpatient clinic in Dallas to serve persons with mental illness after their discharge from the state hospital. In 1959 the clinic was moved to Routh Street since, at the time, this location was in the midst of a number of other medical facilities (Hudson, 1981).

After passage of House Bill 3 in 1965, several abortive attempts were made to establish a community MHMR center in Dallas County. In February 1966, the commissioners court appointed an MHMR planning commission to develop, within 45 days, an administrative and legal structure for a local MHMR center. The commission's report recommended a "county-wide, publicly-sponsored administrative structure and service system of comprehensive mental health and mental retardation services. It is to utilize existing public, voluntary, and proprietary resources and to make services available and accessible, to all residents in need" (DCMHMR, 1968).

In May 1967, the first DCMHMR board of trustees was appointed by the commissioners court. Under the provisions of HB 3, a board of trustees is responsible for the administration of the MHMR center; board members are to serve two-year, staggered terms. As the single sponsoring agency for DCMHMR, the commissioners court appoints all nine members of the board. In addition, the county decided that DCMHMR board members could serve up to six consecutive calendar years (Long, 1981). HB 3 allows, but does not require, local participating or sponsoring agencies to contribute land, buildings, facilities, personnel, and funds to an MHMR center. However, since HB 3 also states that TDMHMR may require that some or all of its state funds to community centers be matched by local support, TDMHMR has historically required varying amounts of local matching funds. Dallas County is one of the few Texas counties that has provided more than token support for its community center.

In February 1968 the Dallas County Commissioners Court allocated its first funds to the new DCMHMR center. In June 1968, the DCMHMR received its first state grant-in-aid funds from TDMHMR. As an early indicator of local priorities, the commissioners court then directed the new board to study and make recommendations for services for mentally ill persons who were in the county jail. As a result of the study, these mentally ill persons were moved to alternate, although temporary, facilities (DCMHMR, 1968).

In order to qualify for federal community mental health center staffing grants, DCMHMR had to divide the county into eight separate catchment areas. Federal regulations defined a catchment area as a geographic area with a population between 75,000 and 200,000. The first federal mental health staffing grant was awarded to DCMHMR in April 1969; the second federal grant was awarded in April 1970. These federal grants, like others under the 1963 CMHC Act, were eight-year declining match grants (i.e., federal funds declined from an initial 80 percent of the total to 30 percent of the total over the eight-year grant period). The two federal grants to DCMHMR funded certain mental health services in only two of the eight catchment areas. The federally required services were inpatient, outpatient, partial hospitalization, emergency, and consultation and education services. In February 1973, DCMHMR received a similar federal grant for child and adolescent mental health services (Long, 1981).

Also in 1973, TDMHMR contracted with DCMHMR for operation of the Routh Street Outpatient Clinic. In 1975, a state statute was amended to allow the Routh Street Clinic to become part of the DCMHMR services, thus eliminating the separate contract with TDMHMR. The clinic's operating funds were combined with a state grant-in-aid (Long, 1981).

DCMHMR opened its drug abuse services in 1974 with funding through the Drug Abuse Prevention Division of the Texas Department of Community Affairs. Federal grants to states for drug abuse services were then channeled through this agency; the grants provided 75 percent in federal funds and required a 25 percent match by the recipient agency (Long, 1981).

The two federal adult mental health service grants expired in 1978 and 1979. The child and adolescent mental health services federal grant ended in 1980. Although state grants-in-aid had increased over the years, the amounts were not sufficient to operate all the services formerly funded under the federal grants. From 1979 to 1981, the DCMHMR suffered severe federal funding losses not fully compensated by local and state funds; retrenchment of services was the only option. DCMHMR had to make severe cuts in staff and mental health services, and consequently in the number of clients served. Some programs were eliminated; others were merged into smaller units. Adult mental health outpatient services were reduced from six to three locations; 101 staff positions, nearly 20 percent of the total, were eliminated (Long, 1981). In 1978, DCMHMR served approximately 14,500 mental health clients; by 1981, this had dropped to about 11,300 clients (DCMHMR, 1989i). The DCMHMR service levels have not yet recovered from those cuts (Puryear, 1989, p. 6).

At the time, many other community mental health centers in the state were experiencing similar cuts in services because of expiring federal grants. In response to the pressures for increased funds, the legislature increased community center appropriations for the 1982-1983 biennium and again in the 1984-1985 biennium.

DCMHMR eliminated the eight catchment area designations as the federal grants expired. The service emphasis was then focused on a centralized concept of service delivery with multiple locations for outpatient services. To more efficiently manage public mental health services for a population of 1.8 million in the 880-square-mile county, DCMHMR has divided Dallas County into four geographical regions for both service and administrative purposes.

DCMHMR plans to eventually provide a full complement of outpatient and related mental health services in each of the four regions. Acute treatment services, such as crisis stabilization, would serve the entire county from a central location. Current funding levels permit the administration of two service regions, identified as "north" and "south" even though most mental health services are presently located in the middle and southern parts of the county (Figure 2.1).

In FY 1988, DCMHMR had a total budget of $23.8 million; its full-time staff of 633 provided mental health and mental retardation services to 13,861 clients. That year, 95.4 percent of DCMHMR's total revenues were public funds; of this, 4.6 percent was federal, 66.65 percent was state, and 28.75 percent was local government funds (Ernst & Whinney, 1988, p. 5). The remaining 4.6 percent of revenues came from client fees, third-party payments, and interest. In FY 1987, DCMHMR ranked 25th of 31 Texas community MHMR centers in total per capita revenues, at $11.95 per capita. The six centers that ranked below DCMHMR are located in El Paso, San Antonio, Houston, the Rio Grande Valley, Johnson County, and Amarillo (ATCMHMR, 1988, p. 5).

Figure 2.1. DCMHMR Adult Mental Health Services: Major Service Locations

(1) Acute Inpatient Treatment Center (AITC)
(2) AMHS, Regions 3 and 4, South Centre Street Clinic
(3) Central Administrative Offices
(4) Parkland Psychiatric Emergency Room, Mental Diagnostic Center (MDC)
(5) Routh Street Clinic
(6) AMHS, Regions 1 and 2, North Ferguson Road Clinic
(7) Independence House (CSP)
(8) Lancaster-Kiest Clinic

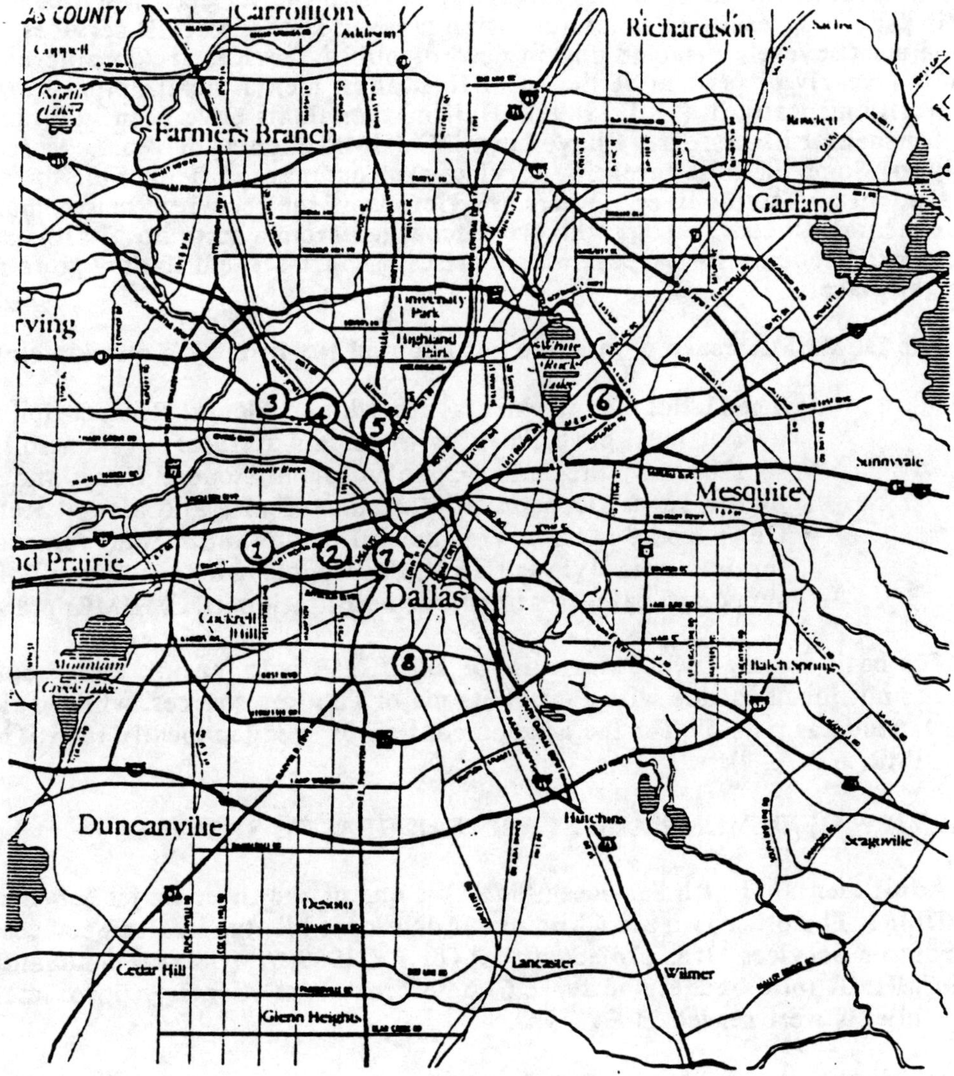

Source: DCMHMR, 1989.

Exacerbating the low level of funding are the often intractable problems of delivering public MHMR services in a metropolitan area: large populations of homeless persons, many of whom are mentally ill, are usually concentrated in metropolitan areas; inner-city poverty areas are more difficult to serve than the more affluent but outlying suburbs; and the political confluence of county, multiple municipal, and special district governments ensure difficulties in coordination, consistency, and accessibility of services.

DCMHMR's residential mental health services, from acute, intensive-care crisis beds to longer-term, apartment-based services, command nearly half of its total budget for mental health services. Most of the remaining half of the mental health budget is allocated to traditional clinic services in four locations. Relatively modest amounts of funds are allocated to more innovative types of services. Substance abuse services are now limited to screening for state hospital admission.

The overall low level of funding, coupled with the service priorities of the major funding sources, results in strict admission criteria for DCMHMR services. Only those who are the most severely disabled and in need of public services are considered eligible for services. Nearly 62 percent of the DCMHMR adult mental health clients are seriously or chronically mentally ill (Gill, 1989a). Half of the clients have been in a hospital at least once for mental illness; many have been DCMHMR clients for years. Most are indigent or nearly so. Some of those receiving services are fortunate in being able to lead relatively independent and stable lives. Others are victims of the recurrent crises characteristic of severe mental illness. Persons who are discharged from a state hospital usually get services; persons experiencing severe psychiatric crises also are served, if they go to or are taken to the right place.

The DCMHMR board of trustees has adopted the following mission statement:

> The Dallas County Mental Health and Mental Retardation Center is a unit of local government with certain statutory responsibilities sponsored by the Dallas County Commissioners' Court and regulated by the Texas Department of Mental Health and Mental Retardation. Our purpose is to provide mental health and mental retardation services to individuals in Dallas County who are in need of publicly supported care, treatment, or habilitation. (DCMHMR, n.d., p. 7)

The basis for the future strategies of DCMHMR is to "ensure that the direction of the center is not incompatible with that of its major funding sources, while maintaining as much latitude as possible for the accommodation of specific locally identified services" (DCMHMR, n.d., p. 2).

OVERVIEW OF DCMHMR ADULT MENTAL HEALTH SERVICES

Adult Mental Health Services (AMHS) is one of the three major service divisions of DCMHMR. The other two are Child and Adolescent Mental Health Services and Mental Retardation Services. It is projected that for FY 1989, AMHS will command 47 percent of the DCMHMR total budget and serve 63.6 percent of its clients. Approximately 8,820 AMHS clients were served in FY 1988.

Under the present structure, the AMHS director oversees three major service areas: Acute Treatment Services, Adult Mental Health Services North Region, and Adult Mental Health Services South Region (Figure 2.2). Other services administered by AMHS include contracted residential services (ADAPT), continuity of care, substance abuse screening, and the forensics program.

Figure 2.2. DCMHMR Organizational Chart

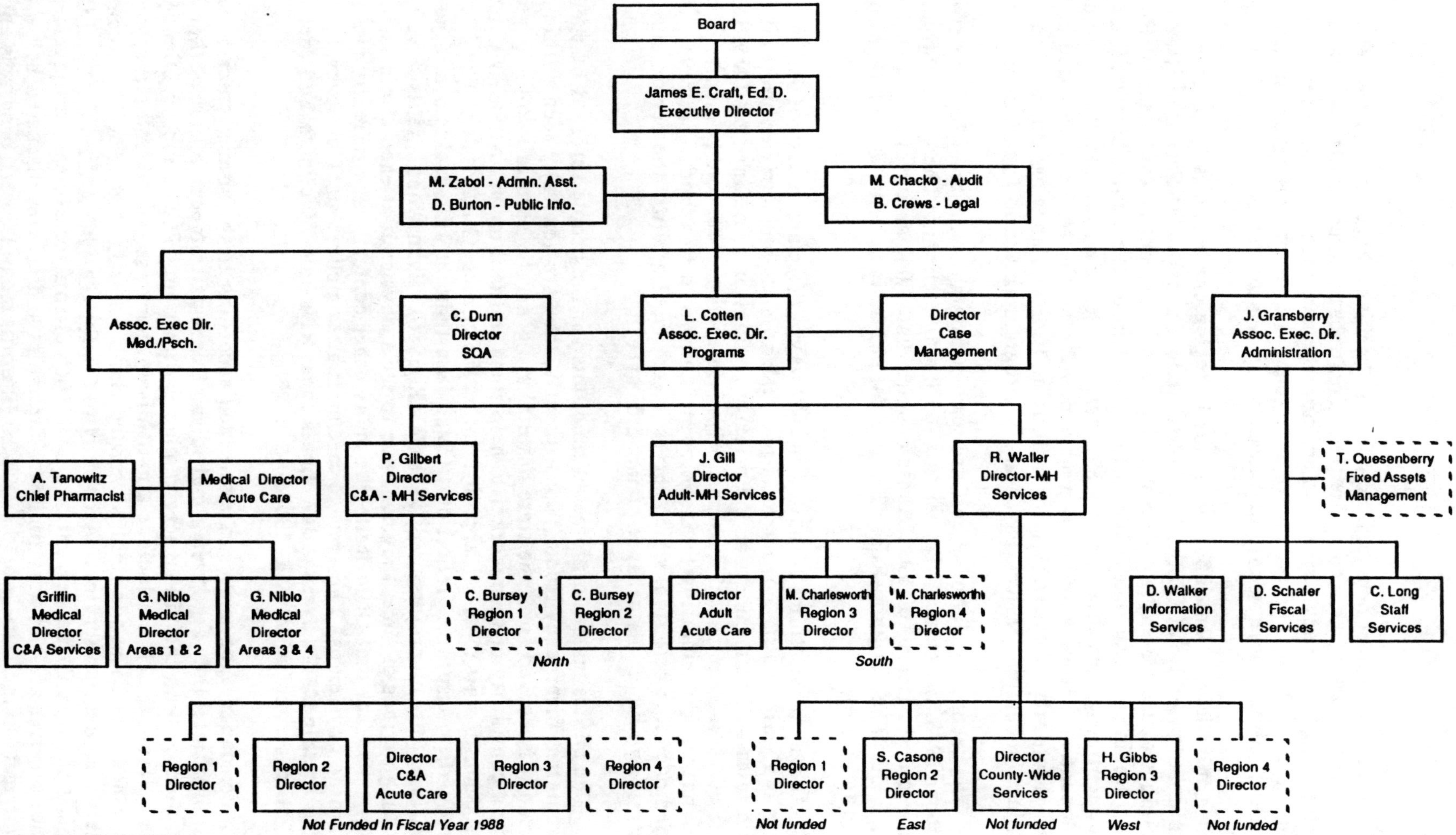

Source: DCMHMR, 1989.

Acute Treatment Services includes the Parkland Psychiatric Emergency Room, two inpatient facilities (the Acute Inpatient Treatment Center and the Mental Diagnostic Center), the Emergency Access System, and the new mobile crisis intervention team. The primary core services delivered are emergency screening, crisis stabilization, multidisciplinary assessments, and medication-related services.

Adult Mental Health Services--North Region encompasses these programs: Routh Street Clinic, Ferguson Road Clinic, the day treatment program at Ferguson Road, forensics, substance abuse screening services, and case management . Adult Mental Health Services--South Region consists of the Lancaster-Kiest Clinic, the Centre Street Clinic, the day treatment program at Lancaster-Kiest, geriatric services, the community support program (Independence House), and case management. The core services provided at the north and south adult MH outpatient clinics include multidisciplinary assessments, case management, medication-related services, psychosocial programming, and family support programs.

The great majority of clients are served through the four outpatient clinics. As of October 1988, the clinics were serving 4,370 active clients. The Centre Street Clinic had an active client caseload of 693, Lancaster-Kiest had 1,042 active clients, and Routh Street had 1,550. The Ferguson Road Clinic had 1,085 active clients, 302 of them in the forensics program.

Access to the clinics is limited in two ways: there are strict admission criteria, and there is a waiting list. For the most part, the admission criteria ensure that those served by the clinics will be members of the priority population as defined by TDMHMR. The person must be 18, have a mental disorder, be presently dangerous and presently dependent, or be in danger of deteriorating to dangerousness and/or dependency. However, DCMHMR added one more criterion, which serves to tighten eligibility: the person must have "extremely severe" disturbance of mood or affect.

The clinics maintain protected time slots for the people referred by the Parkland Psychiatric Emergency Room. Consequently, they are generally seen within a week. Persons discharged from the state hospital are generally seen in two to four weeks, and have a continuity-of-care worker to help them in the interim. All other persons have a one- to six-month wait to get an appointment at the clinics (Gill, 1989a). The 1986 Standards and Quality Assurance report on DCMHMR attributed this backlog in large part to the inefficient use of professionals (TDMHMR, 1986). Even when clients have been stabilized for long periods of time, they continue to see a physician at each clinic visit. This occurs despite the fact that DCMHMR, like many other centers, has difficulty finding and retaining physicians. The average caseloads among clinic staff of several professional levels are high: MDs average 342 clients each, RNs have 80 clients, and caseworkers average 137 clients each (DCMHMR, 1989c).

Persons seeking services are screened according to the admission criteria. If admission is appropriate, they are given a multidisciplinary assessment. A caseworker is assigned to the client and an individual service plan is drawn up. The services a client would typically receive from the clinics include a multidisciplinary assessment and a caseworker to help implement the client's individual service plan. An estimated 98 to 99 percent of the clients receive medication services. According to the Evaluation for Fiscal Year 1988 (TDMHMR, 1988, Appendix C), 9.5 percent of DCMHMR's clients receive case management services. Other services are also very limited. The tables and figures discussed below provide some numerical characteristics of the DCMHMR adult mental health programs and the clients they serve.

Table 2.5 illustrates trends in the major categories of adult mental health services from 1986 to 1988. The number of clients served in the Parkland Psychiatric Emergency Room and in the MDC has steadily declined over the three years. As a result, the unit cost of these services has increased. An increase in the number of clients served is documented for nonacute residential services, case management, psychosocial services, and day treatment. The unit cost for these services has also increased. The number of clients served across the categories should not be totaled, since many clients received more than one service.

Some demographic characteristics of mental health clients served by DCMHMR are listed in Table 2.6. Black and Hispanic clients are underrepresented in comparison to their proportion of the population. The percentage of whites served is slightly less than in the county population. The percentage of adult clients 18 to 64 years is 15 percent greater than their numbers in the population. The proportion of adolescent clients 13 to 17 years old closely matches their proportion in the population, but the numbers of children 12 years old or less are much less representative.

Figure 2.3 illustrates the various diagnoses recorded for adults in DCMHMR mental health services. Diagnosis is unreported for nearly half of the client caseload. A little more than one-quarter of the clients have diagnoses of either schizophrenia or affective disorder (depression). However, DCMHMR staff report that 62 percent of adult mental health clients are seriously or chronically mentally ill.

Even though diagnosis is not reported for a large number of clients, all clients are assigned to one of the TDMHMR service groups, as shown in Figure 2.4. Nearly 54 percent are assigned to service group I, the most chronically disabled group.

Fifty percent of the clients have been hospitalized at least once for mental illness, as Figure 2.5 illustrates. Nearly 37 percent are reported to have no history of hospitalization. Data for the remaining clients were not available.

The service needs which are projected for Dallas County are much greater than are currently being met. The needs estimated by DCMHMR are shown in Table 2.7. More recent estimates place the total adult mental health need, excluding substance abuse, at 61,165 persons in Dallas County (Holzer, 1988).

Table 2.8 compares FY 1988 data about mental health clients served by DCMHMR with those served by the three other large urban centers in the state, Bexar, Harris, and Tarrant counties. Although DCMHMR ranked low in total per capita revenues in FY 1987, new state funds and the heavy emphasis on mental health services by the county increased overall mental health services funds. In FY 1988, of the four large centers, DCMHMR had the highest per capita expenditures for mental health services, and the second highest expenditures per client served. DCMHMR ranked above only Harris County in the number of MH clients served per 100,000 population.

Expenditures for mental health services provided by the four large centers are compared in Table 2.9. DCMHMR allocates a greater percentage of its MH services budget to residential services than do the other centers; only Harris County allocates a smaller percentage of its budget to case management than does DCMHMR. DCMHMR is the only large center that does not provide intermediate beds; it should be noted that Tarrant County provides no structured noncrisis beds. Overall, however, DCMHMR provides more residential beds per 100,000 population than do the three other centers.

Table 2.5. Recent Trends in DCMHMR Adult Mental Health Services

	FY 1986	FY 1987	FY 1988
24 Hour Emergency (Parkland)			
Server Hours*	3,853	3,690	3,212
Cost per Server Hour	$112.44	$118.97	$170.80
Number Served	2,061	2,117	1,793
Mental Diagnostic Center (MDC) (Capacity: 45 beds =16,425 bed days)			
Bed Days	11,824	8,691	9,589
Cost per Bed Day	$183.10	$237.96	$226.83
Number Served	1,541	1,260	1,272
Acute Inpatient Treatment Center (AITC) (Capacity: 20 beds = 7300 bed days)			
Bed Days	5,935	6,099	5,994
Cost per Bed Day	$164.94	$164.49	$187.30
Number Served	421	429	406
Other Residential			
Bed Days	50,188	59,935	57,810
Cost per Bed Day	$7.30	$7.96	$7.89
Number Served	245	305	259
Outpatient Services(Medication)			
Server Hours	66,844	69,824	67,539
Cost per Server Hour	$47.93	$43.92	$54.41
Number Served	6,853	6,663	6,520
Continuity-of-Care			
Server Hours	N/A	5,466	4,410
Cost per Server Hour	N/A	$22.90	$25.60
Number Served	N/A	1,003	908
Case Management			
Server Hours	N/A	18,906	17,681
Cost per Server Hour	N/A	$26.37	$26.87
Number Served	N/A	820	1,891
Psychosocial Services			
Client Hours**	133,412	90,128	82,868
Cost per Client Hour	$3.95	$6.28	$7.24
Number Served	351	360	395
Day Treatment			
Client Hours	14,691	25,816	25,106
Cost per Client Hour	$8.96	$11.12	$11.01
Number Served	43	145	109

Source: DCMHMRC, 1989t

*Server Hours are hours of direct service provided by staff.

**Client Hours are hours of services received by clients.

Table 2.6. DCMHMR Mental Health Clients: Demographic Characteristics

	Number FY 1986	Percent of Total MH Caseload	Percent of Dallas Co. Population
Sex			
Male	4,291	49%	48.90%
Female	4,460	51%	51.10%
Age			
0-12	406	4.60%	19.90%
13-17	496	5.70%	6.70%
18-64	7,034	80.40%	64.60%
65 +	815	9.30%	8.70%
Ethnic Group			
White	4,895	55.90%	67.30%
Black	2,636	30.10%	19.70%
Hispanic	676	7.70%	13%
Other/Unknown	544	6.20%	N.A.
Total	8,751	100%	1,790,330(100%)

Source: DCMHMR, 1989v.

Figure 2.3. Adult Mental Health Clients by Diagnosis
FY 1988 Clients = 8,820

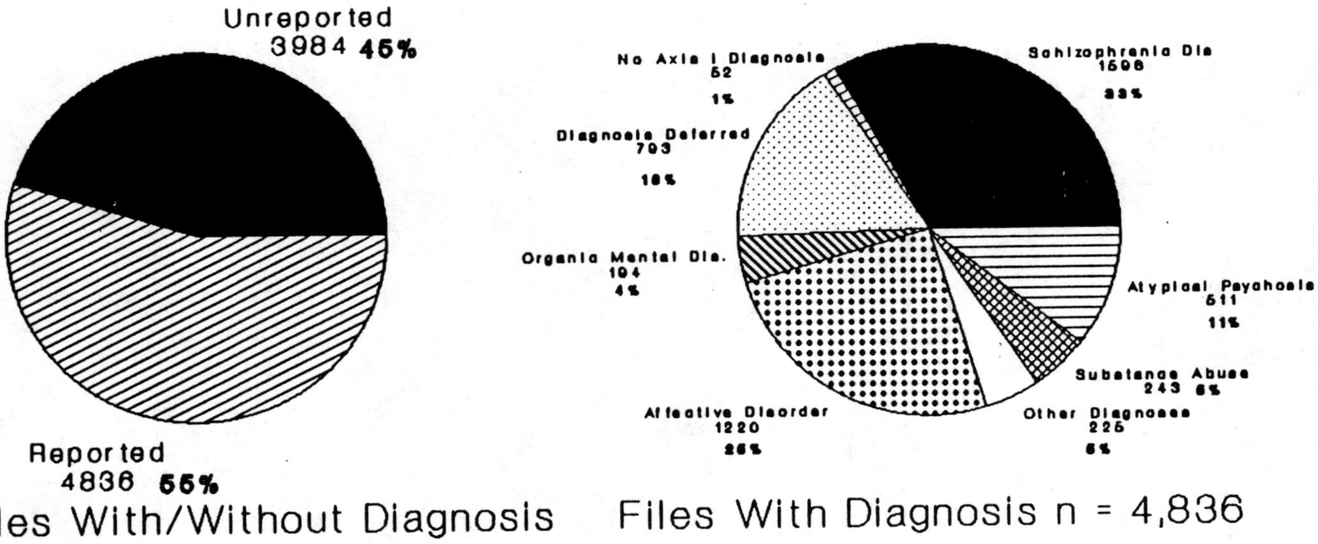

Source: DCMHMR 1989.

**Figure 2.4. Adult Mental Health Clients by Service Group
FY 1988 Total Clients = 8,820**

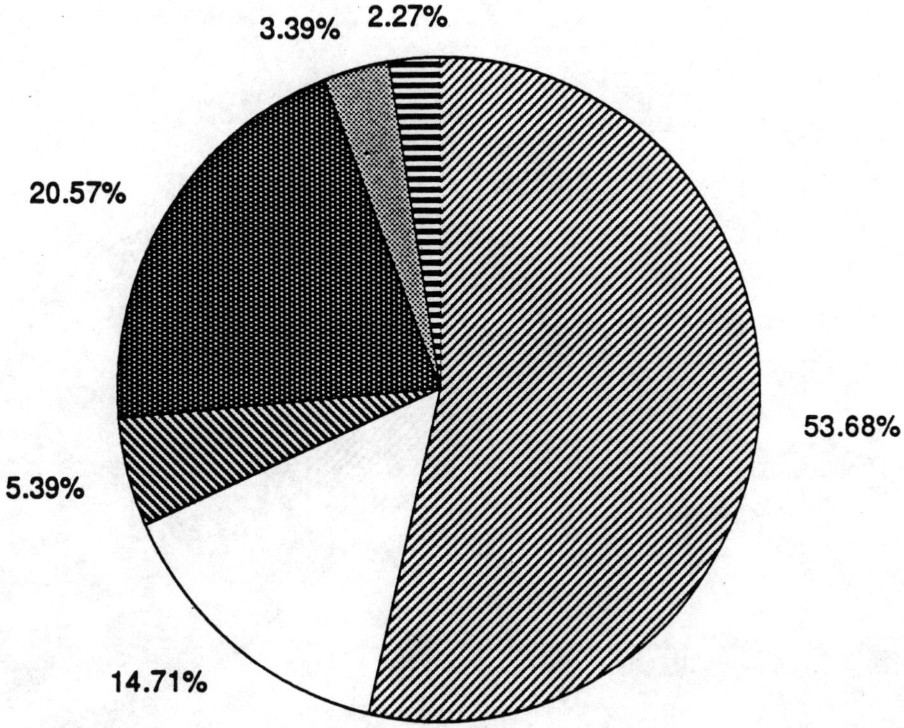

Source: DCMHMR, 1989.

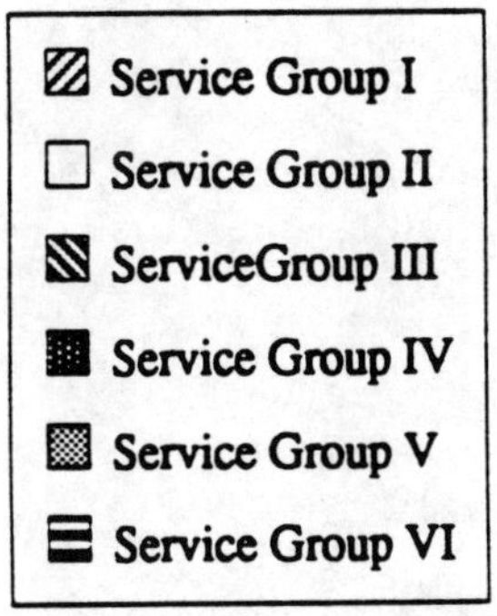

Figure 2.5. Adult Mental Health Clients' History of Hospitalization FY 1988 Total Clients = 8,820

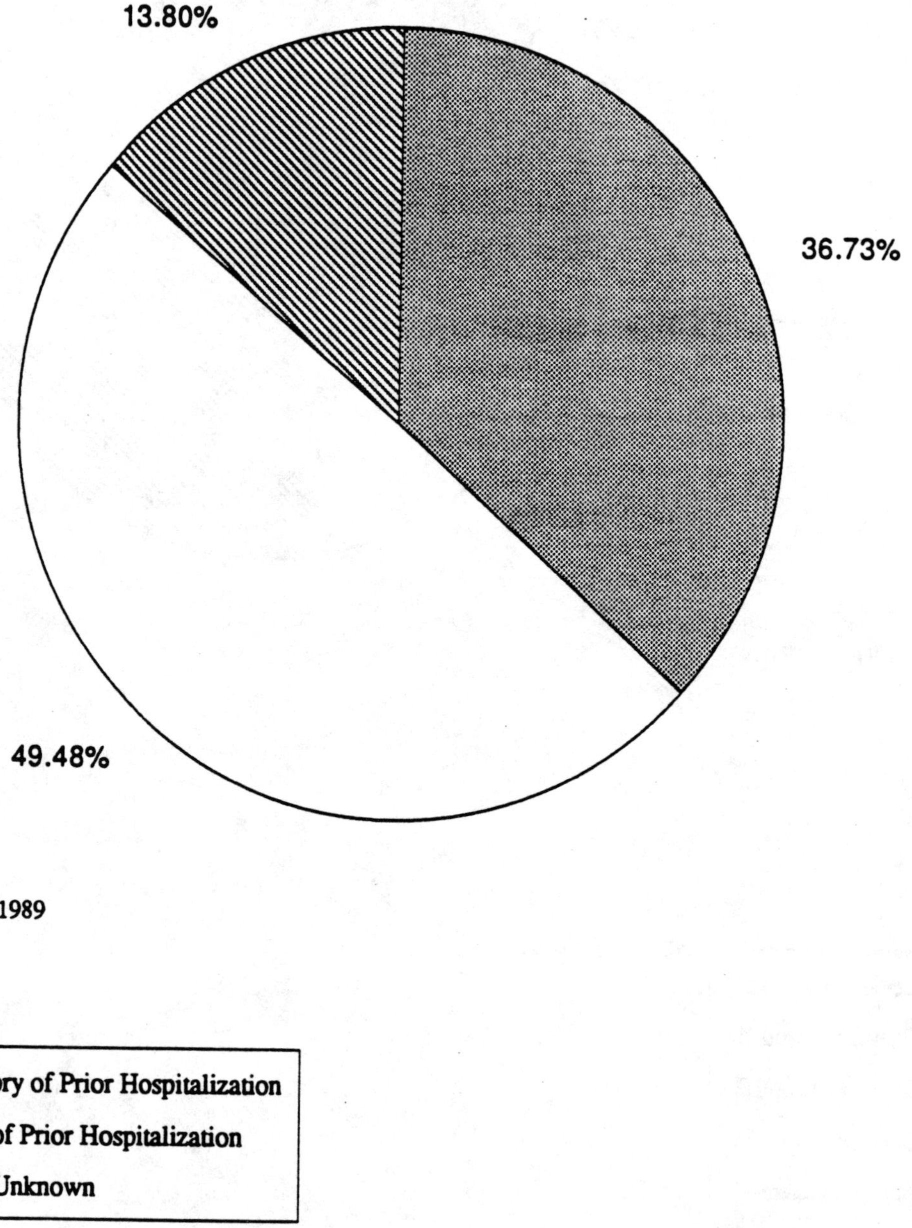

Source: DCMHMR. 1989

Table 2.7. Dallas County Adult Mental Health Client 1988 Need Projections

Disability Level	18-64 years	65+ years	Total
Extreme	1,100	168	1,268
Severe	2,029	309	2,338
Moderate	5,775	880	6,655
Mild	16,455	2,509	18,694
		Total	**29,255**

Source: DCMHMR 1989v, p. 48.
Note: Projections based on a 1976 TDMHMR prevalence and incidence study.

Table 2.8. Mental Health Clients Served by Texas' Four Largest Centers

Fiscal Year 1988	Bexar	Dallas	Harris	Tarrant
County Population	1,158,478	**1,810,294**	3,004,791	1,077,631
Total MH Clients Served*	10,948	**11,441**	13,564	12,529
MH Clients/100,000	945	**632**	451.5	1163
Total Dollars per MH Client	$895.74	**$1,391.42**	$1,799.85	$494.86
Total MH Dollars Per Capita	$8.47	**$8.79**	$8.12	$5.75

Source: TDMHMR, 1989.
*Includes adults and children.

Table 2.9. Mental Health Services in Texas' Four Largest Centers

Fiscal Year 1988	Bexar	Dallas	Harris	Tarrant
Total MH Budget	$9,806,579	$15,919,235	$24,413,130	$6,200,104
MH Residential	$3,686,458	$6,658,103	$9,025,379	$1,381,602
MH Client and Family Support	$4,282,527	$7,188,189	$11,948,753	$3,860,733
MH Case Management	$624,835	$522,499	$718,265	$304,490
MH Management and Support	$1,212,759	$1,550,444	$2,720,733	$653,279
Residential/% of Total Budget	37.60%	41.80%	36.97%	22.28%
Cl. & Fam. S./% of Total Budget	43.67%	45.15%	48.94%	62.27%
Case Mgmnt/% of Total Budget	6.37%	3.28%	2.94%	4.91%
Client & Fam. Sup. $/Client	$585.29	$651.75	$872.04	$304.40
Case Management: $/Client	$505.12	$172.78	$703.49	$749.98
Case Management: Cts. Svrd.	1237	3024	1021	406
Structured Crisis Beds	40	80	294	28
Structured Non-crisis Beds	65	150	91	0
Intermediate Beds	54	0	23	4
Semi-Independent Beds	84	187	95	101
Total Beds	243	417	503	133
Total Beds per 100,000	21	23	16.7	12.4

Source: TDMHMR, 1989.

Like other community centers, DCMHMR provides a variety of services to persons with serious or chronic mental illness. Some of these services are required by state law. These "core" services are emergency screening, crisis stabilization, multidisciplinary assessment, case management, medication-related services, psychosocial rehabilitation services, and family support services. DCMHMR provides other services which, although not required by state law, are essential community services for persons with serious mental illness. The noncore services include residential, hospital liaison, continuity-of-care, income support, and forensics services. Each of the core and noncore services provided by DCMHMR for adults with serious mental illness is discussed below.

CORE SERVICES

Emergency Screening

TDMHMR requires each community center to provide an emergency services program which has a 24-hour crisis hotline and a 24-hour crisis intervention component. Emergency screening programs are designed to assess all persons who are experiencing a psychiatric crisis, or who have the potential to become dangerous to themselves or others, or who are engaging in bizarre behaviors (TDMHMR, 1987).

The DCMHMR emergency screening programs are the Parkland Psychiatric Emergency Room (Parkland ER) and the Emergency Access System (EAS). The four outpatient clinics also provide some emergency screening and crisis intervention services for DCMHMR clients. Generally, when a crisis occurs, the outpatient clinics are the first to be contacted by the client or the client's family. Although the outpatient clinics can dispense medication to stabilize a person in crisis, they are not equipped to handle a very acute crisis (Gonzalez, 1989a). DCMHMR also staffs a Substance Abuse Screening Unit, which works closely with staff of Terrell State Hospital (TDMHMR, 1986, p. 42). However, neither the clinics nor the substance abuse unit meet the 24-hour, seven-day-a-week criterion specified by TDMHMR's definition of emergency screening.

Emergency screening and crisis intervention are provided at the Parkland ER 24 hours a day, seven days a week. Generally, the Parkland ER is used after hours, on weekends, and on holidays when the outpatient services are closed. DCMHMR has a hospital liaison at the Parkland ER who works with the physicians to determine the disposition of a person's case. Another caseworker, at the mental illness court, assists in providing the screening required for court orders of protective custody, as well as consultation and referrals when such orders are not deemed necessary (TDMHMR, 1986, p. 37).

The Parkland ER is located in the Parkland Memorial Hospital. The program began in 1978 with support from the Department of Psychology at the University of Texas Health Science Center, Parkland Memorial Hospital, and DCMHMR (TDMHMR, 1986, p. 37). The purpose of the Parkland ER is to provide short-term, ambulatory emergency and crisis intervention services. This includes identifying precipitating stresses and designing plans to handle them, building up a support network for family and others, ruling out medical problems, and arranging for follow-up care, such as clinic appointments. Persons can also receive drug and alcohol abuse intervention if indicated (Puryear, 1989).

Many persons are brought to the Parkland ER in an acute psychiatric crisis. However, others come because they missed a clinic appointment, want a medication refill, cannot get in touch with their doctor, or cannot get into a clinic within a reasonable amount of time (Puryear, 1989). When a person needs more than crisis intervention, which may or may not include medication, he or she can be transferred to a crisis stabilization (inpatient) program. A person can also be placed in an isolation room if he or she becomes violent . When a person is brought to the Parkland ER by the Dallas Police Department or the Sheriff's Department, and is an involuntary patient, the Parkland ER must get an Order of

Protective Custody (OPC) before it may hold the patient (Puryear, 1989). The Parkland ER may treat patients without an OPC, if the patients are willing. In the rare cases in which a person presents an immediate danger to the emergency room itself, emergency treatment can be provided against the person's wishes (Puryear, 1989).

When a person needs inpatient treatment, the Parkland ER will refer him or her to the DCMHMR Mental Diagnostic Center (MDC) or Acute Inpatient Treatment Center (AITC), Terrell State Hospital, or other area hospitals. Occasionally, persons are referred to Parkland's psychiatric unit, located on the eighth floor of the main building.

Trends in admissions to and referrals from the Parkland ER are shown in Table 2.10. Total visits and total patients brought in on warrants remained relatively constant from 1981 to 1988, despite the county's population growth. The number of persons referred to hospitals, including the MDC, dropped by nearly 50 percent in the time period. The Parkland ER staff have emphasized crisis intervention as a way of avoiding hospitalization since 1981. A specific goal has been to reduce the number of patients hospitalized at MDC or elsewhere (Puryear, 1989). Figure 2.6 is a graphical representation of some of the data in Table 2.10. As shown in Figure 2.7, the number of referrals to the MDC from Parkland has clearly declined since 1981.

If, following emergency services, a person does not require hospitalization but does need follow-up outpatient services, Parkland and the four outpatient clinics use a "protected slot" system (Bursey, 1989a). This system allows appointments to be reserved during a week-long period for clients who have been referred by the Parkland ER (Bursey, 1989a). The client is able to receive follow-up treatment at an outpatient clinic within one week.

The Emergency Access System (EAS) is a 24-hour emergency telephone information and referral service. Generally, it is used by clients and clients' family members when the DCMHMR outpatient services are closed. This would include evenings, weekends, and holidays (Bursey, 1989a). The EAS is staffed by caseworkers with specific training in crisis techniques (Gonzalez, 1989a). Trained telephone counselors, primarily graduate students, respond to the calls from DCMHMR clients, family members, and others (Gonzalez, 1989a). The telephone counselor first assesses the situation and determines whether the client can wait for outpatient services or is in need of immediate crisis intervention services. If the counselor thinks that the caller is indeed approaching a crisis, he or she can contact the assigned backup administrator or physician who is on call (Gonzalez, 1989a).

The four outpatient clinics also provide some screening services for DCMHMR clients. The outpatient clinics are usually the first to be contacted by the clients and the client family members if the crisis occurs during regular working hours. The outpatient clinic will screen the client to determine his or her condition. If the outpatient clinic staff feels that the client is in acute crisis, the client may be sent to the Parkland ER, the AITC, or the MDC (Gonzalez, 1989a).

Another screening service provided by DCMHMR is the Substance Abuse Screening Unit, located at the Routh Street Clinic. This program is designed to assist Dallas County residents who would like to enter the substance abuse program at Terrell State Hospital (TDMHMR, 1986, p. 42). Screening for hospital admission is the only substance abuse service now offered by DCMHMR. The unit has one caseworker who works closely with the Terrell State Hospital staff. Potential clients make intake appointments. The applicants must then fill out a self-questionnaire regarding substance abuse and patterns of

Table 2.10. Parkland Hospital Psychiatric Emergency Room Trends

	1981	1982	1983	1984	1985	1986	1987	1988
Total Patient Visits	7933	9312	9589	10606	11465	11047	10667	9720
Total Patients on Warrants	1124	1020	1134	1237	1419	1279	1288	1191
Total Referred to All Hospitals	2138	1931	1704	1556	1668	1336	1125	1126
Total Referred to MDC	1482	1472	1324	1288	1335	1111	943	922
Patients on Warrants to MDC	732	568	558	610	648	480	465	432
Other Patients to MDC	883	883	766	679	687	631	478	490

Source: Data provided by Parkland Hospital Psychiatric E.R. staff, January 1989.
Note: Readmissions not reported separately.

Figure 2.6. Parkland Hospital's Emergency Room Admission and Referral Trends

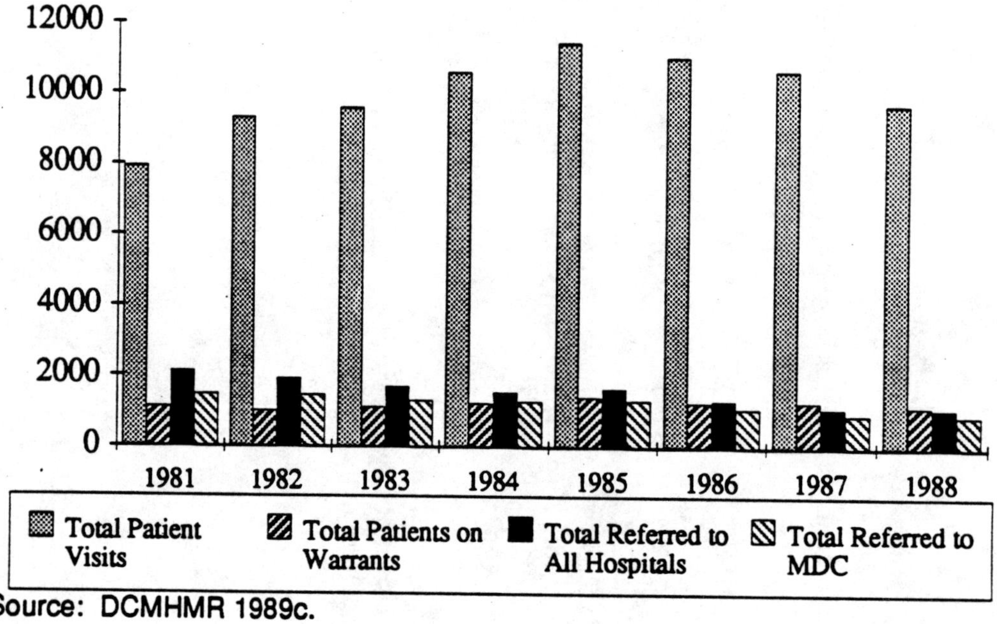

Source: DCMHMR 1989c.

Figure 2.7. Trends in Referrals to the Mental Diagnostic Center from Parkland's Psychiatric Emergency Room

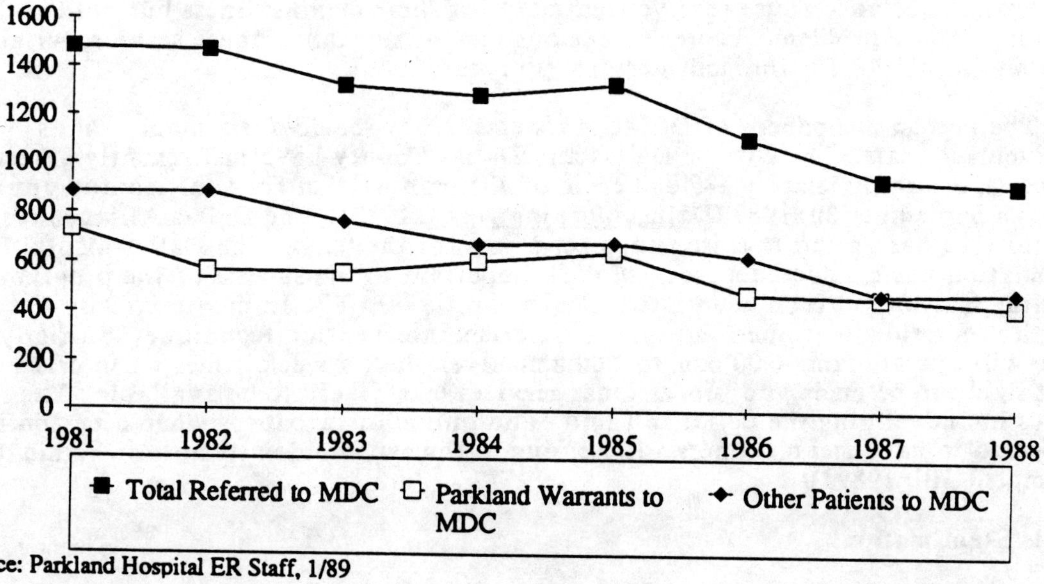

Source: Parkland Hospital ER Staff, 1/89

use. The client must convince the caseworker that he or she is serious about wanting help with a drug or alcohol problem. The client must remain drug- and alcohol-free to be eligible for the program at Terrell State Hospital. At the conclusion of the interview, persons who meet these requirements are placed on the Terrell State Hospital waiting list (TDMHMR, 1986, p. 42). At present, the waiting time is anywhere from 60 days to four months.

Follow-along services are not provided to persons who are awaiting inpatient services for substance abuse problems. The only contact a client receives from the caseworker while on the waiting list is notification when a bed is available at Terrell State Hospital. Once a client has been discharged from Terrell State Hospital's substance abuse program, little aftercare is provided to the patient by DCMHMR (TDMHMR, 1986, p. 42). Reportedly, a major problem is that many clients who have a dual diagnosis of both mental illness and substance abuse receive treatment for their mental illness but not for their substance abuse problem. There is a serious lack of substance abuse services within and without DCMHMR for indigent persons. (Puryear, 1989).

The newest component of DCMHMR's emergency services is a mobile crisis intervention team. The City of Dallas and Dallas County have just recently agreed to split the costs, or approximately $87,000 each, of the mobile team for four months, June 1 through September 30, 1989 (Dallas Morning News, 1989). The Dallas Alliance for the Mentally Ill has agreed to raise funds for a van for the team. The Dallas Mental Health Association has conducted advocacy work important to the success of the program. Future funding has not yet been negotiated (Boardman, 1989). The team will consist of two mental health professionals trained in psychiatric crisis intervention techniques. Initially, the team will operate from 6:00 p.m. to 2:00 a.m. seven days a week, times when crisis calls are most likely to be made and professional services least likely to be available. The team's duties include aiding the police in family and public disturbances when a person is suspected to have mental illness and helping to thwart suicide attempts or homicide attempts (Gill, 1989d).

Crisis Stabilization

Crisis stabilization programs provide short-term (acute) inpatient care in a highly structured and supervised environment (TDMHMR, 1987). The program serves persons who are in a psychiatric crisis and in need of intensive treatment or stabilization. At DCMHMR, the crisis stabilization programs are the Mental Diagnostic Center and the Acute Inpatient Treatment Center.

The MDC is a short-term, licensed psychiatric hospital located behind Parkland Memorial Hospital. The MDC is funded by the Dallas County Commissioners Court and operated by DCMHMR (Long, 1989). DCMHMR contracted with Dallas County to operate the MDC, formerly the Mental Evaluation Center, in 1976, nine years before crisis stabilization was required by the state (Long, 1981). The purpose of the MDC is to provide aggressive crisis stabilization while a patient is being assessed by the courts. All patients are admitted involuntarily and must have an OPC, effective for 14 days (Puryear, 1989). The average length of stay is six days; usually a patient remains in the MDC until the mental illness court decides whether he or she should be committed to the Terrell State Hospital, referred to other community programs, or released to return home to the family. A mental illness court is located on the premises of the MDC (Gill, 1989a).

While at the MDC, a client is assessed by a team of nurses, a general physician, two psychiatrists, and caseworkers to determine the team's recommendation to the court. The client is stabilized with both medication and therapy, and is supervised 24-hours per day (Gonzales, 1989). The staff at MDC also offers classes to assist the client in stress reduction, assertiveness training, communication skills, and goal planning as part of the crisis stabilization program (Gonzalez, 1989b).

Clients are referred to the MDC from a variety of sources, including the Parkland ER, DCMHMR, Terrell State Hospital, private hospitals, the Veterans Administration, and others. The number of referrals to the MDC from the Parkland ER dropped from 70.6 percent to 66.6 percent of total referrals between the first and fourth quarters in calendar year 1988 as shown in Table 2.11. The proportion of patients in the MDC with serious psychoses also dropped from 70 percent to 60 percent of the total over the year. Both the percentage and absolute number of persons referred to Terrell State Hospital by the MDC also dropped. This is viewed as a positive result by DCMHMR (Gill, 1989a).

The MDC serves men and women of all ages, as well as a small number of children and adolescents. Persons who are sent to the MDC have a variety of mental illnesses, often coupled with drug or alcohol dependencies. According to Douglas Puryear, M.D., director of Emergency Services, "patients with drug and alcohol problems, especially patients whose problem is primarily drug and alcohol, are rarely sent to the MDC. There is in fact a serious lack of treatment within or without the MHMR system for drug and alcohol problems for the indigent" (Puryear, 1989, p. 3). Details regarding client referrals, diagnostic categories, and case disposition are shown in Table 2.11.

When the client is stabilized and the mental health court determines that the client can be discharged, the client leaves the MDC. In FY 1988, the MDC served 1,272 clients (Gonzales, 1989a). The average cost per client per day at the MDC is reported to be $226.83. The total annual costs were reported to be $2,175,113. The 45-bed MDC reported 9,589 bed days, which represents a 58 percent occupancy rate (DCMHMR, 1989o). At full occupancy there would be a total of 16,425 bed days. The current occupancy rate of 58 percent (it was 72 percent in 1986) is a concern because the lower occupancy rate increases the cost per client.

The other DCMHMR crisis stabilization program is the Acute Inpatient Treatment Center, (AITC) located at the Hillside Center. Formerly the Beverly Hills Psychiatric Hospital, the facility was acquired by DCMHMR in 1977 through a long-term lease. The facility was initially licensed for 29 beds; this was expanded to 45 beds in 1978, and to 70 beds in 1981 (Long, 1981). It is now licensed for 40 beds but operates only 35 beds (TDMHMR, 1986, p. 56). The 20-bed AITC provides intensive psychiatric care for Dallas County adults. Of the 20 adult beds, 10 are for men and 10 are for women (Gonzalez, 1989b). The 15-bed unit for children and adolescents has recently been temporarily closed, primarily because of funding and staffing problems.

The objective of the AITC is to help stabilize clients to prevent them from returning or transferring to Terrell State Hospital (Gonzalez, 1989b). The clients need to be stabilized quickly so they can be transferred to a less restrictive environment (Gonzalez, 1989). AITC staff will only accept voluntary clients; the staff is reluctant to accept clients who are suicidal, violent, or seriously disturbed. The patient must be able to function in an open but highly protective and therapeutic environment (Gonzalez, 1989b).

The average length of stay in the AITC is 16 days, but a patient can remain until he or she is ready to be transferred to a less restrictive environment (Gonzalez, 1989b). Most patients stay from one to three weeks, depending on their condition (TDMHMR, 1986, p. 57). A variety of activities are provided as part of the crisis stabilization program at the AITC. These highly structured activities focus on skills designed to help the patient reintegrate into society by teaching basic coping, survival, and self-help skills (Gonzalez, 1989b).

Table 2.11. Mental Diagnostic Center Service Characteristics

	1/1/88-3/31/88	10/1/88-12/31/88
Client Referral Source		
Parkland Memorial Hospital	281	237
DCMHMRC	44	25
Home	12	6
Terrell State Hospital	20	26
Private	30	41
Dallas/Waco Veteran's Admin.	7	18
All Other	4	3
Total	398	356
Admissions of Children/Adolescents	15	28
Client Diagnostic Categories		
Schizophrenia	7%	10.10%
Paranoid Schizophrenia	21%	17.10%
Atypical Psychosis	30%	23.30%
Bipolar Disorder	12%	9.60%
Alcohol/Drug Dependence	8%	9.50%
Other Disorders	22%	30.40%
Disposition of Clients		
Terrell State Hospital	39.70%	33.10%
DCMHMRC Adult Inpatient	18.60%	21.60%
DCMHMRC Outpatient	7.30%	6.20%
Home	18.10%	25.60%
Parkland Inpatient	2.50%	3.70%
Shelter/Salvation Army	1.50%	1.70%
Criminal Justice System	1%	1.40%
All Other	11.30%	6.70%
Average Daily Census	24.18	21.81
Average Patient Length of Stay	5.53 days	5.64 days

Source: DCMHMR Quarterly Reports to Dallas County Judge and Commissioners, 1/1/88-3/31/88; 10/1/88-12/31/88.

When patients leave the AITC, they are often released to an intensive follow-up program such as a day treatment or a community support program. Patients with a stable home environment are able to return home. However, the patients usually need a more intensive follow-up than just assignment to an outpatient clinic (Gonzalez, 1989b).

Most patients who come to the AITC are indigent. If the patient has Medicaid or Medicare coverage, it can be used to pay for the services offered at the AITC. Most patients sent to the AITC have no private insurance or their insurance has run out. A majority of the costs are covered by revenue received from TDMHMR (Gonzalez, 1989b).

In FY 1988, the AITC served 406 patients. The unit cost per day was $187.30. Total annual cost was $1,122,652. The AITC reported 5,994 bed days (DCMHMR, 1989o). These figures include services to both adults and children based on the 20 adult beds and 15 child and adolescent beds.

Multidisciplinary Assessment

Multidisciplinary assessment is the assessment or evaluation of a client by a psychiatrist and other psychological, nursing, or social service workers (TDMHMR, 1987). Several DCMHMR programs offer multidisciplinary assessments for adult clients, including the MDC, the AITC, and the four adult outpatient clinics.

According to DCMHMR, the purpose of the MDC is to provide aggressive crisis stabilization while patients are being assessed for the courts (TDMHMR, 1986, p. 47). The MDC staff includes 3 psychiatrists, 1 general physician, 7 caseworkers, 1 psychologist, 2 recreational therapists, 11 registered nurses, and 2 licensed vocational nurses (TDMHMR, 1986, p. 48). This team provides thorough physical, psychological, and social examinations on each client. The client's past medical and psychiatric information is also assessed during admission into the MDC (DCMHMR, 1988c, p. 4). The combined evaluations of the multidisciplinary team constitute the recommendation that is given to the mental illness court to determine the disposition of the client's case.

The AITC also provides multidisciplinary assessments to the clients who are referred to them. The staff at the AITC includes one general physician, one full-time psychiatrist, one half-time psychiatrist, one RN, two LVNs, and four social workers (Gonzalez, 1989b). The client is given a multidisciplinary assessment as part of the crisis stabilization program at the AITC (Gonzalez, 1989b).

Multidisciplinary assessments are provided to clients by the outpatient clinics, which assign clients to the clinics by their zip codes (Bursey, 1989b). The Routh Street Clinic currently has 3.3 psychiatrists, 3 RNs, and 8 caseworkers. The Ferguson Road Clinic has 2.6 psychiatrists, 2 RNs, and 4 caseworkers. The Lancaster-Keist Clinic has 4.5 psychiatrists, 2 RNs, and 8 caseworkers. The Centre Street Clinic currently has 1.5 psychiatrists, 2 RNs, and 5 caseworkers (DCMHMR, 1989c).

If a client has been referred by the Parkland ER, the client is put on a "protected slot" list. The outpatient clinic will see the client within one week (Bursey, 1989b). The hospital liaison contacts the clinic and supplies basic information about the client (Bursey, 1989b). This emergency client can also been seen by the pro bono clinic, which is a volunteer clinic provided every Thursday night by the Dallas chapter of the North Texas Psychiatric Physician Association. Nine time slots are reserved each week for clients referred from Parkland ER (Bursey, 1989b). If the client is not on the "protected slot" list and is not considered to be in crisis, there is often a wait of up to four to six weeks for a multidisciplinary assessment. It can take up to one to six months to be assessed at the larger clinics (Gill, 1989a).

All multidisciplinary assessments at the outpatient clinics basically follow the same procedures. A caseworker sees the client to determine the client's past hospitalizations, social history, environmental factors, family history, vocational history, and past services used (Bursey, 1989b). Other needs of the client are also assessed, including the client's housing, emotional, and financial needs (Bursey, 1989b). Then the client is seen by a psychiatrist to discuss the client's past psychiatric history, emotional problems, and other needs. At this point an RN will check the client's weight, height, blood pressure, heart, and lungs. Since not all of the outpatient clinics have a general physician, the client can be referred for further medical attention to Parkland Memorial Hospital or can wait to see the public health nurse who comes to the clinics once a month (Bursey, 1989b).

Medication-Related Services

In addition to the prescription and dispensing of various medications to clients, medication-related services include laboratory monitoring, medication education, and counseling. Since an estimated 98 to 99 percent of outpatient clinic clients are taking medication, medication-related services constitute a very large share of services.

DCMHMR operates four licensed pharmacies. The pharmacists maintain a manual patient profile for each client receiving medications; this profile includes the medication(s), strength, dosage form, drug sensitivities, and related information. The manual system is to be computerized in the near future, allowing more information to be kept for each client. The pharmacies dispense only psychotropic medications. DCMHMR spends approximately $500,000 each year for medications. Prescribed medications are provided free of charge to indigent clients. Those clients with some financial resources are requested to pay on a sliding fee scale (Tanowitz, 1989).

Medical peer review is conducted monthly by the staff physicians, outside consultants, and others qualified to evaluate client treatment and response. These reviews focus on appropriateness of prescribing patterns, including dosage levels, client response, and adverse drug reaction, and on laboratory work and physical assessments when indicated (Cotten, 1989b).

The DCMHMR physicians see clients who are taking prescribed medications every four to six weeks or, if necessary, once a week. Physicians require weekly appointments for those clients who need a greater degree of monitoring, a possible change in psychotropic medication, or laboratory work. More stabilized clients are seen at least every six months; physical exams, laboratory tests, and mental assessments are conducted when indicated. To help increase flexibility in scheduling appointments, DCMHMR ensures that time slots are available for clients who are drop-ins or for those who have missed appointments. Clients who are delinquent in keeping appointments are referred to their caseworker, who then makes at least three attempts to contact the clients.

The physician, nurse, or case manager meets with individual clients monthly about all aspects of their medication, reinforcing the critical nature of taking medication as prescribed and educating clients about indications of adverse reactions and other side effects. This is an ongoing process to assist the client and the staff in detecting reactions that might dictate medication reappraisal. DCMHMR has a written curriculum for educating clients, both individually and in groups, about stress management, emphasizing techniques for combatting high stress and debilitating anxiety levels. Coping mechanisms, such as biofeedback, support groups, and psychotherapy are often suggested.

The critical role of medication compliance and adequate diet in mental health care is reviewed on a continuing basis. The contribution of support groups, whether friends, family, or peers, in achieving medication compliance and adequate diet is repeatedly sought. Case managers try to assist clients in forming self-help networks, including family advocacy groups. In addition, case managers attempt to help families understand the various facets of mental illness.

Case Management

All priority population clients are assessed for case management at the inpatient units or as they enter the adult outpatient clinics. The primary referral sources for case management are the adult outpatient clinics, the inpatient units, the community support programs, and the continuity-of-care unit. No formal waiting list exists, although all parties agree that the demand exceeds the available slots.

For a client to be admitted to case management, he or she must (1) be eligible for one or more clinical services of DCMHMR; (2) require assistance in specific areas of deficiency to maintain reasonable autonomy in the community, which cannot be provided through other programs or staff of DCMHMR; (3) agree to a specific plan of case management services; and (4) be markedly deficient in one or more of the following areas: basic living skills, appropriate housing, food or public support services, employment or educational skills, the ability to comply with care and treatment plans without ongoing monitoring or support, or an adequate caregiver support system.

Case management provides the client with service referral, linking, coordinating, and monitoring, as well as an individualized service plan, 24-hour accessibility to case managers through beepers or through the Emergency Access System, and case managers who work out in the community.

Clients are discharged from case management when (1) they have reached their stated goals on the individual service plans or have achieved maximum possible benefit from the service and require no further monitoring, support, or advocacy by the case manager; (2) their condition deteriorates to the extent that care in a state facility is needed (clients placed at the MDC and AITC are not discharged from case management); (3) they fail to make progress toward their stated goals despite staff efforts to renegotiate goals, remove barriers, and confront unproductive behaviors over at least a 30-day period; or (4) they choose to discontinue their participation, they move out of the service area, or they die (DCMHMR, 1989e).

Organizational Structure. According to the DCMHMR organizational chart, the director of Case Management Services is within two levels of the executive director, as required by TDMHMR's case management standards. However, this position has been vacant for two years. Presently there are three case management teams, each with their own supervisors, who are administratively supervised by the north and south regional directors. The director of Mental Health Services is the acting director of Case Management Services at DCMHMR and has overall responsibility for the program. In FY 1988, 1,891 clients were served for 17,681 server hours at a cost of $475,100. This is a cost of $251.24 per client or $26.87 per server hour.

Case Management Units. The North Region unit consists of two case managers at the Ferguson Road Clinic, two at the Routh Street Clinic, and a coordinator for the region. The South Region unit consists of two case managers at the Centre Street Clinic, two at the Lancaster-Kiest Clinic, and a coordinator for the region. The residential case management team for the Community Support Program consists of five case managers, one supervisor, and one coordinator. The coordinator takes half a case load and spends the rest of her time on administrative chores.

Of the total 17 case managers, 7 serve the 110 residential clients at Independence House exclusively (Williams, 1989). The other 10 case managers serve those clients eligible for case management from the remaining 8,710 adult mental health clients. The average community center in Texas case manages 9.68 percent of its total MH clientele at any one point in time (TDMHMR, 1988, Appendix C). If this same percentage were to hold for Dallas, these 10 case managers would be managing 843 clients for an average caseload size of 84.3. Since the clinic case managers are reporting caseload sizes of between 22 and 24, DCMHMR case management is obviously serving a smaller percentage of its clients than the average community center is at any given point in time. If 24 is accepted as the average caseload size, then the total number of clients being case managed at any one time at DCMHMR is approximately 350 (240 and 110), or 4 percent of the total clients being served.

According to data issued for the first and second quarter of FY 1988 by Case Management Services at Central Office, DCMHMR reported that 706 of 7,423 MH clients were receiving ongoing case management. Taken at face value, this would mean huge caseload sizes (42 if all clients were divided equally and 59.6 if the seven case managers assigned to Independence House and their 110 clients are factored out). These numbers do not agree at all with the caseload sizes the case managers are reporting. One interpretation is that the figure 706 was reported incorrectly and reflects not the number of ongoing clients receiving case management but, instead, the total served by case management in the first and second quarter. A reasonable conclusion that can be drawn from these numbers is that although the proportion of clients who receive case management at DCMHMR is similar to the proportion of clients receiving case management at other community centers, the DCMHMR clients receive the service for shorter periods of time. DCMHMR has a large turnover of clients in case management; the number, 706 clients, is in line with what DCMHMR would serve over a six-month period.

In its long-range plan, DCMHMR estimated that 15 percent of the clinic population needs case management services at any one time. As of October 1988, the clinics had 4,370 active clients. Fifteen percent of this would be 656 clients, a number significantly higher than the approximately 240 being served. The center requested four new case managers (one for each clinic) in its FY 1989 budget proposal to their board; the request could not be funded.

A discussion of case management at DCMHMR must take into account the two different forms of case management being practiced. The residential case management team that is part of the Community Support Program at Independence House operates very differently from the teams at the clinics. The seven case managers at Independence House (actually one of the seven has a reduced caseload, since the coordinator divides her time between clients and administrative tasks) deal exclusively with the 110 clients who live in the Community Support Program (CSP) apartments. The only exception to this is when they occasionally deal with other nonresidential CSP clients, in preparation for their joining the apartment program. Case management of the apartment residents is very intense; it even involves teaching clients how to defrost their freezers. The case managers totally manage their clients' environment and are credited with keeping their clients out of the state hospital. Their case management is long-term; they have clients who have been on their caseloads for four or more years. The average caseload size is 17. In many ways, this is the classic definition of case management according to TDMHMR. But there is one important difference: this is a <u>residential</u>-based case management team. Admission to case management is based on where the clients live; only those clients living in the CSP apartments are eligible to receive this service.

The remainder of this section will deal with the case management teams at the clinics. There are two distinctive aspects to clinic-based case management services. The first is that they are decentralized. The advantages of this decentralized approach are (1) the case manager is closer to the population base he or she serves and to other members of the treatment team; (2) there is less friction between case managers and caseworkers because caseworkers see that, while case managers have smaller loads, they deal with them more intensely and operate "out in the field"; and (3) the clinic has greater flexibility to use the case managers where they are most needed. A result of this flexibility is that case managers are occasionally used by the clinics for tasks other than case management, a practice that does not comply with TDMHMR's standards. An example of this is using case managers to help secure income support for clients who are not eligible for case management. Another disadvantage is that, although each clinic has exactly two case managers, they have vastly different numbers of active clients. For instance, Routh Street Clinic has 1,550 active clients; the Centre Street Clinic has only 693 active clients. Assuming they have the same client profile, with the same percentage of clients needing case management services, then case management is less accessible to clients at Routh Street than at Centre Street.

The second, and probably more important, distinction of clinic-based case management at DCMHMR is that while Central Office envisions case management as ongoing, long-term support, DCMHMR expects clinic-based case management to focus on concrete issues with measurable objectives and to be time-limited. Before admission into the program, the client, the assessment team, and the case manager agree to a specific case management service plan. For the most part, these service plans call for three months or less of targeted intervention (according to the DCMHMR Long-Range Plan, it is 1 to 12 weeks). Generally targeted are housing, income support, and other services essential to living in the community. While the service plan may not exceed 90 days, it may be renewed or modified. Once the goals are met or if progress toward the goals is not occurring because of the client's "unproductive behavior," the client is dismissed (DCMHMR, 1989e).

DCMHMR staff realize that some clients may require further monitoring after specific goals are met. In fact, a two-tier system is in existence, with a majority of the clients passing through case management in the three-month period while others remain much longer. These two tiers represent very different philosophies and practices of case management, and they demonstrate the philosophical differences between DCMHMR and Central Office when it comes to case management.

DCMHMR, in many ways, epitomizes the Hobson choice available to many of the large urban centers when it comes to case management. The staff agrees, in concept, with the idea of long-term case management and, in fact, views this as the ideal state of affairs. However, it has so many clients in need of case management and it has so few resources, in terms of funds and personnel, to service this need that it opts for shorter, targeted case management in order to provide a critical service to a larger number of people. "If you have ten people in front of you, each of whom needs case management, but you only have the resources to provide pure long-term case management to one of them, you can either opt to provide it to the one and tell the others that you can't help them or you can give all of them at least a have-to-have level of service" (Gill, 1989c). DCMHMR, by and large, opts for the latter.

Psychosocial Programs

TDMHMR defines psychosocial programs as an array of services designed to help clients acquire and maintain life skills. Required components include ongoing social support activities, independent living skills (learning to manage money, purchasing and preparing food, using community resources such as public transportation, libraries, and public health clinics, and adopting appropriate social behavior through personal-social adjustment training), prevocational training, and vocational training.

DCMHMR has some exemplary psychosocial programming, but service availability falls far short of demand. At any one time, approximately 383 adult mental health clients are involved in some form of psychosocial programming at DCMHMR: 250 in the community support programs, 32 in the day treatment programs, and 101 in ADAPT, a private contractor of a vaiety of psychosocial services. This is approximately 4.7 percent of the total adult mental health clients being served. In the FY 1989 budget proposal to its board, DCMHMR staff requested a new psychosocial rehabilitation program for 200 clients and 14 FTEs at a cost of $452,596. The program would have included prevocational training, social and educational training, supported employment and vocational training, and semi-independent apartment living (20 beds). There were insufficient funds for granting the request (DCMHMR, 1988a).

There are three psychosocial programs at DCMHMR. The Community Support Program (Independence House) meets all of TDMHMR's standards, providing programs in all four required areas of psychosocial services. The Community Support Program is the only program identified in the DCMHMR's budget as a psychosocial program. The day treatment programs, despite the name and the fact that DCMHMR lists this service as noncore, clearly have psychosocial elements. ADAPT is listed in the budget as structured noncrisis residential, according to the TDMHMR contract budget structure. But ADAPT provides more than 30 hours per week per client of psychosocial programming.

Community Support Programs at Independence House. Started in 1977, Independence House is based on a clubhouse model in which the clients are "members" and services are provided in an atmosphere of comfortable informality. Independence House is not one but five "programs," although these are not identified as separate services. The five program components are prevocational, vocational, social/educational, transitional (cluster) apartment living, and long-term apartment living. Clients are "members" and help to plan the services. Staff and members work together in a "partnership model." The emphasis is on encouraging clients to take responsibility for themselves. In general, Independence House clients are less dysfunctional than those referred to ADAPT.

There are approximately 250 members at any one time. A member is someone who is enrolled in one of the CSP programs or is a resident of the CSP apartments. Apartment residents have priority access to the CSP programs and use approximately 50 percent of the available slots (Blegen-Sola, 1989). To be eligible for the CSP program, a client must be at least 18 years old, and have a two-year history of chronic mental illness, with at least one psychiatric hospitalization. The prevocational and vocational programs have additional admission criteria.

The primary referral sources for the CSP programs are the DCMHMR adult outpatient clinics, the MDC and AITC, DCMHMR's Case Management Services, the DCMHMR day treatment programs, Terrell State Hospital, and other CSP service units. In FY 1988, 395 clients were served, for 82,868 client hours at a cost of $600,296 or $1,520 per client or $7.24 per client hour.

The social/educational program is open to the entire membership, but because of limited physical space only 80 clients can participate in any one activity. The program consists of planned social activities such as holiday celebrations, plays, movies, trips, and campouts, as well as less structured activities at the clubhouse like games, TV, and music. The educational/information groups include a formal curriculum in basic community living skills as well as rotating classes such as GED classes, and classes on income tax preparation, voter registration, orientation to community recreational resources, leisure-time management, and communication skills. The social/educational activities are held Monday through Thursday from 3:00 p.m. to 8:00 p.m., on Fridays from 3:00 p.m. to 10:00 p.m., and Saturdays from 11:00 a.m. to 6:30 p.m. (DCMHMR, 1989g).

In the prevocational day program, clients join one of three work activity units available from 9:00 a.m. to 3:00 p.m. Monday through Friday. The program capacity is 36 (12 per work unit). The program admits clients who have been recently discharged or are about to be discharged from inpatient facilities and who need the structure of a daily program to make a successful transition back to independent community living. DCMHMR reports that clients with a primary diagnosis of schizophrenia or major depression benefit most from the program (DCMHMR, 1989f).

In the clerical work activity unit, members answer the phone, type, file, order supplies, distribute the mail, and produce the "Independence House Flyer" newsletter. In the food services unit, members plan menus, grocery shop, and prepare and serve two meals a day, in addition to special holiday refreshments. The maintenance and grounds work unit crew is responsible for cleaning the clubhouse, landscaping and keeping the grounds, making minor repairs, and attending to special projects such as the greenhouse.

To join this program a client must (1) be presently stabilized on psychotropic medications and in need of a structured day program to maintain stability, avoid rehospitalization, or to develop a readiness for work or job training; (2) be willing to attend a minimum of three days per week and to become actively involved in a work unit; (3) not be presently abusing street drugs or alcohol; (4) have self-control to the extent that behavior does not pose a hazard to self or others; and (5) have transportation to and from the program (DCMHMR, 1989f).

The vocational program provides a continuum of vocational evaluation, training, and paid employment opportunities "designed to develop the work potential of adults with a history of chronic mental illness" (DCMHMR, 1989h). The program has a capacity of 80 clients, and preference is given to clients who have no other income source and are thus at significant risk for rehospitalization, with first priority going to CSP residential clients who must work to remain in their apartment.

Clients are involved in one or more of the following services according to their individual needs :

1. Vocational evaluation: The client's skills, abilities, work tolerance, training needs and vocational interests are assessed through a battery of formal and informal tests and work samples. The McCarron-Dial Vocational Evaluation Battery is a part of this assessment.

2. Job readiness classes: The client receives up to 30 hours of intensive instruction in those practical skills and behaviors that lead to obtaining and keeping a job. The curriculum for these classes is certified by the Texas Rehabilitation Commission (TRC).

3. Contract employment: Work-ready clients are placed on small work crews. Workers are supervised by familiar CSP vocational staff, and they earn minimum wage. There are currently two work crews. One crew works up to 30 hours a week keeping Dallas highways litter-free under a contract with the Texas Department of Highways and Public Transportation. Another crew works 3 hours a night providing janitorial services to two agency clinics.

4. Transitional employment: Clients who need up to one year of work training or experience in a supportive setting are placed in jobs within the DCMHMR housekeeping, canteen, or food service departments, again at minimum wage.

5. Job placement: Clients with demonstrated readiness are placed in a variety of competitive community jobs by CSP job placement specialists. They receive the same salary and benefits as any employee. CSP vocational staff remain involved with the client and community employer indefinitely to ensure the best chance for ongoing success.

6. Worker recognition: Many working clients function as role models and leaders in other CSP Independence House programs. The clubhouse fosters recognition through special events such as vocational awards banquets which draw together workers, employers, and civic leaders.

To participate in the vocational program, clients must be presently stabilized on psychotropic medication and willing to comply with the medication plan, have adequate physical stamina and willingness to participate in vocational programming, and not be presently abusing street drugs or alcohol or demonstrating destructive behavior that would pose a hazard at a job site (DCMHMR, 1989h).

These community support programs at Independence House received much praise in the 1986 Standards and Quality Assurance report and justly so. The clients interviewed expressed the opinion that, but for these programs, they would have no reason to go on. Unfortunately, the demand for these programs exceeds the program's capacity. The director of the South Region said she could easily fill three more Independence Houses.

A major obstacle to CSP's growth is the inadequacy of its facilities, which are old and cramped. Inadequate facilities also limit CSP in other ways. Both the prevocational and vocational programs might be eligible for TRC funds if the facilities at Independence House were handicapped-accessible. Because the facilities are not, CSP receives monies from TRC only when that agency specifically refers someone to CSP for job training classes (Williams, 1989). If and when new facilities are secured, TRC money can be more vigorously pursued.

Day Treatment Programs. Day treatment services operate from 8:30 a.m. to 4:30 p.m. Monday through Friday at the Ferguson Road Clinic for the North Region and the Lancaster/Kiest Clinic for the South Region. Each of the two programs has a capacity for 16 clients. With only 32 places, the capacity is severely limited. This program is designed as therapeutic intervention within a day program for individuals at risk for hospitalization or in need of continued support and structured treatment after hospitalization. Clients may stay up to 90 days based on individual need. Treatment is based on a combination of stabilization and psychoeducational models. Clients with primary diagnoses of schizophrenia and affective disorders tend to do best in this program (DCMHMR, 1989a).

Each client has an individual service plan and is involved in structured activities and groups based on his or her individual needs. The psychoeducational groups and activities are offered based on current client population needs. These groups include but are not limited to the following: mental illness and medication education, stress management, relaxation, hygiene and grooming, nutrition and cooking, use of community resources, public transportation, constructive leisure, goal planning, vocational resources, job readiness, communication skills, and assertiveness training. The program is based on social support activities and independent living skills; there is no formal prevocational or vocational training in the day treatment programs.

The primary referral sources for the day treatment programs are the adult outpatient clinics, the inpatient units, the CSP programs, and continuity-of-care services. To participate in this program the client must (1) be an active DCMHMR mental health client who is at least 18 years of age and in need of structured daily programming to prevent hospitalization or make a smooth transition from the hospital back into community living; (2) be willing to attend a minimum of three days per week, to become active in the program, and to take psychotropic medications as prescribed; (3) be free from current abuse of alcohol or street drugs; (4) be ambulatory and free from acute or chronic medical conditions that would pose a hazard in the program; (5) be able to maintain at least minimal self-care without individual supervision; and (6) have transportation or be willing and capable of learning to ride a bus, with assistance when necessary, if not residing in the program pickup area.

Psychosocial Services at ADAPT. ADAPT is a privately run program, whose corporate headquarters are in St. Louis, Missouri, that contracts with DCMHMR to provide structured residential and psychosocial programming for 101 DCMHMR clients. A description of ADAPT and its residential component follow later in this report. This section will deal only with the psychosocial component.

DCMHMR contracts with ADAPT to provide a minimum of 30 hours per week of psychosocial programming at a cost of $25 per day per client. The contract is monitored by the director of Special Projects for DCMHMR and two caseworkers who are full-time liaisons with ADAPT. Clients are picked up at their residential facilities and taken to Chez Harbor, the psychosocial rehabilitation facility.

ADAPT uses a highly structured programming system designed to accommodate a variety of client functional levels. On paper, the program is impressive and conceptually sound. In practice, however, the 30 hours of programming is skewed toward recreational and leisure activities. The ADAPT team acknowledges this gap and attributes it to the fact that enrollment for the program was less than anticipated. Enrollment would need to reach 200 to financially support the staff necessary to fully implement the program (Heinrichs, 1988).

ADAPT's clients participate in the planning of the month's social activities, which include church, bowling, movies, field trips, dances, and nights out on the town. ADAPT's group classes cover basic education skills, prevocational skills, social and leisure skills, and functional skills. One month's group schedule included classes in money management, personal-social adjustment, communication, relaxation, community management, budgeting, shopping coordination, prevocational skills, GED classes, and preparation of the ADAPT newsletter (ADAPT Institute of America, 1989).

ADAPT's vocational program, the Employment Training Program, allows work-ready clients to join (for pay) one of four activity units. These include housekeeping (12 hours per week), groundskeeping (8 hours per week), and dietary (8 hours per week) at Tejas Center and janitorial (12 hours per week) at Chez Harbor. This 40 hours of available work is divided into many work slots to maximize the number of paid work opportunities for clients (ADAPT Institute of America, 1989). Clients may participate in the Employment Training Program for three months at a time. This allows other clients to rotate into the limited work areas available.

Family Support Services

TDMHMR specifies two categories of programs under this heading. The first is the noncore, in-home respite program. DCMHMR discontinued its in-home respite care in 1986 because of a lack of funds. The second is the required core family support program, which includes sponsoring of advocacy meetings, counseling of family members, and self-help groups for family members. Family support programs are not a prominent feature of DCMHMR's array of services. Funds are sufficiently limited that DCMHMR must concentrate on providing services to its clients, not their families. Moreover, the Alliance for the Mentally Ill (AMI) is very active in the Dallas area and tends to fill this need (Charlesworth, 1989b). The following activities constitute the family support program at DCMHMR:

1. Advocacy meetings: DCMHMR does not sponsor any advocacy meetings but it does network with AMI, advising its clients and their families of AMI's existence and supplying information about AMI and its upcoming events.

2. Counseling family members: Counseling of family members is often an adjunct to continuity-of-care services, case management services, and casework services. However, counseling is generally limited to the amount necessary to ensure the care of the client. It is generally centered around educating the family about the client's illness and medication needs, and advising them about available services. Therapists rarely have the time to offer true ongoing support to the family.

3. Groups for family members: Independence House has recently begun a family support group for the families of clubhouse members. The first few events were potluck dinners which were, unfortunately, poorly attended, with only one or two families represented. The poor attendance is attributed to the fact that most of their members are estranged from their families (Blegen-Sola, 1989).

The day treatment programs have established family support groups for family members of clients enrolled in the programs. However, since there are only 32 spots open in day treatment, only 32 families are potentially eligible to participate.

The clinics periodically offer family education and support groups for families of active clients. They are usually conducted by the caseworkers or therapists. These groups have been offered periodically throughout the years, but only recently has the effort been made to schedule them more frequently. These groups still primarily follow the family education model, educating the family about mental illness, medication management, and strategies for living with and helping their family members. However, plans are being made to eventually enlist AMI members to help conduct these groups and expand their basis (Charlesworth, 1989b).

NONCORE SERVICES

Residential Services

As in every Texas county, Dallas County is experiencing a critical shortage of housing available to adults with serious mental illness. TDMHMR established a minimum target of 25 community residential beds per 100,000 population for FY 1988; this was increased to 30 per 100,000 population for FY 1989. Based on current population estimates, there is a need for 438 community beds in Dallas County in FY 1988 and an additional 87 beds in FY 1989 (Dyer, 1987, p. 33). TDMHMR's estimates are considered to be quite conservative. The Texas legislature has recognized that there is a need for 60 beds per 100,000.

Currently, DCMHMR has 105 beds available for residential placement and 65 inpatient beds (Beard, 1988). According to TDMHMR estimates, Dallas County immediately needs an additional 96 housing units for the adults who are chronically mentally ill. A minimum of 20 beds should be designated for transitional residential care, at an estimated cost of $182,400 (38 apartments, 2 residents each, at $200 per bed per month) (Dyer, 1987, p. 33). The costs of community-based residential services average $30 per day as contrasted with $150 per day in a state hospital.

According to the Dallas Community Outreach Coalition, there are between 4,000 and 5,000 homeless people in the streets of Dallas at any given time. Out of this group, an estimated 1,000 to 1,500 are mentally ill (English, 1988). Other experts estimate that 30 to 40 percent of the homeless are persons with serious mental illness. Table 2.12 lists costs associated with care for the homeless persons who are mentally ill.

Table 2.12. Comparison of Costs to Public for Jail versus Hospital Care

JAIL COSTS	
Sheriff pick up	$ 46.00
Officer pick up	$ 27.60
Lunacy Warrant	$ 55.20
Placed in jail	$ 13.80
Transfer from city to county jail	$ 7.93
Transfer from Parkland	$ 40.00
HOSPITAL COSTS	
Terrell State Hospital	$ 156.00
Emergency Room Parkland	$ 60.00
Overnight Parkland	$ 95.00
MDC per day	$ 225.00
Average MDC stay of 6 days	$ 1500.00

Source: North Dallas Shared Ministries, 1988.

DCMHMR has recently started a new program for persons who are homeless and mentally ill in cooperation with the Community Outreach Coalition. Called the Community Living Skills Training Center for Homeless Mentally Ill, the program offers psychiatric treatment, case management, psychoeducational groups, socialization and daily living skills training, prevocational assessment and basic work skills training, vocational training, including supported employment, and permanent housing assistance. The total cost of the program in FY 1988 was $382,020. Of this, $305,616 was Stewart B. McKinney Act (federal) funds provided through TDMHMR, $48,680 was an in-kind match provided by the City of Dallas in building space and utilities, and $27,724 was an additional local match from DCMHMR. The program staff projected serving 500 homeless mentally ill individuals during its first year (DCMHMR, 1987).

A majority of adults with serious mental illness in Dallas live with their families. Another large number live in board and care homes (Beard, 1988). DCMHMR has not begun to register these board and care homes, as required by state law, because of the large number of board and care homes and the great expense of the registration process. A list of 36 of the more commonly used and known board and care homes in Dallas was provided by staff. This list represents only a small part of the total number of board and care homes in Dallas. The board and care homes listed are the facilities that DCMHMR case managers suggest, even though they cannot make recommendations or placements. Dallas County directly contracts with approximately 20 board and care home operators in the Dallas area for care of mentally handicapped and seriously physically disabled persons. The county pays the operators $11 per day per person served; 8,000 to 9,000 persons are served annually. The operators homes are inspected by the county welfare division and Dallas Neighborhood Housing Services (Seymore, 1989). The number of DCMHMR clients in these facilities is undetermined.

Independence House, which is located in Oak Cliff, offers two types of apartment-based programs: a short-term, transitional program and a long-term program. In addition, Independence House offers a variety of other services that include vocational training, prevocational training, and social and educational opportunities (Beard, 1988). Independence House currently has 400 members and has housed over 100 members (Beard, 1988). The clients housed in the transitional and the long-term apartments are given priority in participating in the various community support programs offered at Independence House.

No one actually lives at Independence House. The staff lease apartments around Dallas and sublease them to Independence House members. The apartments are located near bus stops, shopping centers, and the Independence House clubhouse. A case manager works closely with resident members to help them acquire needed services and daily living skills. The case managers also provide resource information, counseling, and monitoring of the members' medication. Staff who are familiar with each member are available 24 hours a day by phone (Beard, 1988).

The transitional apartments, which are available to clients for up to eight months, are designed for persons newly discharged from Terrell State Hospital. Currently, there are seven units with 28 beds. Each residential member shares a low-cost, two-bedroom furnished apartment with three others. A staff person stays on site at the apartments and works closely with all the residents on an ongoing basis.

Independence House has several eligibility requirements for participation in the transitional apartment program. A member must be at least 18 years of age and have a history of at least two years of mental illness, with at least two psychiatric hospitalizations. The client should be presently in Terrell State Hospital or at risk for rehospitalization unless a stable living situation is provided. The client must also be stabilized and on psychotropic medication and be willing to comply with the medication plan (Beard, 1988). The program primarily accepts persons discharged from Terrell State Hospital, but also accepts a few community referrals (Beard, 1988).

The long-term apartment program is designed for clients who can function at a somewhat higher level than those in the transitional program. The program offers 20 units with 77 beds. Compatible groups of four male clients or four female clients share each two-bedroom apartment. The apartments all have central heat and air and are in various complexes, most of which are in the Oak Cliff or Oak Lawn areas. No staff stay on site at the apartments, but staff work closely with all residents on an ongoing basis. The length of stay is essentially indefinite, based on clients' needs and their progress to greater independence. Clients in the transitional program often graduate to the long-term program.

In both programs, rent and utilities are charged at a current rate of $125 a month. The members cover the costs of food, transportation, and personal care items. For clients who meet TRC eligibility, up to two months of $50 per week maintenance monies are available for a maximum of ten weeks. Limited money for other emergency needs is also available if a client has absolutely no resources. Most of the Independence House clients are eligible for food stamps (Beard, 1988).

Phoenix House is a Fairweather Lodge program operating in Dallas. Phoenix House receives referrals from Terrell State Hospital, DCMHMR, the community, and TRC. Sixty percent of the lodge members receive SSI, and 5 percent receive SSDI. Phoenix House is funded by TRC and DCMHMR. The lodge supports itself by doing janitorial work. Phoenix House currently has a work contract with DART, which is the mass transportation system in Dallas County. Ten other Fairweather Lodges in the Dallas area, which are affiliated with Phoenix House, provide approximately 50 beds (Texas Fairweather Association, n.d.).

ADAPT is a for-profit residential program which started contracting with DCMHMR and Terrell State Hospital in 1984. ADAPT has a contractual relationship with two nursing homes and operates one nursing home directly in various parts of Dallas County. In the spring of 1989, 101 clients were housed in these three residential facilities, which are the Sunnyvale and Segoville Manor nursing homes and Tejas. In mid-1989 all clients of DCMHMR and Terrell State Hospital who were housed in the Segoville Manor nursing home were moved to the Sunnyvale facility (Gill, 1989b).

Tejas is licensed as a nursing home and is owned by ADAPT. This facility has 62 beds, of which 55 are used to house clients in the ADAPT program (Gill, 1989b). The average age of the persons with mental illness in Tejas is 39 years. This group is not Medicaid-eligible for inpatient or custodial mental health services in an institute for mental disease. The DCMHMR pays $27.50 per day per client to cover housing costs. DCMHMR pays an additional $25 per day for psychosocial programs. These funds are reimbursement monies from the R. A. J. v. Jones settlement (Gill, 1989). Terrell State Hospital also has a separate contract for a few non-Dallas County client beds (Gill, 1989b).

Sunnyvale houses a number of clients of DCMHMR and Terrell State Hospital. This nursing home is in south Dallas. Sunnyvale received patients from Segoville Manor, which served primarily geriatric patients from Terrell State Hospital, with an average age of 73. All of these clients are eligible for Medicaid, which paid Segoville for nursing home expenses. The Medicaid payment was approximately $37 per bed day. DCMHMR advances funds to the nursing home until the Medicaid paper work is complete (Gill, 1989b). DCMHMR paid ADAPT $25 per bed day for psychosocial rehabilitation for each client (Gill, 1989b).

Terrell State Hospital and DCMHMR became involved in this program to enable eligible clients to take advantage of available community-based services instead of remaining in the state hospital. Almost all referrals to the ADAPT program are from Terrell State Hospital (Gill, 1989). Terrell State Hospital, DCMHMR, and ADAPT must all agree upon the participants in this program. To be eligible for ADAPT, a client must not be dangerous to self or others, be at least 18 years of age, be a Dallas County resident, and need a long-term highly structured environment to help cope with daily living needs (DCMHMR, 1988c, p. 31).

The ADAPT program is DCMHMR's experiment with privatization. So far this program has been quite successful. DCMHMR is now negotiating with the ADAPT Institute to increase the daily allowance, which would help ADAPT to more adequately meet some of the high costs of housing seriously mentally ill persons in Dallas County (Gill, 1989b).

Continuity of Care (Hospital Liaison)

Continuity-of-care workers serve as an interface, on behalf of clients, between the state hospital and DCMHMR community-based services, aiding in discharge planning and serving as the party responsible for the client from the time of hospital discharge until admission by adult outpatient or other services. Although technically not a required core service, continuity of care is required under the Texas Mental Health Code. TDMHMR offically calls this service Hospital Liaison.

There are five continuity-of-care workers at DCMHMR who handle between 1,100 and 1,200 hospital referrals a year. Two of the five workers work at the state hospitals (usually Terrell), where DCMHMR generally has between 300 and 400 clients at any one time. The workers follow these clients through treatment and assist with their discharge planning. The other three continuity-of-care workers follow clients from hospital discharge to admission by adult outpatient services two to four weeks later. Most clients who leave the hospital are discharged with a discharge plan. The only clients who leave without such a plan are those who leave by unauthorized departure and some of those who leave against medical advice (Baughman, 1989). The FY 1988 fourth quarter report from DCMHMR indicates that only 42 percent of Dallas County residents discharged from all Texas state hospitals were discharged with a discharge plan. The continuity-of-care coordinator took "strong exception to the 42 percent figure" and did not know its source (Baughman, 1989).

During the site visit, the DCMHMR staff examined a random sample (N=24) of 215 persons discharged from Terrell State Hospital and assigned to DCMHMR from January 1 to June 30, 1988. All 24 had received a discharge plan and continuity-of-care services; 15 received medication-related services, and 1 received case management (DCMHMR, 1989p).

At any one time, there are 50 to 100 continuity-of-care clients in the community. During the two to four weeks between a client's hospital discharge and subsequent outpatient clinic admission, the worker responsible for implementing the client's discharge plan performs case management-type activities for the client, monitoring the client's psychological well-being, assessing his or her nonclinical support needs, and sometimes initiating the income support process. The worker can access a psychiatrist if necessary, the CSP program at Independence House if warranted, and, less frequently, the day treatment program or help from case management (particularly with income support eligibility). Clients are generally discharged with 30 days of medication, but if it is lost or the supply runs low, the continuity-of-care worker can obtain a refill.

The continuity-of-care worker's responsibility for a particular client usually ends when the client is admitted to adult outpatient services. At this point, the responsibility for the client transfers to an outpatient clinic caseworker, designated before the client left the hospital. Sometimes, if the continuity-of-care worker has already initiated a service for the client, such as income support, he or she will remain involved with the client until the service is completed.

Income Support

In theory, a client's eligibility for income support, such as SSI, SSDI, Medicaid, Medicare, and food stamps, is checked at all entry points to the system through the screening and assessment process. In reality, income support is not vigorously pursued unless a client is incapable of financially maintaining himself or herself in the community; that is, unless the need is apparent and compelling (Gill, 1989c; Baughman, 1989). The reason for this is that securing income support for the client usually means that a caseworker must accompany the client to the Social Security office and help him or her to fill out the forms. Caseworkers, burdened with large caseloads, do not have the time for this tedious, time-consuming process.

Before a client is discharged from the state hospital, a discharge plan is drawn up and a continuity-of-care worker is assigned to ensure that it is carried out. These plans will often include securing income support if necessary. It is not unusual, then, to see continuity-of-care workers down at the Social Security office initiating this process for their clients. Their services, however, are time-limited. If the process is nearing completion at the time of admission to the adult outpatient services, they will stay involved until it is complete. In most cases, however, they will recommend that these clients be referred to case management.

For clients who enter adult outpatient services through other avenues (Parkland, the inpatient units, or directly through the clinics), income support is assessed at the time of the multidisciplinary assessment. Demonstrated need of entitlement is one reason for referral to case management. Sometimes, case managers will be asked to assist clients, who are not otherwise eligible for case management, in securing entitlements. However, the majority of clients who are not eligible for case management will simply be directed to the Social Security offices and left to their own devices to get there and fill out the forms. Rarely does a caseworker have the time to accompany a client. For the 9.51 percent of clients who are admitted into case management, income support eligibility will be rigorously pursued. Case managers are the income support "specialists" of the center.

Finally, it should be noted that DCMHMR does maximize entitlements for its clients who participate in the ADAPT program, and has been very successful at doing so. (ADAPT's ability to operate depends on securing these entitlements.) In fact, it is the advent of this program which has demonstrated to DCMHMR just how many of its clients would be eligible for entitlements if they were more vigorously pursued (Gill, 1989c; Baughman, 1989). Unfortunately, DCMHMR remains too short of funds and personnel to launch the same intensity of effort for its remaining clientele. DCMHMR had no centrally available information about the number of its clients who receive income support.

Under the state's In-Home and Family Support program (HB 1154), DCMHMR had $125,021 budgeted for mental health clients in FY 1988. Since the program itself was late in being implemented that year, the funds not spent were rolled over to FY 1989. Twenty mental health clients had requested support for a variety of services from the program in FY 1988. Items requested included eyeglasses, in-home attendant care, transportation, temporary rent and utilities payments, legal expenses, and entertainment for the homebound. In FY 1988, DCMHMR spent $12,975 for 14 clients under the HB 1154 program (DCMHMR, 1988b).

Diagnostic, Assessment, and Treatment Services (DATS/Forensics)

DATS provides screening, psychological assessments, medication maintenance, individual and/or group therapy, psychoeducational groups, and referral services for individuals who have a history or recent diagnosis of major mental illness and who are concurrently involved with the criminal justice system for any criminal activity not related to drugs or alcohol (DCMHMR, 1989l). Individuals are referred to DATS by the judicial system, parole or probation departments, the Dallas County Community Corrections Residential Facility, the DCMHMR inpatient units, continuity-of-care services (for individuals discharged from state hospitals who were previously DATS clients), and the Parkland ER. DATS targets individuals who have committed major, violent, or other felonious crimes as well as individuals with "antisocial personality disorders" as the primary diagnosis.

DATS is housed in the Ferguson Road Clinic. As of October 1988, there were 302 active DATS clients (DCMHMR, 1989o). The average length of participation is one to six months, although individuals on probation or parole are eligible to continue for as long as they want to. Most individuals participate in 60-minute to 90-minute weekly group sessions for no less than 16 weeks. DATS clients are reevaluated at the end of 16 weeks.

The director of Psychiatric Emergency Services at Parkland Hospital has identified some specific deficiencies in the DATS program. These include specific programs for sexual offenders, programs designed especially for violent individuals, and medication clinics for drug abusers. Nevertheless, he states that "the forensics clinic has been a major and critical resource for the emergency room" (Puryear, 1989, p. 6).

DATS was started at the request of the Dallas County Commissioners Court (Cotton, 1989). Except for a contract with the Dallas County Community Corrections Residential Facility to provide service for its residents, DCMHMR is totally unreimbursed for this service. In addition to the building space, DCMHMR provides the following staff for the DATS unit: a unit coordinator (100 percent), a Psychologist II (100 percent), an Associate Clinical Psychologist IV (50 percent), a psychiatrist (25 percent), and two secretaries (150 percent).

DALLAS COUNTY MENTAL HEALTH SERVICES BUDGET

Overview

Over the past 20 years total annual revenues for DCMHMR have increased from $1 million in 1970 to $26 million in 1989, as shown in Figure 2.8. In its early years, DCMHMR's primary revenue source was federal grants, supplemented by some state and some local funds. By 1978, approximately 53 percent of DCMHMR revenues were from state grants-in-aid and county tax funds; by 1988, funds from these two sources accounted for 61 percent of total revenues. Figures 2.8 and 2.9 illustrate these comparisons.

Today federal funds comprise less than 5 percent of the DCMHMR budget. In 1988, 44.4 percent of the DCMHMR revenues were from state grants-in-aid and 16.4 percent from county tax funds. The remaining funds come from 38 other revenue sources. The growth of state and county funding of DCMHMR from 1978 to 1989 is shown in Figure 2.9.

Table 2.13 illustrates the DCMHMR's total annual revenues by source for fiscal years 1984 through 1988. It should be noted that local county tax funds, as a proportion of total revenue, declined from a high of 19.8 percent in 1986 to 16.4 percent in 1988. Also, as a proportion of the DCMHMR total revenue, state grants-in-aid have declined from 57.1 percent in 1984 to 44.4 percent in 1988. When TDMHMR funds from the staff-to-patient and staff-to-client programs are added to grant-in-aid, it is found that the total TDMHMR funds to DCMHMR have remained relatively constant over these five years as a proportion of the budget, from 57.1 percent in 1984 to 59.6 percent in 1988. The center has also increased revenues from other state sources by more than 50 percent. In absolute dollars, the total DCMHMR budget increased by 50 percent from 1984 to 1988.

DCMHMR has significantly increased collections from Medicare and Medicaid since 1984, although direct patient fees and other insurance collections have declined. DCMHMR collected 3.6 percent of its total annual revenues through third-party and client fee collections, as illustrated in Table 2.14. In 1987, DCMHMR ranked fourth among all Texas centers in total dollar amounts in fees collected. However, the mean for fees collected by all Texas centers in 1987 was 5.46 percent of total budget. In this respect, DCMHMR ranked sixth from last among the centers in fees collected as a percentage of total budget. DCMHMR does not maintain centrally available data on client income sources or on client eligibility for new income sources.

Table 2.14 shows that private insurance is the greatest source of collections for inpatient services. Fees collected from Medicaid for adult outpatient services and case management should increase considerably under provisions of the recently amended state Medicaid plan. While direct client fees collected declined from FY 1987 to FY 1988, collections from Medicare and Medicaid increased sufficiently to offset the decline. However, DCMHMR collected $34,113 less than it had expected in FY 1988 (DCMHMR, 1989m).

Table 2.15 illustrates total revenues received in FY 1987, and budgeted and actual revenues for FY 1988. DCMHMR is one of the very few centers in the state that can meet TDMHMR's average 20 percent local match requirement with true "local" funds. In FY 1988, DCMHMR was required to contribute a 25 percent local match, or $2,694,918. The center actually budgeted a 62 percent match, or $6,730,026, its total "local" revenues for FY 1988, which included not only county tax funds but also other funds designated as local (DCMHMR, 1987). It should be noted that only a few of the line items listed under "Local Revenue" in Table 2.15, primarily county tax funds and patient fees, were actually "local" funds. The other line items under "Local Revenue" are state and federal government funds which were considered "earned income" for the purposes of local match. Under former TDMHMR guidelines, many centers budgeted all such items as local revenues in

Figure 2.8. Dallas County MHMR Center Gross Annual Budgets

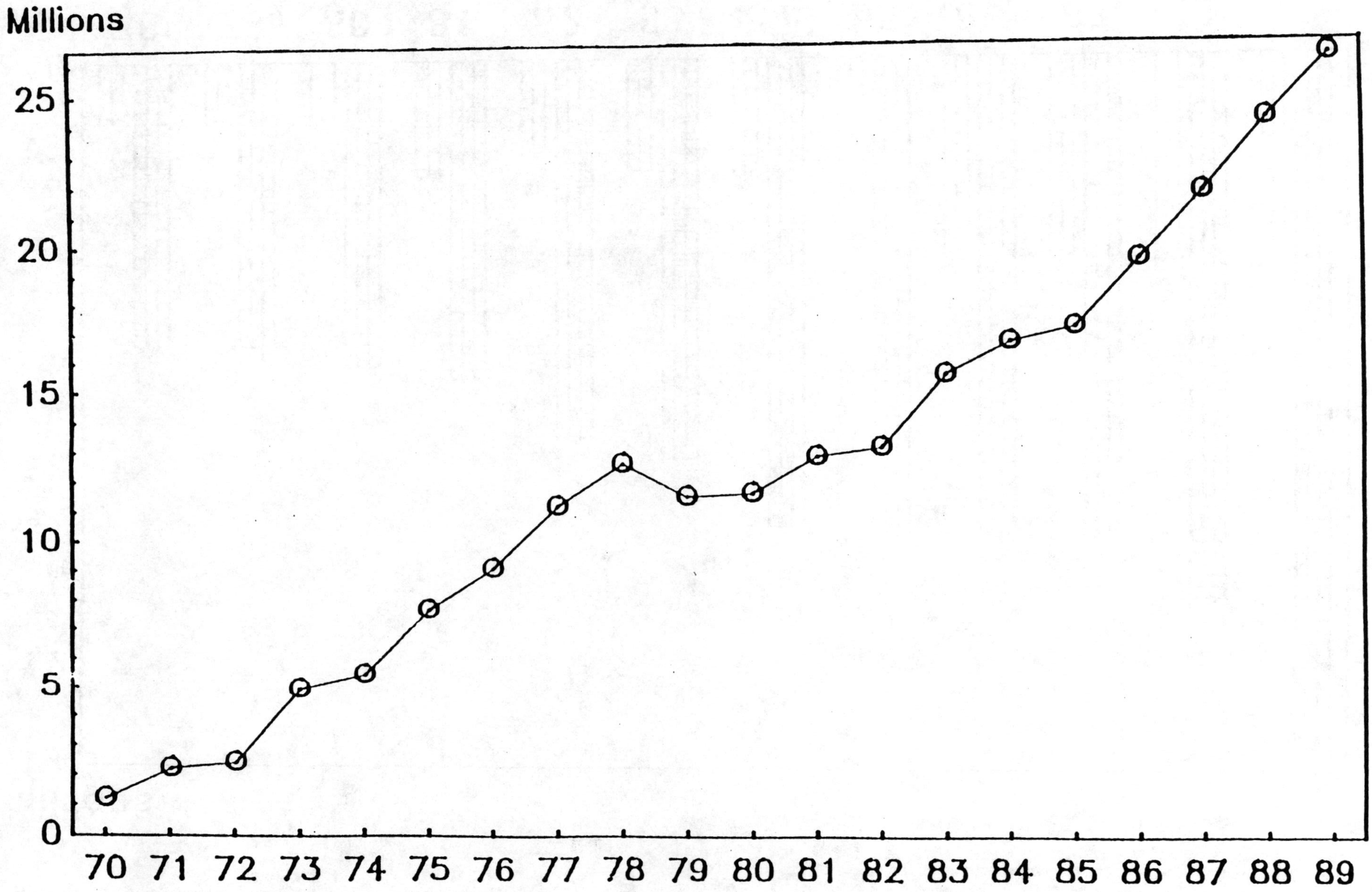

Source: DCMHMR, 1989.

Figure 2.9. Dallas County Contribution and State General Revenue

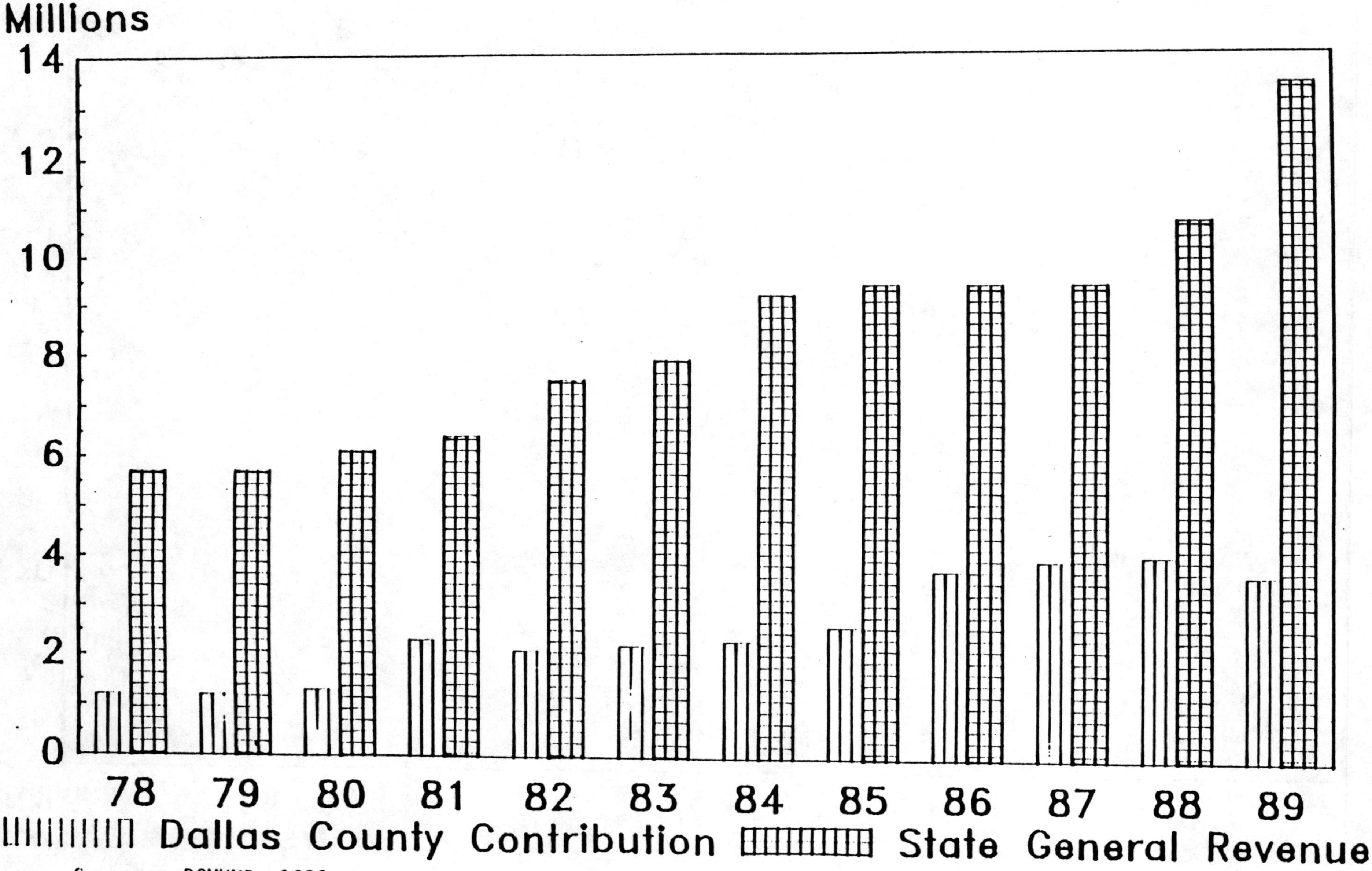

Source: DCMHMR, 1989.

Table 2.13. DCMHMR Total Revenues by Source: FY 1984-1988

Total Revenue By Source	FY 1984	FY 1985	FY 1986	FY 1987	FY 1988
Local Revenue					
Tx. DHS (Geriatrics)	$83,924	$84,662	$94,327	($182)	
Tx. DHS (Title IV B)			$66,775	$52,015	$162,419
ICF-MR	$985,425	$847,316	$773,999	$773,206	$763,389
Tx Rehab. Comm.	$17,516	$8,227	$11,298	$12,888	$17,599
Title XVIII Medicare	$40,767	$36,761	$44,842	$51,784	$68,089
Title XIX Medicaid	$45,179	$37,969	$78,008	$85,974	$103,910
Patient fees/insurance	$944,446	$952,457	$739,964	$749,988	$874,246
County Tax Funds	$2,280,229	$2,610,492	$3,658,277	$3,886,097	$3,963,138
DISD (Autism)			$60,238	$157,088	$164,172
Interest		$355,761	$178,598	$151,853	$237,013
Workshop Contracts		$178,793	$289,876	$261,735	$254,522
Designated Reserves					$150,000
Miscellaneous	$643,225	$163,328	$407,468	$569,260	$185,750
Sub-Total: Local Revenue	**$5,040,711**	**$5,275,766**	**$6,403,670**	**$6,751,706**	**$6,944,247**
State Revenue					
State Grant-in-aid (TDMHMR)	$9,224,223	$9,363,394	$9,363,394	$9,371,145	$10,729,112
Staff-to-Patient Program (TDMHMR)		$181,228	$534,737	$1,703,432	$2,313,226
Staff-to-Client Program (TDMHMR)			$291,693	$930,092	$1,365,663
Other State Funds	$1,023,849	$1,186,285	$1,029,302	$1,271,824	$1,692,814
Sub-Total: State Revenue	**$10,248,072**	**$10,730,907**	**$11,219,126**	**$13,276,493**	**$16,100,815**
Federal Revenue					
Tx. DHS (Liaison Workers)	$381,849	$387,117	$396,145	$376,661	$401,330
TEA (Chapter 1-Handicapped)	$50,953	$51,002	$61,874	$53,531	$68,647
Mental Health Block Grant	$309,113	$436,268	$307,993	$346,244	$346,244
Dallas Co. Community Co. (Title IIIB	$81,846	$89,734	$96,615	$103,015	$104,135
TRC (MSS)					$191,057
U.S. Probation	$36,287	$34,419	$400		
DHHS		$66,897			
Sub-Total: Federal Revenue	**$860,048**	**$1,065,437**	**$863,027**	**$879,451**	**$1,111,413**
Total Revenues	**$16,148,831**	**$17,072,110**	**$18,485,823**	**$20,907,650**	**$24,156,475**

Source: DCMHMR Independent Financial Audits, 1984-1988.

Table 2.14. DCMHMR FY 1988 Third-Party and Client Fee Collections

Service Area	Medicare	Medicaid	Private Insurance	Client Fees	Total
Acute MH Treatment	$14,808	$26,455	$175,070	$47,257	$263,590
Less Passthrough*	$4,886	$6,476	$54,011	$19,324	$84,697
Net for Acute MH	$9,921	$19,979	$121,059	$27,934	$178,893
Adult Outpatient	$56,841	$79,015	$20,045	$237,216	$393,117
Child & Adolescent	$32	$3,818	$103,841	$34,502	$142,193
MR Services				$160,754	$160,754
Adapt	$1,295	$1,098	$36		$2,428
Total: FY 88	**$26,167**	**$103,910**	**$244,981**	**$460,406**	**$877,386**
Total: FY 87	**$13,941**	**$85,974**	**$224,432**	**$514,971**	**$877,160**

Source: DCMHMR, 1989r.

*By agreement, Dallas County is reimbursed half of all fees collected by the MDC.

Table 2.15. FY 1988 Budgeted and Actual Revenues by Source

Total Revenue By Source	FY 1987 Actual	Percent of Total	FY 1988 Budgeted	FY 1988 Actual	Percent of Total
Local Revenue					
Tx. DHS (Geriatrics)	($182)	0.00	$0	$0	0.00
Tx. DHS (Title IV B)	$52,015	0.25	$186,735	$162,419	0.67
ICF-MR	$773,206	3.70	$772,224	$763,389	3.16
Tx Rehab. Comm.	$12,888	0.06	$12,500	$17,599	0.07
Title XVIII Medicare	$51,784	0.25	$53,500	$68,089	0.28
Title XIX Medicaid	$85,974	0.41	$85,000	$103,910	0.43
Patient fees/insurance	$749,988	3.59	$780,255	$874,246	3.62
County Tax Funds	$3,886,097	18.59	$4,200,338	$3,963,138	16.41
DISD (Autism)	$157,088	0.75	$168,000	$164,172	0.68
Interest	$151,853	0.73	$0	$237,013	0.98
Workshop Contracts	$261,735	1.25	$242,300	$254,522	1.05
Designated Reserves	$0	0.00	$150,000	$150,000	0.62
Miscellaneous	$569,260	2.72	$138,225	$185,750	0.77
Sub-Total: Local Revenue	$6,751,706	32.29	$6,789,077	$6,944,247	28.75
State Revenue					
State Grant-in-aid	$9,371,145	44.82	$10,929,673	$10,729,112	44.42
Staff-to-Patient Program	$1,703,432	8.15	$1,974,068	$2,313,226	9.58
Staff-to-Client Program	$930,092	4.45	$1,346,036	$1,365,663	5.65
Other State Funds	$1,271,824	6.08	$1,722,361	$1,692,814	7.01
Sub-Total: State Revenue	$13,276,493	63.50	$15,972,138	$16,100,815	66.65
Federal Revenue					
Tx. DHS (Liaison Workers)	$376,661	1.80	$385,686	$401,330	1.66
TEA (Chapter 1-Handicapped)	$53,531	0.26	$68,647	$68,647	0.28
Mental Health Block Grant	$346,244	1.66	$346,244	$346,244	1.43
Dallas Co. Community Co. (Title III	$103,015	0.49	$97,796	$104,135	0.43
TRC (MSS)	$0	0.00	$204,453	$191,057	0.79
Sub-Total:Federal Revenue	$879,451	4.21	$1,102,826	$1,111,413	4.60
Total Revenues	$20,907,650		$23,864,041	$24,156,475	

Source: Ernst & Whinney, 1988, p. 5.

order to meet their minimum local match requirement, since their local city or county tax funds were insufficient.

As they were defined before June 1989, the dollar amounts for local match in center contracts were not limited to the actual support of local governments or local communities for community mental health services. Moreover, the local match definition obscured the value of some significant local government support for community mental health which is off-budget. For example, in Dallas, the county contributes funds supporting the Parkland Psychiatric ER, the MDC, and other services which are not included in the DCMHMR budget. The in-kind contribution by the City of Dallas to the program for homeless mentally ill persons is off-budget. Similar situations exist for many other community centers.

Mental Health Services Revenues

DCMHMR's total revenue for mental health services has increased by 41.7 percent from 1984 to 1988, as shown in Table 2.16. Within this overall increase, local funds increased by 17.4 percent and state general revenue increased by 23.4 percent. Funds earned under the staff-to-patient line item accounted for 11 percent of all revenues for mental health services in FY 1988. The bulk of the increase in "Other State" funds is from Terrell State Hospital (TSH) for various adult mental health residential programs. The DCMHMR FY 1988 TSH contract for $822,833 funded 71 structured noncrisis beds ($671,613); 17 Fairweather Lodge beds ($33,720); 28 supervised apartment beds ($79,500); and medication-related services ($38,000) (DCMHMR, 1987). Total state funds in FY 1988 (almost all through TDMHMR) constituted 68.4 percent of the mental health services budget, an increase from 61.2 percent of the total in FY 1984.

Table 2.17 summarizes the proportion of the major mental health services budget categories funded by each of the primary revenue sources. DCMHMR has chosen to use 90 percent of its staff-to-patient earnings for residential services. The relatively small amount budgeted for case management is nearly all from state general revenue funds. Local funds pay for 54 percent of the costs of residential services and 42 percent of all client and family support services. From FY 1988 to FY 1989, DCMHMR received $913,665 in "per capita increase" in state general revenue funds for mental health services. Called equalization funds, these new state funds were provided to "equalize" the low per capita centers. Of this amount, $263,000 was earmarked for the In-Home and Family Support program. The DCMHMR received an additional $248,277 in state funds, designated as an across-the-board increment for mental health services in FY 1989. Dallas County reduced its allocation to DCMHMR by $716,970 from FY 1988 to FY 1989. The county applied its own 5 percent across-the-board cut to the DCMHMR request; further, it then reduced its allocation to children and adolescent services by an additional $500,000 (Boardman, 1989). According to DCMHMR staff, the county reduced its funding after learning of the new state funds to be available (Gill, 1989).

Mental Health Services Expenditures

Table 2.18 lists DCMHMR expenditures for FY 1988 adult (excluding children's services) mental health services by revenue source for the required core and noncore services. In Table 2.18, the required core services listed are those core services required by state law; therefore, management and support is not included under core services. However, in the FY 1988 contracts, TDMHMR defines management and support as a core service. Funds from all state sources accounted for 68.4 percent of total adult mental health expenditures. State funds paid for 70.6 percent of the costs of the mandated core services and 94.6 percent of the noncore services costs at DCMHMR. All available federal funds were used for core services. Local funds supported 24.2 percent of the costs of core services and 5.4 percent of the costs of the noncore services.

Table 2.16. Allocations of Local, State, and Federal Revenues to Mental Health Services FY 1984 - FY 1988

	FY 1984	FY 1985	FY 1986	FY 1987	FY 1988
Local Funds	$3,922,616	$3,943,431	$5,548,994	$5,181,103	$4,606,909
State General Revenue	$6,727,619	$6,914,730	$7,034,733	$6,827,483	$8,302,944
Staff to Patient-MH			$534,737	$1,660,715	$1,763,255
Other State	$178,301	$138,566	$220,178	$477,955	$869,754
Federal MH Block Grant	$309,113	$436,268	$307,993	$346,244	$346,244
Other Federal	$149,953	$89,735	$210,281	$103,014	$104,135
Total Actual	$11,287,602	$11,522,730	$13,856,916	$14,596,514	$15,993,241
Budgeted	$11,663,099	$12,014,982	$14,396,971	$14,045,043	$16,452,742

Source: Main Hurdman, 1984, 1985, 1986; Peat Marwick, 1987; Ernst & Whinney, 1988.

Table 2.17. FY 1988 Revenue Allocation by Type of Mental Health Service

			Service	Type					
Revenue Source	Residential Services	Percent of Row Total	Client and Family Support	Percent of Row Total	Case Management	Percent of Row Total	Management and Support	Percent of Row Total	Total
Local Funds	$2,465,243	53.51	$1,939,465	42.10	$42,316	0.92	$159,885	3.47	$4,606,909
General Revenue	$1,918,852	23.08	$4,584,750	55.15	$480,183	5.78	$1,330,118	16.00	$8,313,903
Staff-to-Patient	$1,584,229	89.85	$118,585	6.73	$0	0.00	$60,441	3.43	$1,763,255
Other State	$774,744	89.08	$95,010	10.92	$0	0.00	$0	0.00	$869,754
MHBG	$0	0.00	$346,244	100.00	$0	0.00	$0	0.00	$346,244
Other Federal	$0	0.00	$104,135	100.00	$0	0.00	$0	0.00	$104,135
Column Total	$6,743,068		$7,188,189		$522,499		$1,550,444		$16,004,200

Source: Ernst & Whinney, 1988, p. 25.

Table 2.18. DCMHMR FY 1988 Expenditures for Core and Noncore Adult Mental Health Services

Revenue Source	Core Services	Percent of Row Total	NonCore Services*	Percent of Row Total	Row Total	Percent of Col. Total
State	$5,816,746	78.16	$1,624,880	21.84	$7,441,626	59.13
General Revenue	$206,028	13.14	$1,361,645	86.86	$1,567,693	12.46
$35.50 Program	$52,630	6.36	$774,745	93.64	$827,375	6.57
Terrell State Hospital						
Sub-Total	$6,075,404		$3,761,270		$9,836,694	78.16
Federal	$450,379	100.00	$0	0.00	$450,379	
MHBG, Other Federal						
Sub-Total	$450,379		$0		$450,379	3.58
Local	$1,921,849	100.00	$0	0.00	$1,921,849	15.27
Dallas County	$2,690	2.06	$127,941	97.94	$130,631	1.04
Client Fees, Third-Part	$158,914	64.84	$86,156	35.16	$245,070	1.95
Other Local**						
Sub-Total	$2,083,453		$214,097		$2,297,550	18.26
Grand Total	$8,609,236		$3,975,367		$12,584,623	

Source: DCMHMR, 1989o.

* Includes Management and Support.
** Sublease income, donations, reserves, contract income, interest income, TRC.

Allocation of funds to specific services from the various revenue sources is not arbitrary in most cases; a notable exception is staff-to-patient funds, which, to date, have had no strings attached to their use. Like other centers, DCMHMR attempts to build a budget, within all the applicable restrictions, that will allow its board the greatest possible degree of choice in decisions for funding programs.

Table 2.19 lists DCMHMR total expenditures for 1987 and 1988 by object of expense. Personnel costs absorbed 60.7 percent of 1988 expenditures, down from 63.8 percent of the 1987 budget. For DCMHMR, as for most Texas centers, building rent has been a fairly significant object of expense, with no recoupment of dollars spent. Until recently, it was the opinion of TDMHMR that centers, as agents of the state, could not incur debt; therefore centers were technically unable to mortgage property. The result was that, each year, millions of community center dollars were spent on building rent ($12 million in 1987 alone). Many centers established nonprofit corporations in the 1970s, which were, at least theoretically, separate from the centers and could finance mortgaged property. Since then, the Texas statute has been amended to allow centers to purchase property; with this and other initiatives discussed later, many centers are gradually acquiring land and buildings.

For DCMHMR, general fixed assets, less accumulated depreciation and amortization, were valued at $2,929,597 in 1984; by 1988 this value had increased to $4,940,456 (Main Hurdman, 1984; Ernst & Whinney, 1988). This ranks DCMHMR at or near the top of Texas centers in value of fixed assets. In FY 1988, DCMHMR owned, free and clear, the Hillside Center (site of the AITC) and two clinics, a total of 74,653 square feet of space dedicated to adult mental health services. The Hillside Center, formerly the privately operated Beverly Hills Psychiatric Hospital, was first leased by DCMHMR in 1977. Initially licensed for 29 beds, the Hillside Center now has 20 adult beds (the AITC) and 15 beds for children and adolescents (Long, 1981).

In late 1988, DCMHMR was allocated $8,620,000 under a new tax-exempt bond program sponsored by the Texas Council of Community MHMR Centers. This program, the Community MHMR Center Facilities Acquisition Program, made available nearly $38 million through bond issues to 15 Texas community centers. About half of the 20-year series bond revenues are to be used to refinance existing property loans at lower interest rates, from 6.25 percent in 1990 to 7.875 percent in 2009. The other half of the revenues are to be used to acquire new facilities or major equipment items. Of the $8,620,000 available to DCMHMR, most will be used to purchase new property (three sites), construct new facilities (four sites), renovate other properties (four sites), and refinance loans on five additional sites. The remainder of the funds will be used for a greatly needed upgrade of computer hardware and software and for purchase of vehicles (Gill, 1989a).

For DCMHMR, the maximum net effective interest rate under this program is 8.75 percent (Ernst & Whinney, 1988, p. 20). DCMHMR reduced its general long-term debt from $1.3 million in FY 1987 to $1.2 million in FY 1988; the net book value of the collateral was $1.5 million. Refinancing its notes and bonds payable under the new program will save significant amounts in interest payments over the life of the program, since the long-term interest rates that DCMHMR paid in FY 1988 ranged from 9.0 percent to 11.25 percent (Ernst & Whinney, 1988, p. 15).

Table 2.20 lists the DCMHMR FY 1988 expenditures for its various adult mental health programs. Most of the DCMHMR $35.50 earnings and the funds from Terrell State Hospital are used to fund the ADAPT program (discussed earlier), a noncore service. ADAPT expenditures account for 31.5 percent of total expenditures on mental health residential services for adults.

Under "Client and Family Support," DCMHMR spent 69 percent of all funds in this category on traditional outpatient clinic services, listed as medication-related in Table 20.

Table 2.19. DCMHMR FY 1987-1988 Expenditures by Object of Expense

Total Expenditures	FY 1987 Actual	Percent of Total	FY 1988 Budgeted	FY 1988 Actual	Percent of Total
	$11,266,222	53.82	$12,309,698	$11,979,808	51.81
Personnel	$1,728,968	8.26	$1,902,720	$1,765,404	7.64
Salaries and wages	$362,449	1.73	$309,100	$277,723	1.20
Fringe Benefits	$362,449	1.73	$156,652	$137,266	0.59
Consultant/Professional Fees					
Travel	$421,419	2.01	$445,002	$434,693	1.88
Consumable Items	$206,253	0.99	$206,429	$205,274	0.89
Drugs	$228,267	1.09	$269,687	$265,513	1.15
Food					
Other	$334,499	1.60	$273,215	$250,195	1.08
Equipment/ Furniture	$172,626	0.82	$187,478	$193,975	0.84
Purchase	$1,123,297	5.37	$1,225,367	$1,356,251	5.87
Rental, repair, service	$502,835	2.40	$166,440	$146,592	0.63
Buildings	$157,298	0.75	$202,499	$201,295	0.87
Repairs/ Maintenance	$3,334,605	15.93	$4,877,985	$4,886,863	21.14
Vehicles					
Service Agency Contracts	$202,527	0.97	$223,141	$219,932	0.95
Other	$173,938	0.83	$184,997	$173,118	0.75
Utilities	$114,456	0.55	$127,086	$124,074	0.54
Postage/telephone	$184,229	0.88	$56,324	$53,426	0.23
Insurance	$315,137	1.51	$740,221	$449,248	1.94
Client wages/workshop supplies					
Other	$20,933,916		$23,864,041	$23,120,650	
Total Expenditures	($26,266)			$1,035,825	

Source: Ernst & Whinney, 1988, p. 6.

Table 2.20. DCMHMR FY 1988 Adult Mental Health Services Summary

	Core Service	Non-Core Service	Dallas Co. Match*	Row Total Expenditures	Percent of Total MH	Unit of Service	Number of Units	Cost Per Unit	Number Served
Residential Services									
Mental Diagnostic Center	$2,175,113		$431,781	$2,606,894	20.03	Bed-Days	9,589	$271.86	1,272
Acute Inp. Treatment Center	$1,122,652			$1,122,652	8.62	Bed-Days	5,994	$187.30	406
Sub-Total: Structured Crisis				$3,729,546	28.65		15,853	$239.33	1,422
Adapt(Structured Non-Crisis)		$1,922,479		$1,922,479	14.77	Bed-Days	44,637	$43.07	152
Semi-Independent Residential		$459,644		$459,644	3.53	Bed-Days	58,285	$7.89	259
Sub-Total: Residential				$6,111,669	46.95				
Client & Family Support									
24 Hour Emergency	$548,618			$548,618	4.21	Server Hrs	3,212	$170.80	1,793
Hospital Liaison		$209,414		$209,414	1.61	Server Hrs	8,181	$25.60	908
HB 1154 (income support)	$12,975			$12,975	0.10			$926.79	14
Medication-Related	$3,674,482			$3,674,482	28.23	Server Hrs	67,539	$54.41	6,520
Psychosocial Rehabilitation	$600,296			$600,296	4.61	Client Hrs	82,868	$7.24	395
Day Treatment		$276,390		$276,390	2.12	Client Hrs	25,109	$11.01	109
Sub-Total: Client & Family				$5,322,175	40.89				
Case Management	**$475,100**			**$475,100**	**3.65**	Server Hrs	**17,681**	**$26.87**	**1,891**
Management & Support		**$1,107,460**		**$1,107,460**	**8.51**				
Grand Total				**$13,016,404**					

Source: DCMHMR, 1989t.

*Support services, facility space estimated value.

DCMHMR spent $12,975 in HB 1154 funds for 14 clients, an average of $926.79 per client. The DCMHMR FY 1988 contract lists an original budget of $125,021 for HB 1154 mental health services; this amount was specially designated out of the new general revenue equalization monies. Under a special contract provision, those centers receiving HB 1154 funds were not permitted to spend any of the funds "prior to the establishment of guidelines for said programs without the express written approval of the Department" (DCMHMR, 1987, Attachment V). Since the guidelines were not issued until April of FY 1988 (mid-way through the third quarter), the program was late getting started and funds budgeted for the year could not all be used. Unspent funds were rolled over to the next fiscal year for this program. As listed in Table 2.20, the number of clients served is a duplicated count and should not be totaled.

Comparison with Other Large Urban Centers

Table 2.21 compares mental health services revenues and expenditures by type of service for Texas' four largest centers. It should be noted that state expenditures for the Harris County and Tarrant County psychiatric hospitals are not reflected in those centers' budgets. Moreover, federal mental health block grant funds cannot be spent on inpatient services, so no center has the option of using those funds for structured crisis and noncrisis beds.

Local funds support 52.7 percent of Harris County's mental health budget, the highest proportion in the state. By contrast, for the other large centers, local funds comprise 28.4 percent (DCMHMR); 22.6 percent (Tarrant County); and 16. 4 percent (Bexar County). Excluding state funds for the two psychiatric hospitals mentioned above, general revenue from TDMHMR accounts for more than 50 percent of total mental health revenues for the four centers: DCMHMR, 52.2 percent; Harris, 52.7 percent; Bexar, 56.8 percent, and Tarrant, 61.5 percent. Harris County receives considerably more federal block grant funds. Harris and Tarrant counties receive far less in staff-to-patient MH funds, which is primarily a result of placements in their respective psychiatric hospitals instead of the state hospitals. These two hospitals are not part of the $35.50 reimbursement program; therefore, reductions of their bed days do not earn the $35.50 funds.

The four centers spent roughly 10 percent of their budgets on management and support. All spend a very small percentage of their budgets on case management, from a high of 6.4 percent in Bexar County to a low of 2.9 percent in Harris County. DCMHMR spends the greatest proportion of its budget (41.8 percent) for residential mental health services, even though it provides no intermediate beds; both Bexar and Harris counties allocate 37 percent, while Tarrant County expends only 22.2 percent. Tarrant County does not provide structured noncrisis beds.

Among the four centers, costs per client served vary dramatically, although a significant amount of the variance is an artifact of budget practices. The clients served and the available beds in the Harris and Tarrant county hospitals are "counted" in the workload measures for the two centers; however, the major state expenditures for the hospitals are not included in the costs . For all FY 1988 mental health residential services in the four centers, costs per client per day vary by more than 100 percent: Tarrant County: $36.41; Bexar County: $41.64; DCMHMR: $54.51; and Harris County: $73.78 (TDMHMR, 1989).

Budgeting practices for client and family support services are more consistent among the centers, but the FY 1988 costs per client also vary widely: Tarrant County, $304.40; Bexar County, $585.29; DCMHMR, $651.75; and Harris County, $872.04 (TDMHMR, 1989). Even greater differences are noted in FY 1988 costs per mental health client in case management services: DCMHMR, $172.78; Bexar, $505.12; Harris County, $703.49; and Tarrant County, $749.98 (TDMHMR, 1989). Since case management is the most cleanly

Table 2.21. Mental Health Revenues and Expenditures in Texas' Four Largest Urban Centers

Fiscal Year 1988	Bexar	Dallas	Harris	Tarrant
MH Residential				
Structured Crisis: Total	$1,822,562	**$4,275,981**	$6,058,480	$402,878
Local	$697,729	**$2,282,686**	$5,285,676	$90,592
General Revenue	$835,477	**$1,727,213**	$772,804	$11,461
Other State	$289,356	**$0**	$0	$0
Other Federal	$0	**$0**	$0	$300,825
MHBG	$0	**$0**	$0	$0
RAJ-$35.50	$0	**$266,082**	$0	$0
Structured Non-Crisis: Total	$473,088	**$1,922,478**	$1,985,964	$0
Local	$79,344	**$21,683**	$919,659	$0
General Revenue	$0	**$150,000**	$976,735	$0
Other State	$0	**$658,328**	$0	$0
Other Federal	$0	**$0**	$71,222	$0
MHBG	$0	**$0**	$0	$0
RAJ-$35.50	$393,744	**$1,092,467**	$18,348	$0
Intermediate Beds: Total	$1,058,832	**$0**	$361,006	$74,315
Local	$129,670	**$0**	$134,171	$34,650
General Revenue	$343,560	**$0**	$214,573	$39,665
Other State	$186,468	**$0**	$0	$0
Other Federal	$0	**$0**	$0	$0
MHBG	$76,118	**$0**	$0	$0
RAJ-$35.50	$323,016	**$0**	$12,262	$0
Semi-Independent Beds: Total	$331,976	**$459,644**	$619,929	$904,409
Local	$0	**$75,909**	$162,293	$0
General Revenue	$0	**$41,639**	$372,675	$594,853
Other State	$26,596	**$116,416**	$64,690	$52,232
Other Federal	$0	**$0**	$0	$0
MHBG	$0	**$0**	$0	$236,689
RAJ-$35.50	$305,380	**$225,680**	$20,271	$21,711
Client & Family Support				
Total	$4,282,527	**$7,188,189**	$11,948,753	$3,860,733
Local	$489,960	**$1,939,465**	$4,332,908	$1,163,854
General Revenue	$3,111,172	**$4,584,750**	$6,340,542	$2,440,231
Other State	$347,169	**$95,010**	$0	$2,733
Other Federal	$0	**$104,136**	$0	$21,017
MHBG	$73,542	**$346,244**	$1,162,742	$185,572
RAJ-$35.50	$260,684	**$118,585**	$112,561	$47,326
Case Management				
Total	$624,835	**$522,499**	$718,265	$304,490
Local	$5,206	**$42,316**	$194,759	$136
General Revenue	$468,333	**$480,183**	$523,506	$185,325
Other State	$0	**$0**	$0	$0
Other Federal	$0	**$0**	$0	$0
MHBG	$0	**$0**	$0	$53,011
RAJ-$35.50	$151,296	**$0**	$0	$66,018

Table 2.21. Mental Health Revenues and Expenditures in Texas' Four Largest Urban Centers (continued)

Fiscal Year 1988	Bexar	Dallas	Harris	Tarrant
Management & Support				
Total	$1,212,759	$1,550,444	$2,720,733	$653,279
Local	$206,899	$159,885	$1,832,991	$112,692
General Revenue	$816,245	$1,330,118	$887,742	$540,587
Other State	$47,334	$0	$0	$0
Other Federal	$20,280	$0	$0	$0
MHBG	$20,995	$0	$0	$0
RAJ-$35.50	$101,006	$60,441	$0	$0
Total MH Revenues	$9,806,579	$15,919,236	$24,413,130	$6,201,180
Local	$1,608,808	$4,521,944	$12,862,457	$1,401,924
General Revenue	$5,574,787	$8,313,903	$10,088,577	$3,812,122
Other State	$896,923	$869,754	$64,690	$54,965
Other Federal	$20,280	$104,136	$71,222	$321,842
MHBG	$170,655	$346,244	$1,162,742	$475,272
RAJ-$35.50	$1,535,126	$1,763,255	$163,442	$135,055

Source: TDMHMR, 1989.
Note: All amounts are for adult and children's mental health services.

defined and budgeted of all the service categories, the cost variations (334 percent across the four centers) are most likely the result of differing practices in case management services.

CURRENT SERVICE NEEDS AND RELATED ISSUES

Linkages Between Community and Hospital Services

A widespread criticism of community centers in the 1970s was their failure to reduce admissions to state hospitals and to provide community care for persons discharged from state hospitals. The current performance contract used by TDMHMR for community centers includes a number of performance measures related to screening state hospital admissions and to the effectiveness of linkages between centers and hospitals for discharged patients.

The performance of DCMHMR on some of these measures is compared with the other three large centers in Table 2.22. The data show that although actual numbers of state hospital admissions and readmissions are relatively low compared to the population base, no center performs adequately on all the screening and discharge measures.

DCMHMR is one of a number of centers which do not meet the performance criteria in one or more areas. Variables which can influence a center's performance on any of the measures, and which should be taken into account in comparing relative performance, include the admission, length of stay, and discharge policies of the state hospitals, over which centers have little to no control. In addition, there are often other extenuating circumstances in local communities. For example, many persons from Harris County no longer go to a state hospital but to the Harris County Psychiatric Hospital. Since these admissions don't "count" in calculations of the performance measures, Harris County has a low rate of inpatient admissions to state hospitals, even though admissions to all inpatient services may be high.

A further look at the DCMHMR continuity-of-care capacity provides some interesting data, but few definite clues leading to an explanation of the relatively low performance level. DCMHMR is located in the service region of Terrell State Hospital. Four other community centers and four outreach units operated by TSH are also in this region. Table 2.23 lists some of the FY 1988 performance measures for the centers in the TSH region. The outreach units do not report such data. DCMHMR has almost the lowest number of admissions per 100,000 of all the centers in the region, but it also has the lowest rate of screening hospital admissions. Of the 1,400 persons from Dallas County admitted to all state hospitals in FY 1988, 1,061 were admitted to TSH. The other 339 persons were admitted to hospitals elsewhere in the state. These totals are for all hospital admissions, regardless of diagnosis.

Figures 2.10 and 2.11 depict trends in admissions to TSH from Dallas County and all the other counties in its region from 1984 to 1988. What is immediately apparent is that the net reduction in TSH admissions over time has come almost exclusively from Dallas County. Total admissions from all other counties have remained relatively constant.

Tables 2.24 and 2.25 further examine admissions over time by length of stay and type of admission (voluntary or involuntary). Although the total number of admissions has decreased since 1984, it is clear from the tables that short-term admissions from all counties have increased as a proportion of total admissions. For Dallas County, the number of short-term (14 days or less) voluntary admissions has increased while Dallas County involuntary commitments have decreased. This is also true in most cases for the other counties.

Table 2.22. FY 1988 Performance Measures of the Four Large Urban Centers

	TDMHMR Minimum	TDMHMR Suggested	Bexar	Dallas	Harris	Tarrant
Number of SH Admissions	--	--	1695	**1400**	706	539
SH Admissions/100,000	--	155	146	**77**	23	50
No. Screened/SH Admissions	--	--	1163	**716**	674	304
% Screened/SH Admissions	70%	--	69%	**51%**	95%	56%
Number of SH Readmissions	--	--	872	**641**	299	207
SH Readm/100,000	--	100	75	**35**	10	19
No. Screened/SH Readmission	--	--	590	**293**	287	65
% Screened/SH Readmissions	70%	--	68%	**46%**	96%	31%
% of SH disch w/joint plan	85%	--	100%	**42%**	81%	90%
% of SH disch assign to Ctr	70%	--	41%	**45%**	77%	62%
% disch/assign/svd. in 7 days	40%	--	68%	**45%**	83%	72%
% disch/assign/svd. in 15 days	90%	--	75%	**60%**	84%	84%
% disch/assign/to case man.	90%	--	100%	**42%**	57%	89%

Source: TDMHMR, 1989.

Table 2.23. FY 1988 Hospital Admissions from Mental Health Authorities in Terrell State Hospital's Service Region

Mental Health Authority	Number of Admissions	Admissions per 100,000	Number Screened	Percentage Screened
Dallas Co. MHMR Center LSA Number 10 Population: 1,810,294	1400	77	590	51%
East Texas MHMR Center LSA Number 12 Population: 291,746	277	95	237	60%
Hunt Co. MHMR Center LSA Number 62 Population: 67,180	113	168	81	58%
Navarro Co. MHMR Center LSA Number 19 Population: 39,992	80	200	44	95%
Northeast Texas MHMR Ctr. LSA Number 21 Population: 130,915	99	76	76	80%
Post Oak-TSH LSA Number 49 Population: 206,224	N/A	N/A	N/A	N/A
Camp County-TSH LSA Number 50 Population: 11,246	N/A	N/A	N/A	N/A
Ellis County-TSH LSA Number 51 Population: 71,981	N/A	N/A	N/A	N/A

Source: TDMHMR, 1989.
Note: Hospital outreach centers do not report performance measures.

Figure 2.10. FY 1984-FY 1988 Admissions to Terrell State Hospital from Dallas County

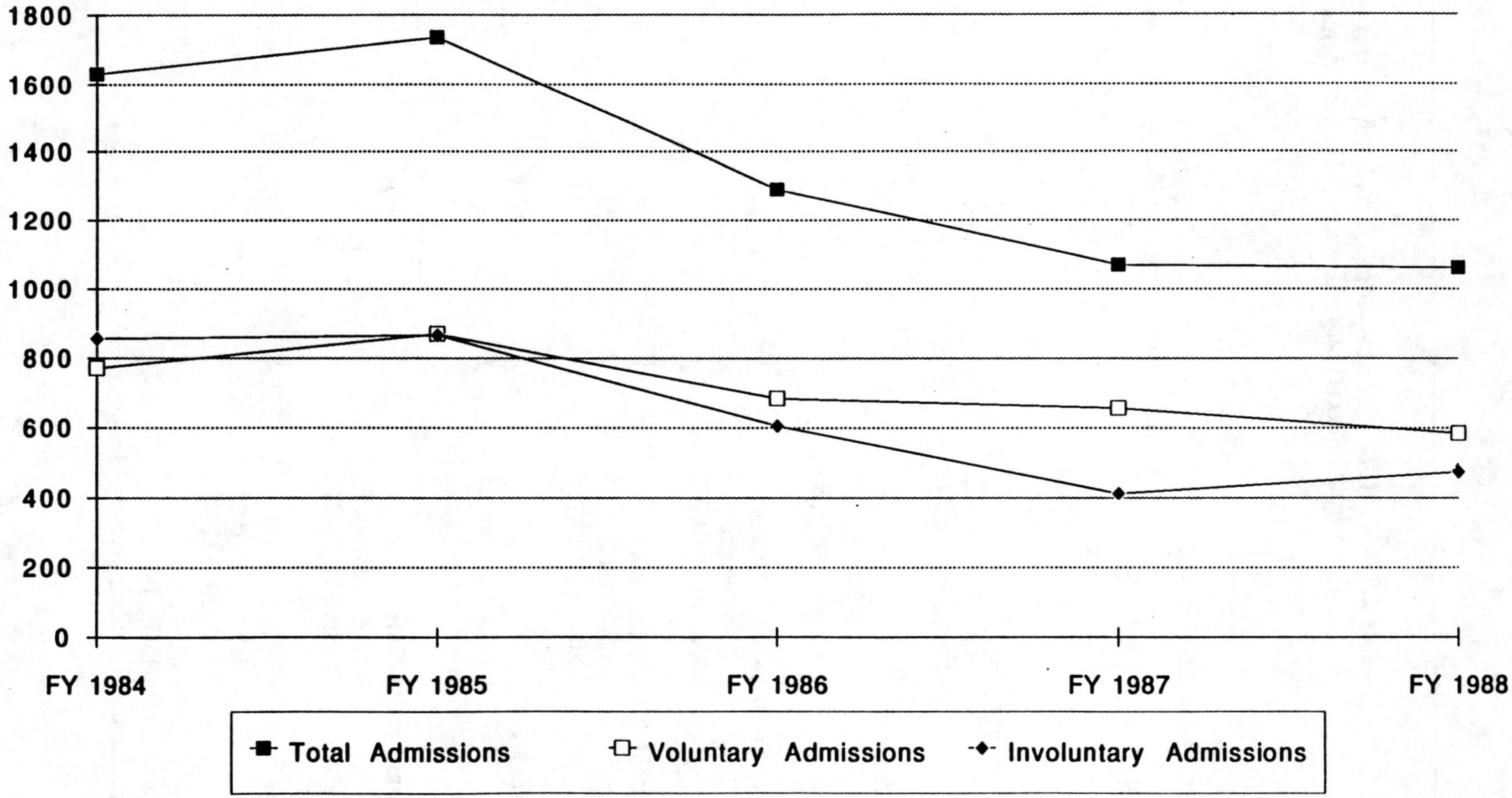

Source: TDMHMR CARE data 1984-1988

Figure 2.11. FY 1984-FY 1988 Admissions to Terrell State Hospital from All Other Counties in Service Region

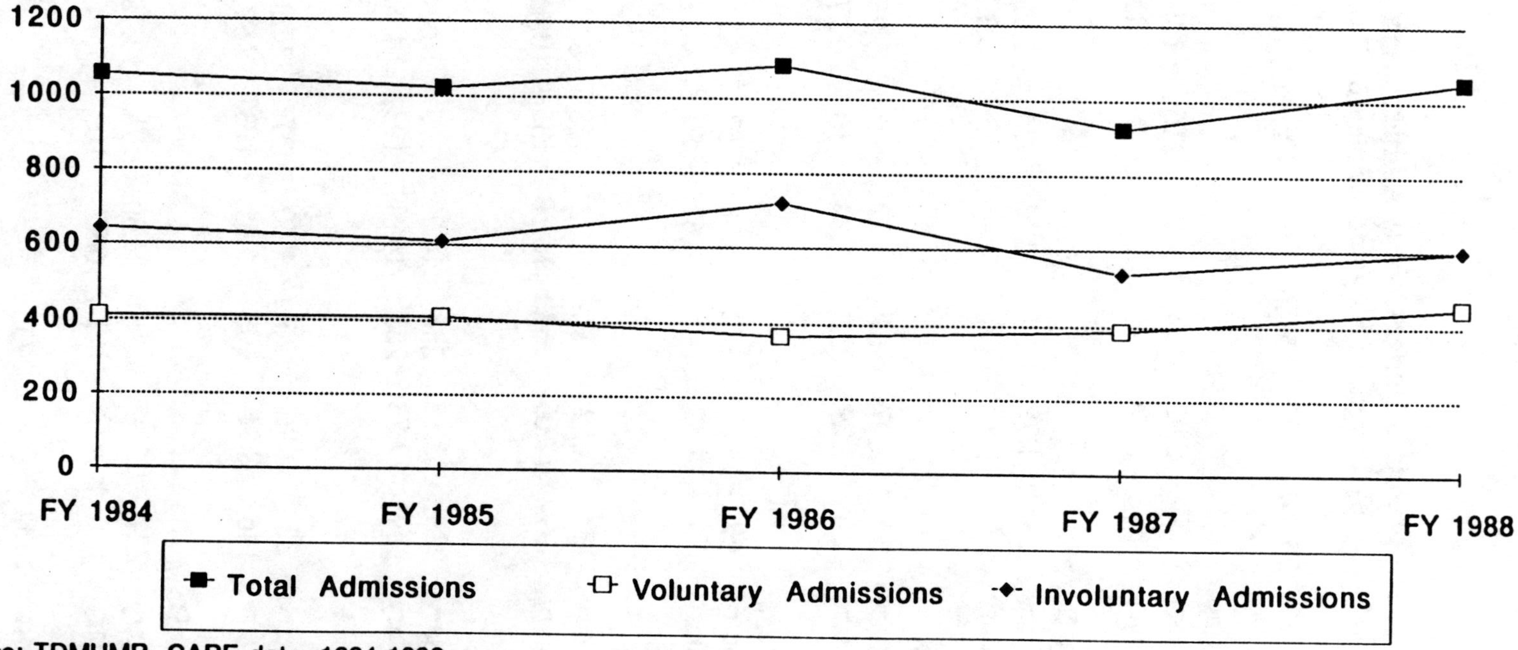

Source: TDMHMR, CARE data, 1984-1988.

Table 2.24. Trends in Dallas County Admissions to Terrell State Hospital by Length of Stay and Admission Type

	FY 84	%	FY 85	%	FY 86	%	FY 87	%	FY 88	%
24 Hours or Less										
Voluntary	15	0.92	22	1.27	16	1.24	24	2.24	12	1.13
Involuntary	3	0.18	6	0.35	2	0.15	3	0.28	3	0.28
Two or Three Days										
Voluntary	29	1.78	37	2.13	25	1.93	30	2.80	23	2.17
Involuntary	2	0.12	8	0.46	5	0.39	0	0.00	6	0.57
Four to Seven Days										
Voluntary	50	3.07	64	3.69	42	3.25	30	2.80	43	4.05
Involuntary	21	1.29	32	1.84	10	0.77	7	0.65	10	0.94
Eight to 14 Days										
Voluntary	63	3.87	102	5.88	69	5.34	64	5.98	64	6.03
Involuntary	73	4.48	81	4.67	59	4.57	23	2.15	44	4.15
15 to 30 Days										
Voluntary	134	8.22	134	7.72	113	8.75	99	9.25	97	9.14
Involuntary	197	12.09	262	15.10	135	10.45	80	7.48	118	11.12
31 to 60 Days										
Voluntary	223	13.68	248	14.29	215	16.64	238	22.24	218	20.55
Involuntary	289	17.73	251	14.47	193	14.94	138	12.90	166	15.65
61 to 90 Days										
Voluntary	32	1.96	26	1.50	27	2.09	19	1.78	28	2.64
Involuntary	146	8.96	105	6.05	103	7.97	62	5.79	76	7.16
More Than 90 Days										
Voluntary	227	13.93	236	13.60	178	13.78	141	13.18	100	9.43
Involuntary	126	7.73	121	6.97	100	7.74	100	9.35	53	5.00
Total	**1630**		**1735**		**1292**		**1070**		**1061**	

Source: TDMHMR CARE data, 1984-1988.

Table 2.25. Trends in Other County Admissions to Terrell State Hospital by Length of Stay and Admission Type

	FY 84	%	FY 85	%	FY 86	%	FY 87	%	FY 88	%
24 Hours or Less										
Voluntary	6	0.57	10	0.98	9	0.83	9	0.97	8	0.76
Involuntary	18	1.70	26	2.54	23	2.11	12	1.30	31	2.95
Two or Three Days										
Voluntary	19	1.80	19	1.86	21	1.93	12	1.30	18	1.71
Involuntary	20	1.89	28	2.73	24	2.20	9	0.97	12	1.14
Four to Seven Days										
Voluntary	38	3.60	44	4.30	35	3.21	36	3.90	48	4.57
Involuntary	39	3.69	51	4.98	46	4.22	22	2.38	37	3.52
Eight to 14 Days										
Voluntary	46	4.35	55	5.37	48	4.41	35	3.79	51	4.85
Involuntary	75	7.10	93	9.08	86	7.90	74	8.01	62	5.90
15 to 30 Days										
Voluntary	95	8.99	95	9.28	67	6.15	71	7.68	86	8.18
Involuntary	163	15.42	136	13.28	146	13.41	129	13.96	138	13.13
31 to 60 Days										
Voluntary	102	9.65	85	8.30	89	8.17	115	12.45	147	13.99
Involuntary	189	17.88	185	18.07	249	22.87	191	20.67	233	22.17
61 to 90 Days										
Voluntary	19	1.80	20	1.95	21	1.93	24	2.60	20	1.90
Involuntary	69	6.53	41	4.00	60	5.51	45	4.87	56	5.33
More Than 90 Days										
Voluntary	87	8.23	83	8.11	78	7.16	85	9.20	72	6.85
Involuntary	72	6.81	53	5.18	87	7.99	55	5.95	32	3.04
Total	**1057**		**1024**		**1089**		**924**		**1051**	

Source: TDMHMR CARE data, 1984-1988.

The increase in short-term voluntary admissions to TSH from Dallas County at the same time that DCMHMR is building up its local crisis stabilization services was an anomaly. DCMHMR staff have offered a partial explanation, but all the reasons are not known at this time. DCMHMR's voluntary AITC stays full; in addition, some persons, who do not meet the criteria for involuntary admission at the Parkland ER, then present themselves at TSH where, presumably, some are admitted (Gonzalez and Charlesworth, 1989). Reportedly, it is difficult for persons to gain voluntary admission to TSH; persons officially referred to TSH for voluntary admission by the Parkland ER find it hard to gain admission (Puryear, 1989).

Table 2.26 illustrates TSH admission trends, by length of stay and diagnosis, from all counties. In all but three of the length of stay categories, the number of persons admitted with a primary diagnosis of mental illness has decreased as a proportion of all admissions since 1984. Similarly, for almost all length of stay categories, the number of persons admitted with a primary diagnosis of alcohol or drug abuse has increased as a proportion of total admissions since 1984.

The lack of community-based alcohol and drug abuse services in Dallas County is likely the most significant cause of the increase of substance abuse admissions to TSH. The one-person substance abuse screening unit at DCMHMR is probably unable to keep up with the rapidly increasing number of substance abuse hospital admissions. This may partly explain the very low performance by DCMHMR in screening hospital admissions. The increase in the short-term admissions unrelated to substance abuse should also be examined. The earlier discussion of the utilization of the DCMHMR crisis stabilization services indicates that the MDC has too many beds and AITC insufficient beds. Shifting bed capacity (and funds) from the MDC to the AITC may help reduce the rate of increase in short-term, voluntary admissions to TSH.

Lack of Adequate Community Services

A major issue for all Texas centers is insufficient funds to provide adequate mental health services in the community for a real and lasting impact on reduction of the use of state hospitals. The lack of adequate services is probably the most significant factor in inhibiting centers' performance.

In August 1985, a Dallas-based task force of mental health professionals and other interested persons was formed to develop a comprehensive model for community mental health services. Now called the Dallas Model, the 1987 work product identified certain current and projected needs for services for seriously mentally ill adults in Dallas County. The Dallas Model estimates are listed in Table 2.27.

The task force assumed that a partnership of local, state, and federal entities, as well as of public and private agencies, is required to create a comprehensive community mental health system in Dallas County. Further, the report stated that "the public mental health system as it exists today in Texas is institutionally based and anachronistic. Reallocation of public funding to support the development of an effective community-based system is imperative" (Dyer, 1987, p. 4)

The Dallas Model report identified certain critical services which were needed immediately in Dallas County. These were an interagency data retrieval system, mobile crisis response team, medication clinics, housing, respite care, and case management. The task force estimated that an additional $3,911,251 was necessary to fund minimally adequate amounts of the identified critical services in Dallas County (Dyer, 1987, p. 35). These critical services were included in the DCMHMR long-range plan for FY 1988-FY 1993.

Table 2.26. Trends in All Admissions to Terrell State Hospital by Length of Stay and Diagnosis

	FY 84	%	FY 85	%	FY 86	%	FY 87	%	FY 88	%
24 Hours or Less										
Mental Ilness	22	1.93	27	0.98	27	1.13	17	0.83	12	0.54
Alcohol Abuse	6	0.22	14	0.51	6	0.25	11	0.54	8	0.36
Drug Abuse	5	0.19	12	0.43	13	0.55	13	0.64	18	0.82
Men. Retardation	0	0.00	0	0.00	0	0.00	0	0.00	0	0.00
No Diagnosis	9	0.33	11	0.40	4	0.17	7	0.34	17	0.77
Two or Three Days										
Mental Ilness	33	1.23	34	1.23	36	1.51	24	1.18	32	1.45
Alcohol Abuse	8	0.30	19	0.69	14	0.59	4	0.20	5	0.23
Drug Abuse	13	0.48	18	0.65	19	0.80	20	0.98	20	0.91
Men. Retardation	0	0.00	0	0.00	0	0.00	0	0.00	0	0.00
No Diagnosis	16	0.60	21	0.76	6	0.25	11	0.54	25	1.13
Four to Seven Days										
Mental Ilness	88	3.27	95	3.44	72	3.02	51	2.50	59	2.67
Alcohol Abuse	22	0.82	45	1.63	24	1.01	13	0.64	13	0.59
Drug Abuse	18	0.67	36	1.30	29	1.22	31	1.52	38	1.72
Men. Retardation	0	0.00	0	0.00	0	0.00	1	0.00	0	0.00
No Diagnosis	21	0.78	15	0.54	8	0.34	13	0.64	33	1.49
Eight to 14 Days										
Mental Ilness	158	5.88	191	6.92	136	5.70	99	4.85	146	6.61
Alcohol Abuse	52	1.93	81	2.93	66	2.77	39	1.91	26	1.18
Drug Abuse	31	1.15	51	1.85	51	2.14	56	2.74	49	2.22
Men. Retardation	1	0.04	0	0.00	0	0.00	0	0.00	0	0.00
No Diagnosis	15	0.56	8	0.29	10	0.42	3	0.15	11	0.50
15 to 30 Days										
Mental Ilness	437	16.26	483	17.49	318	13.34	241	11.81	327	14.81
Alcohol Abuse	98	3.65	80	2.90	64	2.68	66	3.23	32	1.45
Drug Abuse	48	1.79	57	2.06	74	3.10	73	3.58	78	3.53
Men. Retardation	1	0.04	1	0.04	0	0.00	0	0.00	0	0.00
No Diagnosis	5	0.19	6	0.22	5	0.21	3	0.15	9	0.41
31 to 60 Days										
Mental Ilness	482	17.93	443	16.04	384	16.11	288	14.11	358	16.21
Alcohol Abuse	228	8.48	193	6.99	183	7.68	170	8.33	142	6.43
Drug Abuse	88	3.27	118	4.27	173	7.26	223	10.93	264	11.96
Men. Retardation	0	0.00	1	0.04	0	0.00	0	0.00	0	0.00
No Diagnosis	5	0.19	14	0.51	6	0.25	4	0.20	2	0.09
61 to 90 Days										
Mental Ilness	244	9.08	184	6.66	194	8.14	131	6.42	165	7.47
Alcohol Abuse	14	0.52	6	0.22	6	0.25	12	0.59	11	0.50
Drug Abuse	8	0.30	1	0.04	10	0.42	9	0.44	6	0.27
Men. Retardation	0	0.00	0	0.00	0	0.00	0	0.00	0	0.00
No Diagnosis	0	0.00	1	0.04	1	0.04	1	0.05	2	0.09
More Than 90 Days										
Mental Ilness	485	18.04	476	17.24	402	16.86	365	17.88	255	11.55
Alcohol Abuse	15	0.56	9	0.33	17	0.71	12	0.59	16	0.72
Drug Abuse	10	0.37	7	0.25	22	0.92	27	1.32	20	0.91
Men. Retardation	1	0.04	1	0.04	0	0.00	1	0.05	0	0.00
No Diagnosis	1	0.04	2	0.07	4	0.17	2	0.10	9	0.41
Total	2688		2761		2384		2041		2208	

Source: TDMHMR, CARE data 1984-1988.

Table 2.27. Dallas County Mental Health Service Availablity and Projected Needs

Service Category	Program Type	Current Service Level	Projected Service Need
Pre-entry	Telephone Services	960 contacts/yr	Unknown
	Mobile Crisis Response	720 visits/yr*	2028 visits/yr
	Emerg. Evaluation & Treatment	11,500 contacts/yr	13,224 contacts/yr
Acute	Intensive Care-Hospital	65 beds	123 beds
	Temporary Respite	None	88 beds
	Respite Relief	None	9 FTE Staff
	Walk-in Clinic	None	52,897 contacts/yr
	Day Treatment	None	176 slots
Maintenance	Transitional Residential Care	None	88 beds
	Long-Term Residential Care	None	229 beds
	Outpatient Clinics	52,000 contacts/yr	143,263 contacts/yr
	Partial Hospital	36 Slots	353 Slots
	Volunteer Companion	None	N.A.
Independence Training	Supervised Residence	72 beds	282 beds
	Semi-independent residences	101 beds	353 beds
	Socialization Services	116 Slots	3256 Slots
	Vocational Services	168 Slots	2645 Slots
Continuity	Case Management	1000 clients	7053 clients

Source: Dyer, 1987, pp. 25-29.
*Provided by Dallas Police Department Social Services

In February 1989, the DCMHMR asked the Dallas City Council to provide $90,000 per year toward the total annual $188,191 Phase I budget for a mobile crisis intervention team. The City Council agreed, pending an allocation of funds from the Dallas County Commissioners Court. The Dallas AMI group has agreed to provide a van for the crisis team. The city and county have recently agreed to share the costs of the crisis team for four months. Funding beyond that time has not been negotiated (Boardman, 1989).

In response to a TDMHMR questionnaire sent to community centers with instructions for the FY 1990-1991 budget request, DCMHMR submitted a list of costs for additional mental health services that would be funded if DCMHMR received mental health services funding at $11.77 per capita. The $11.77 per capita level did not represent an ideal or adequate funding level; it only represented the highest per capita funding any Texas center received during the FY 1988-1989 biennium. As stated earlier, DCMHMR received mental health funds at $8.79 per capita in FY 1988. If funded at the higher per capita level, DCMHMR would receive $14,564,645 for mental health services in FY 1990. This amount still would not be sufficient to adequately fund the state-mandated core services or other essential community services for Dallas County (Craft, 1988).

Relationships with the Private Sector

Dallas County has a large number of psychiatrists, virtually all in private practice. Historically, the private psychiatrists and DCMHMR have operated almost wholly independently, in part because the Dallas County Commissioners have instructed DCMHMR not to compete with the private sector for clients or funds. This is a major reason that DCMHMR is so completely dependent on public funds, without income from some possible entrepreneurial efforts (Cotten, 1989). Others think that entrepreneurial efforts by DCMHMR would be welcomed within the private sector; direct competition between the two sectors is unlikely since the populations served and the services offered are almost completely different (Puryear, 1989).

The first substantial linkages between the public and private practice of psychiatry in Dallas County are described in the DCMHMR long-range plan. Both efforts involve expanding psychiatric coverage for DCMHMR clients at nominal cost to DCMHMR. In the first, the North Central Texas Society of Psychiatric Physicians operates a pro bono clinic for DCMHMR clients. This may be only a temporary stop-gap for the primary problem of DCMHMR's inability to recruit and retain physicians (Puryear, 1989). The second option with the society is the establishment of a voucher program in which the more stable DCMHMR clients would be assigned to private practice psychiatrists, who would be reimbursed at a rate similar to the costs for psychiatric services provided at DCMHMR (DCMHMR, n.d., p. 38). Since physician recruitment and retention has long been a problem for DCMHMR, as for public mental health services everywhere, this may represent a solid first step toward necessary cooperation with the private psychiatric sector and a beginning solution to the physician manpower problem.

CONCLUSION

Because of the geographic size and the burgeoning population of Dallas County, DCMHMR hopes to be able to provide a complement of core and other essential services in each of the four areas of the county that DCMHMR has designated as service regions. Right now, only two regions are operational.

Dallas County has a number of positive forces which could work to expand the mental health services available. Dallas County has a number of medical facilities, Southwestern Medical School, and a relatively affluent population. Only one other Texas county (Harris) provides more in local financial support for public mental health services. Until recently, DCMHMR has received very few funds from the City of Dallas. In FY

1988, the City of Dallas and community organizations provided $76,404 worth of space, utilities, and related in-kind matching for $305,616 in federal funds for services to mentally ill homeless persons. The local Mental Health Association and the Alliance for the Mentally Ill are active and supportive. DCMHMR could conceivably increase its revenues from fee collections through more aggressive pursuit of client entitlements and related sources of funds.

DCMHMR is perhaps uniquely situated to foster further development of a public-private partnership in Dallas County, not only with the private psychiatric sector, but with others in the private sector, such as general practitioners, apartment associations and other real estate investors, employers, and schools and colleges. In 1966, the planning commission appointed to study the creation of a MHMR center in Dallas recommended that the new center "utilize existing public, voluntary, and proprietary resources" (DCMHMR, 1968). Although community centers in other states have developed similar public-private relationships, a broad partnership of this sort would be a unique model for Texas.

How well does community mental health work in Dallas County? Probably at least as well as can be expected, given the extremely low levels of funding. However, the current structure of mental health services budgets and the current official service definitions cannot support an accurate analysis of community mental health services in Dallas County or any other county. Mental health budgets do not reflect many of the dollars that are actually spent, particularly locally, for some services. Further, budgets are tied to specific programs. The discussion of core and noncore services at DCMHMR clearly shows that the required core and other essential services are generic services, elements of which are provided across programs. The mental health client data system at DCMHMR is inadequate. Under these conditions, it is not possible, for example, to establish current costs for emergency screening services provided to a specific number of clients, nor project the costs of services which would be adequate for identified local needs.

Generic community mental health services are system-interdependent; the inadequacy of one or more services diminishes the effectiveness of all the others. The limited public dollars for community mental health services are stretched too thinly; the inevitable result is that many services are inadequate for the need. Each mandated service is an irrevocable decision on the allocation of already scarce resources. Virtually all of the adult mental health services provided by DCMHMR are those which are required by one level of government or another. And these may not be all the types of services which are necessary and most appropriate to the needs of persons with serious mental illness. Perhaps a continuing dilemma for public mental health services is that the consumer is not the one who pays.

References

ADAPT Institute of America. 1989. An Employment Training Program Manual. St. Louis, Mo.

Austin-Travis County MHMR Center (ATCMHMR). 1988. FY 1987 Summary Data Book for Community MHMR Centers. Austin, Texas.

Baughman, Jon. 1989. Coordinator of Continuity-of-Care Services, DCMHMR, Dallas, Texas. Telephone interview by Lynn Parish, February 16 and 27.

Beard, Jonathan. 1988. Director of Residential Services, Independence House, DCMHMR, Dallas, Texas. Personal interview by Jana Blasi, November 23.

Blegen-Sola, Mary. 1989. Independence House Clubhouse Supervisor, DCMHMR, Dallas, Texas. Telephone interview by Lynn Parish, February 20.

Boardman, Diane. 1989. Fiscal Services, DCMHMR, Dallas, Texas. Telephone interview by Jan Rienstra, June 22.

Bursey, Cynthia. 1989a. North Regional Director, Adult Mental Health Services, DCMHMR, Dallas, Texas. Personal interviews by Jana Blasi, Charles Blissitt, Lynn Parish, and Jan Rienstra, January 26 and January 27.

_______________. 1989b. North Regional Director, Adult Mental Health Services, DCMHMR, Dallas, Texas. Telephone interview by Jana Blasi, March 24.

Charlesworth, Marilyn. 1989a. South Regional Director, Adult Mental Health Services, DCMHMR, Dallas, Texas. Personal interviews by Jana Blasi, Charles Blissitt, Lynn Parish, and Jan Rienstra, January 26 and January 27.

_______________. 1989b. South Regional Director, Adult Mental Health Services, DCMHMR, Dallas, Texas. Telephone interview by Lynn Parish, February 16.

Cotten, Larry. 1989a. Associate Executive Director, Program Services, DCMHMR, Dallas, Texas. Personal interviews by Jana Blasi, Charles Blissitt, Lynn Parish, and Jan Rienstra, January 26 and January 27.

_______________. 1989b. Associate Executive Director, Program Services, DCMHMR, Dallas, Texas. Telephone interview by Charles Blissett, February 16.

Craft, James. 1988. Executive Director, DCMHMR, Dallas, Texas. Letter to Tom Suehs, Deputy Commissioner for Management and Support, TDMHMR, June 2.

Dallas County MHMR Center (DCMHMR). 1968. "Historical Outline." Dallas, Texas.

_______________. 1987. FY 1988 Contract for Services. Austin, Texas: TDMHMR.

_______________. 1988a. "Adult Mental Health Services FY 1989 Budget Proposal." Dallas, Texas. (May 20.)

_______________. 1988b. "DCMHMR In-Home and Family Support Program Report as of July 21, 1988." Dallas, Texas.

_______________. 1988c. Directory of Services. Dallas, Texas. (Informational Handout.)

_______________. 1989a. "Adult Day Treatment Programs." (Informational Handout.)

_______________. 1989b. "Adult Mental Health Outpatient Clinics Services". (Informational Handout.)

_______________. 1989c. "AMH Outpatient Average Caseload per FTE." (October.)

_______________. 1989d. "An Introduction to Independence House." (Informational Handout.)

_______________. 1989e. "Case Management Services in Adult Mental Health." (Informational Handout.)

_______________. 1989f. "CSP Prevocational Day Program." (Informational Handout.)

_______________. 1989g. "CSP Social/Educational Program." (Informational Handout.)

_______________. 1989h. "CSP Vocational Program." (Informational Handout.)

_______________. 1989i. "DCMHMR Clients Served, FY 1973-FY 1988." (Handout.)

_______________. 1989j. "DCMHMR Core/Noncore Services for Adult Mental Clients FY 1986-FY 1988." (Handout.)

_______________. 1989k. DCMHMR FY 1988 Unaudited Revenue Analysis by Source." Dallas, Texas.

_______________. 1989l. "Diagnostic, Assessment, and Treatment Services (Forensics)."

_______________. 1989m. "Fourth Quarter Report of Third Party and Client Fee Collections, June 1988-August 1988." Dallas, Texas.

_______________. 1989n. "FY 1988 Core and Non-core Funding, Adult Mental Health." Dallas, Texas.

_______________. 1989o. "FY 1988 Cost per Unit of Service, Core and Non-core Services, Adult Mental Health." Dallas, Texas.

_______________. 1989p. "Services Provided AMH Clients Discharged from Terrell State Hospital, 1/1-6/30/88." (Handout.)

_______________. n.d. "Long Range Plan: Fiscal Years 1988-1993." Dallas, Texas.

Dallas Morning News. 1989. Editorial. (June 26.)

Dyer, Dolores. 1987. "The Dallas Model: A Community Based System of Treatment for People with Long-Term Mental Illness." In Background Papers, Vol. I. Sixth Sutherland Seminar in Mental Health, Austin, Texas: Hogg Foundation for Mental Health. University of Texas.

English, Matt. 1988. Executive Director, North Dallas Shared Ministries, Dallas, Texas. Personal interview by Jana Blasi, November 23.

Ernst & Whinney. 1988. DCMHMR FY 1988 Annual Independent Financial Audit Report. Dallas, Texas.

Gill, John. 1989a. Director of Adult Mental Health Services, DCMHMR, Dallas Texas. Personal interviews by Jana Blasi, Charles Blissitt, Lynn Parish, and Jan Rienstra, January 26 and January 27.

____________ 1989b. Director of Adult Mental Health Services, DCMHMR, Dallas, Texas. Telephone interview by Jana Blasi, March 27.

____________ 1989c. Director of Adult Mental Health Services, DCMHMR, Dallas, Texas. Telephone interview by Lynn Parish, February 16 and February 27, April 24.

____________ 1989d. "Mobile Crisis Intervention Team: Executive Summary." Dallas, Texas: DCMHMR. (January 23.)

Gonzalez, Florence. 1989a. Director, Acute Treatment Services, DCMHMR, Dallas, Texas. Personal interviews by Jana Blasi, Charles Blissitt, Lynn Parish, and Jan Rienstra, January 26 and January 27.

____________. 1989b. Director, Acute Treatment Services, DCMHMR, Dallas, Texas. Telephone interview by Jana Blasi, March 24.

Gonzalez, Florence, and Marilyn Charlesworth. 1989. DCMHMR, Dallas, Texas. Letter to Jan Rienstra, March 17.

Heinrichs, Douglas. 1988. "Project ADAPT Site Visit." Twelfth Report to the Court, RAJ Review Panel. (January 20.)

Holzer, Charles, et al. 1988. "Estimates of Need for Mental Health Services in Texas Counties." In Background Papers, Vol. II. Sixth Sutherland Seminar in Mental Health. Austin, Texas: Hogg Foundation for Mental Health, University of Texas.

Hudson, Catherine. 1981. DCMHMR Services Description. Dallas, Texas: DCMHMR. (January 28.)

Long, Carolyn. 1981. "A History of Dallas County MHMR Center." Dallas, Texas: DCMHMR.

____________. 1989. Director of Personnel, DCMHMR, Dallas, Texas. Personal interview by Jana Blasi, January 27.

Main Hurdman. 1984. DCMHMR FY 1984 Annual Independent Financial Audit Report. Dallas, Texas.

____________. 1985. DCMHMR FY 1985 Annual Independent Financial Audit Report. Dallas, Texas.

____________. 1986. DCMHMR FY 1986 Annual Independent Financial Audit Report. Dallas, Texas.

Peat Marwick. 1987. DCMHMR FY 1987 Annual Independent Financial Audit Report. Dallas, Texas.

Puryear, Douglas. 1989. Director of Psychiatric Emergency Services, Parkland Memorial Hospital, Dallas, Texas. Letter to David Warner, April 7.

Seymore, Kathy. 1989. "Private Homes Help the Needy," Dallas Times Herald. (June 25.)

Tanowitz, Alan. 1989. Chief Pharmacist, DCMHMR, Dallas, Texas. Telephone interview by Charles Blissett, February 16.

Texas Almanac, 1988-89. 1987. Dallas Texas: Dallas Morning News.

Texas Department of Commerce. 1988. Projections of the Population of Texas and Counties in Texas by Age, Sex, and Race/Ethnicity for 1990-2025. College Station, Texas: Department of Rural Sociology, Texas Agricultural Experiment Station, Texas A & M University. (December.)

Texas Department of Mental Health and Mental Retardation (TDMHMR). 1986. Program Review Report on DCMHMR. Austin, Texas: Office of Standards and Quality Assurance, TDMHMR. (June 23-June 27.)

__________________. 1987. "FY 1988 Mental Health Service Definitions." Austin, Texas.

__________________. 1988. Case Management Services: Evaluation for Fiscal Year 1988. Austin, Texas. (October 3.)

__________________. 1989. "Preliminary Data, FY 1988 Contracts for Services; Fourth Quarter Reports." Austin, Texas. (Computer printout.)

Texas Fairweather Association. n.d. Fairweather Lodge Directory. Houston, Texas.

Timms, Ed. 1989. "Revolving Door: Justice System Often Unable to Help the Mentally Ill." Dallas Morning News. (February 19.)

Williams, Marvin. 1989. CSP Coordinator, DCMHMR, Dallas, Texas. Telephone interview by Lynn Parish, February 20.

Chapter 3. Tri County MHMR Services

Joellen Harper, Carolina Martinez, Timothy J. Tompkins

INTRODUCTION

Tri County MHMR Services was chosen as the subject of a case study for this project for two reasons: it has made great strides since its establishment in reducing the state hospital bed day utilization of its clients, and it has been innovative in securing various sources of income to fund its programs. The following is a description of its history, programs, and financing as well as a discussion of some of the issues that are unique to Tri County.

Table 3.1 provides selected statistics from fiscal year 1988 for Tri County MHMR Services. Of Tri County's $9.2 million budget, approximately 50 percent was expended for mental health services. A total of 2,262 clients were served, at an average cost per client for the year of $2,016.45. This amounts to approximately $14.00 per capita for the population of the Tri County service area. The mental health portion of Tri County's budget finances residential, client and family support, case management, and management and support services. Client and family support, which includes a variety of core mental health services, received 57.4 percent of the mental health (MH) budget. Tri County has limited resources for residential beds: 26.7 percent of the MH budget was expended on 66 residential beds of varying degrees of supervision. This amounts to 20 beds per 100,000 population in the service area.

BACKGROUND

Local Service Area

As of 1988, the total population for the Tri County service area, which consists of Liberty, Walker, and Montgomery counties, was 325,852 (TDMHMR, 1987b, p. 32). Walker, a rural county, had a population of 58,943 in 1988, covering 786 square miles, resulting in population density of 75 persons per square mile. Walker County earns income from cattle, horses, and hogs; cotton, grains, and hay; and the timber industry (Kingston, 1987, p. 253). The business economy is based on education, state employment, agribusiness, lumbering, and tourism (Kingston, 1987, p. 253). Huntsville, which is the county seat, is the Texas Department of Corrections headquarters. Other towns include New Waverly and Riverside.

Liberty County, also characterized as rural, had a population in 1988 of 58,427 covering 1,174 square miles. Population is somewhat less dense in Liberty than Walker, approximately 50 persons per square mile. Much of Liberty County's income is from crops such as rice and soybeans (Kingston, 1987, p. 211). There is also a cattle and timber industry that provides jobs. The business sector is composed of agribusiness, chemical plants, varied manufacturing, tourism, and forest industries (Kingston, 1987, p. 211). Liberty is the county seat; other towns include Cleveland, Dayton, Hardin, and Devers.

Montgomery is the largest, most densely populated county of the three in the Tri County service area. In 1988 it had a population of 208,482 over 1,047 square miles, with a population density of 199 persons per square mile. The county earns income from horses, cattle, hay, nursery and greenhouse products, and timber products (Kingston, 1987, p. 222). The southern portion of the county consists of affluent suburbs such as the Woodlands and a portion of Kingwood. Many people work in Houston and also in lumber industries and oil products (Kingston, 1987, p. 222). In addition to Conroe, the county seat, towns in Montgomery County are Willis, Magnolia, and Oak Ridge.

Table 3.1. Tri County MHMR Services Selected Statistics (FY 1988)

	Expended/ Achieved FY 1988
1988 Population	325,852
Total Budget	$9,194,151
Mental Health Budget	$4,561,202
MH Budget as Percentage of Total Budget	49.6%
Mental Health Clients Served	2,262
MH Clients Per 100,000 Population	694.00
Average Cost Per MH Client Served	$2,016.45
Total Expended MH Dollars Per Capita	$14.00
MH Program Budgets	
MH Residential	$1,216,803
MH Client and Family Support	$2,619,044
MH Case Management	$186,108
MH Management and Support	$539,247
MH Programs as Percentage of Total MH Budget	
MH Residential	26.7%
MH Client and Family Support	57.4%
MH Case Management	4.1%
MH Management and Support	11.8%
MH Residential Cost per Client Day	$89.62
Client and Family Support Average Cost per Client per Year	$1,159.38
Case Management Average Cost per Client per Year	$1,148.81
Case Management Clients Served in FY 1988	162.00
Residential Beds	
Structured Crisis	41.00
Structured Noncrisis	5.00
Intermediate	14.00
Semi-Independent	6.00
Total Residential Beds	66.00
Beds per 100,000 Population	20.00

Source: Tri County MHMR Services, 1988a.

History of Tri County MHMR Services

Tri County MHMR Services began serving the mentally ill and mentally retarded on September 1, 1983. The formation of Tri County was in response to the conditions in the Montgomery County Jail, where mentally ill persons were being incarcerated because of the lack of any alternative. A volunteer group, consisting of nine businessmen, attorneys, teachers, and other local citizens, was appointed by the local commissioner's court to investigate the problem. This group comprised the board that contacted TDMHMR and suggested that some type of MHMR center be opened. Walker, Liberty, and Montgomery counties together formed Tri County MHMR Services. A $60,000 planning grant was awarded to Tri County to begin providing at least basic services for the mentally ill and mentally retarded who were not being served through the TDMHMR system. The initial budget at Tri County was approximately $800,000; the center in 1989 operated under a budget of approximately $10.5 million and employs about 270 people.

Leon Evans, who had experience as the assistant executive director at the MHMR Regional Center of East Texas and as MR director at Heart of Texas in Waco, was hired as the executive director two months prior to the opening of the center. A five-year plan of goals for the center to accomplish was established based on a report by an outside consultant. These goals specifically outlined the provision of an alternative for the people who were being placed in jails and the establishment of a crisis unit. In one year the center reached the goals that were targeted for the five-year period with a small staff who were transferred from Rusk State Hospital. Tri County assumed a number of programs from TDMHMR, including the outreach programs of Rusk State Hospital for Huntsville, Conroe, Cleveland, Liberty, and New Caney. Two years later it assumed the four sheltered workshops and the four early childhood intervention programs.

The mission statement of the Tri County board states that Tri County will provide comprehensive MHMR services for the local service area. Tri County MHMR Services includes Tri County Industries, the former Tri County Associates, and other service components. The role of Tri County Associates, now known as LifeSync, was to provide services to all Tri County clients and counseling services for the nonpriority population. LifeSync continues to provide some screening, counseling, and crisis services to priority population clients. The majority of outpatient services for the priority population have been assigned to newly formed intake and support units. In addition, it offers counseling services for fee-paying clients at five locations in the Tri County service area.

Tri County Industries obtains work contracts on behalf of the center to provide employment for Tri County clients. Currently, Tri County Industries has contracts with both state and county highway departments. It serves as a vocational program that is less restrictive and provides at least a minimum wage for activities such as highway cleanup. The program also has much smaller contracts involving activities such as yardwork or janitorial services.

CLIENTS

Tri County serves clients with varying ethnicities, incomes, ages, and diagnoses. Table 3.2 presents summary centerwide client data from FY 1988. Tri County served a total of 3,295 predominantly white clients, the majority of which had MH diagnoses. Only 17.2 percent had a prior history of hospitalization. Of these clients, 1,110 fell into the age group 26-40, and 1,499 were supported by an income of less than $8,000. The male-to-female ratio was very close to 50 percent.

Table 3.2. Tri County MHMR
Centerwide Clients and Client Characteristics

Total Clients	3,295
Clients with State Facility History	566
Percentage with State Facility History	17.2%
Clients Not Registered *	545

Service Group by Program Category

	MH	MR	ECI/DD	Sub. Abuse
I	329	73	2	79
II	262	7	1	29
III	177	73	4	27
IV	383	45	3	83
V	257	4	139	75
VI	456	2	1	105

Ethnicity	
White	2,243
Black	421
Hispanic	72
Nat. Amer.	0
Oriental	4
Other	3

Cty. of Residence	
Montgomery	1,409
Liberty	786
Walker	413
Other	143

Sex	
Female	1,304
Male	1,446

Age	
0 - 10	207
11 - 18	281
19 - 25	429
26 - 40	1,110
41 - 65	625
66 -	70

Income	
$ 0 - 8,000	1,499
$ 8,001 - $12,000	0
$12,001 - $24,000	472
$24,001 +	320

Source: Tri County MHMR Services, 1989.

Note: Numbers in statistical categories may not sum to equal total clients.

* "Clients Not Registered" are included in "Total Clients" but are not counted in the statistical profiles.

Table 3.3 includes information on those Tri County clients who received outpatient mental health services in FY 1988. Of these clients, 16.1 percent had prior hospitalization history. The characteristics of the clients in this group very closely parallel those of the centerwide clients. Table 3.4 describes those clients who used Tri County residential services during FY 1988. These clients were somewhat more likely to have had a prior hospitalization. Nearly 35 percent of the clients included were served in Tri County's Crisis Resolution Unit for substance abuse problems. Table 3.5 characterizes Tri County's mental health case management clients for FY 1988. As might be expected, a much higher proportion of these clients, 68.1 percent, had a prior history of hospitalization.

PROGRAMS AND SERVICES

Traditionally, there have been many different points of access for services at Tri County, which was recognized by the staff to be confusing and inefficient (Thompson, 1989). Beginning March 13, 1989, a new process for screening clients began. Tri County has established "intake units" which are responsible for screening all clients and handling initial crisis intervention. There are now several intake units in each of Tri County's two regions. Region 1 includes west and south Montgomery County and Walker County (Conroe, Huntsville, and the Woodlands), and Region 2 covers east Montgomery and Liberty counties (New Caney, Cleveland, and Liberty).

Under the new intake and support (I&S) system, there are intake units in Cleveland, Conroe, Huntsville, Liberty, and New Caney. These I&S units handle client registration and perform the initial client assessment, which includes obtaining the client's past history of hospitalization. In addition, specific program eligibility is determined by the staff of the I&S units. Focus on the client during the screening process has always existed, but now it is more concentrated in the system. Under the new system, all clients will be screened at the intake units. (This does not include clients in the nonpriority population. The assessments for these clients are performed at the LifeSync offices.) The screening staff (intake specialists and caseworkers) first must consider how a client is functioning. Next, they must determine what the client needs, whether it be housing, work, a support system, or psychosocial or vocational training. Finally, the staff must decide what Tri County and community services are available to meet the needs of the client.

The screening staff of the intake and support units may refer priority population clients to LifeSync for screening, counseling, or crisis services. For example, the staff of LifeSync perform the client assessment that determines the need for 24-hour care.

All clients receive a multidisciplinary assessment from a team consisting of a caseworker, nurse, and psychiatrist. In addition, each client has a client program coordinator (CPC). It is the CPC's job to have knowledge of all of Tri County's programs and other community resources. The CPC's recommendations for services are based on what is appropriate and necessary for each individual client.

Another component to Tri County's screening system is a contract with Southeast Regional Texas Medical Center in Conroe. Tri County's crisis team is on call to the Medical Center emergency room to screen persons considered to be experiencing a mental health crisis. Each time the crisis team is called to screen an individual, the Medical Center pays Tri County $90 (Young, 1989d).

Tri County does not have a waiting list for the intake of clients. Persons in crisis always receive services immediately. At the busiest time, those not in crisis may have to wait two weeks for an initial appointment (Thompson, 1989). Tri County targets services to those in its three-county service area. However, the center will serve a person living outside the service area under two circumstances: if the person is a transient in a mental health crisis or if the person can be served on a full fee-for-service basis.

Table 3.3. Tri County MHMR Outpatient Mental Health Clients and Client Characteristics

Outpatient MH Clients	2,915
Clients with State Facility History	470
Percentage with State Facility History	16.1%
Clients Not Registered *	527

Service Group by Program Category

	MH	MR	ECI/DD	Sub. Abuse
I	313	25	2	79
II	247	2	0	23
III	172	16	0	24
IV	372	19	1	78
V	257	2	2	73
VI	447	1	0	104

Ethnicity	
White	1,968
Black	356
Hispanic	51
Nat. Amer.	0
Oriental	4
Other	1

Cty. of Residence	
Montgomery	1,250
Liberty	679
Walker	343
Other	117

Sex	
Female	1,140
Male	1,248

Age	
0 - 10	69
11 - 18	262
19 - 25	365
26 - 40	1027
41 - 65	589
66 +	66

Income	
\$ 0 - \$ 8,000	1,259
\$ 8,001 - \$12,000	0
\$12,001 - \$24,000	418
\$24,001 +	293

Source: Tri County MHMR Services, 1989.

Note: Numbers in statistical categories may not sum to equal total clients.

* "Clients Not Registered" are included in "Total Clients" but are not counted in the statistical profiles.

Table 3.4. Tri County MHMR Mental Health Residential Clients and Client Characteristics

MH Residential Clients	577
Clients with State Facility History	167
Percentage with State Facility History	28.9%
Clients Not Registered *	36

Service Group by Program Category

	MH	MR	ECI/DD	Sub. Abuse **
I	77	2	0	50
II	52	1	0	16
III	53	0	0	25
IV	85	1	0	41
V	50	0	0	33
VI	34	0	0	21

Ethnicity	
White	444
Black	89
Hispanic	6
Nat. Amer.	0
Oriental	0
Other	0

Cty. of Residence	
Montgomery	337
Liberty	139
Walker	54
Other	11

Sex	
Female	231
Male	310

Age	
0 - 10	2
11 - 18	17
19 - 25	114
26 - 40	289
41 - 65	111
66 +	7

Income	
$ 0 - $ 8,000	369
$ 8,001 - $12,000	0
$12,001 - $24,000	51
$24,001 +	18

Source: Tri County MHMR Services, 1989.

Note: Numbers in statistical categories may not sum to equal total clients.

* "Clients Not Registered" are included in "Total Clients" but are not counted in the statistical profiles.

** Substance Abuse clients in this category received services in the D.E.A.R. unit (now the detoxification side of the Crisis Resolution Unit).

Table 3.5. Tri County MHMR Mental Health Case Management Clients and Client Characteristics

MH Case Management Clients	163
Clients with State Facility History	111
Percentage with State Facility History	68.1%
Clients Not Registered *	1

Service Group by Program Category

	MH	MR	ECI/DD	Sub. Abuse
I	63	1	0	1
II	24	0	0	1
III	21	0	0	0
IV	40	0	0	0
V	8	0	0	0
VI	3	0	0	0

Ethnicity	
White	105
Black	54
Hispanic	3
Nat. Amer.	0
Oriental	0
Other	0

Cty. of Residence	
Montgomery	105
Liberty	30
Walker	24
Other	3

Sex	
Female	72
Male	90

Age	
0 - 10	2
11 - 18	0
19 - 25	17
26 - 40	86
41 - 65	51
66 +	3

Income	
$ 0 - $ 8,000	139
$ 8,001 - $12,000	0
$12,001 - $24,000	8
$24,001 +	4

Source: Tri County MHMR Services, 1989.

Note: Numbers in statistical categories may not sum to equal total clients.

* "Clients Not Registered" are included in "Total Clients" but are not counted in the statistical profiles.

RESIDENTIAL SERVICES

Structured Residential Programs

Structured Crisis Stabilization Residential Programs. These programs offer 24-hour care under intensive staff supervision to clients who are experiencing demonstrable mental health crises of moderate to severe proportions. Clients in these programs are in need of intensive treatment or stabilization services in a highly structured and supervised environment.

Following the TDMHMR mental health service definitions, Tri County's Crisis Resolution Unit (CRU) offers 24-hour residential services that are short-term in nature and are available to clients who are unable to cope successfully in the community or in less restrictive residential programs. These clients are usually in a significant psychiatric crisis or are in need of substance abuse detoxification. The CRU enables persons to remain in or near their home community when they otherwise would be sent away for hospitalization. Clients may be court-committed into these programs and are those who might otherwise be candidates for hospitalization. Typically, these programs are licensed by TDMHMR and are nonhospital (but with strong medical components), free-standing units located in the community. Each community center is required by TDMHMR to offer either this service or contracted inpatient beds, which are described below. Tri County's CRU services are available for anyone who is 18 years of age or older and who is deemed by a professional screening staff to be experiencing a mental health crisis or in need of substance abuse detoxification, and thus unable to function in a normal environment. Those with outstanding criminal warrants that cannot be dismissed at the time of the admission will not be admitted. Individuals are not admitted with handicapping conditions or medical problems requiring intensive medical supervision or treatment. The standard fee for CRU care is $250 per day plus psychiatric fees, but the actual fee is based on each individual's ability to pay. There are 12 beds for detoxification patients and 18 for MH patients. During the admission process, the forms are completed, a room is assigned, and a physician is contacted so that medical treatment can be given when needed. The client is examined to determine the severity of the case. The admission process at the CRU is on a strictly voluntary basis. All clients are evaluated either at the intake offices or at the center itself. Other professionals can be consulted if needed. If the admission occurs after working hours, the client is still screened by a professional and a joint decision is made by the physician and the mental health workers. If a screener chooses to release a person, it is only after gaining approval from the physician.

According to the staff at Tri County, there are times when the police are involved in bringing people to the center who will not voluntarily seek services; some are transients who have lost all support systems that were previously available to them. These people have often been involved in misdemeanor offenses such as loitering, trespassing, or intoxication, especially on the weekends. Other people are residents whose family calls the police because they are unable to cope and want the family member to seek services. The police officers in the Tri County area assess these situations and bring the person directly to the offices under a warrantless apprehension. Upon arrival, they are screened by professional staff.

A person's stay in Tri County's CRU will be terminated when the crisis has been resolved or detoxification has been completed. Dismissal will also take place if the client is there on an involuntary basis and the legal authority to detain the client expires or commitment requires transfer to more appropriate services.

A detoxification center aims at restoring the normal physiological functioning for persons experiencing problems with alcohol or drugs. Alcoholism treatment programs must be licensed by the Texas Commission on Alcohol and Drug Abuse (TCADA) except if they are part of a crisis stabilization unit. Tri County is voluntarily licensed with TCADA even though it is not required to be. Programs operated by components of the TDMHMR system require 24-hour-per-day on-duty nursing staff and 24-hour on-call medical coverage. As discussed above, Tri County has 12 beds in its CRU that are for individuals needing to recover from alcohol or substance abuse. A detoxification center is not defined by TDMHMR as a required core service.

Tri County combines mental health crisis and detoxification services in one Crisis Resolution Unit that has 30 beds. During FY 1989, the CRU expects to serve 416 clients for a total of 7,582 client days. The estimated cost per client day in the CRU is $133.42 (Tri County MHMR Services, 1988b, p. 33). The staff at Tri County feel their CRU is the model for the state of Texas (Tri County MHMR Services, 1989). The CRU is located on the third floor of the old county hospital where Tri County originally began its MHMR services. It is designed specifically for short-term emergency care. It is split into two distinct units. Detoxification is for use with voluntary patients, while the MH unit can be used on a voluntary basis or by those who have been sent there by a judge. The goal is to stabilize the individual and then work with the court to determine an appropriate level of care.

TCADA pays the CRU $75 per day per client and will fund a maximum of 5 days for alcohol and 11 days for other substances. If Tri County decides to keep the patient longer, it must do so with its own funds. If the patient has insurance or income, $250 per day is charged for CRU care, but the actual fee is based on the ability to pay. During the first five months of FY 1989, however, only about $5,000 had been collected from client fees and insurance (Tri County MHMR Services, 1989). Certified alcohol and drug abuse counselors (CADACs) are employed through LifeSync. One CADAC serves at the CRU.

Tri County's CRU, located in Montgomery County, is the center for emergency screening and assessment for Tri County's service area. It attempts to treat clients based on immediate need rather than just diagnosis. The fact that Tri County gets paid for this service enhances its capacity to handle difficult cases. When a patient is discharged from the CRU, a working record is kept and the complete record is transferred to the program providing aftercare. No one is discharged from Tri County through the CRU, meaning that efforts are made to coordinate aftercare services for all clients of the unit. Follow-up visits are scheduled before the client leaves. If the patient misses an appointment, letters are sent out encouraging the person to reschedule. TDMHMR standards mandate that attempts be made to contact and serve "hard-to-reach" clients up to 90 days after discharge. There must be documentation in the client's record showing these follow-up attempts, such as letters, phone calls, and home visits. The incidence of missed appointments at Tri County for substance abusers is much higher, due partly to the fact that MH clients often maintain contact if only to receive their medication.

The problem in dealing with low-functioning clients (those who require the most attention) is that it is very hard to mix them with the high-functioning clients (those who require minimal attention). Because of this wide range of functioning among the clients, beginning March 31, 1989, the CRU implemented a wider variety of programs to meet the needs of the different levels of clients. Each client will have an individualized program to take into account the wide range of functioning levels.

Contracted inpatient beds are another type of structured crisis stabilization residential program. These beds are contracted to provide stabilization of an acute psychiatric crisis on an inpatient basis in a licensed general or psychiatric hospital. These beds must be available to clients in each service area unless the local mental health authority (MHA) provides community-based crisis services through a crisis stabilization unit, such as the one at Tri County. At Tri County, inpatient beds are not made available by contract for payment but by arrangement with local psychiatric hospitals to make bed days available as part of a reciprocal agreement (Tri County MHMR Services, 1988b, p. 17).

Structured Noncrisis Residential Programs. These programs offer 24-hour on-site intensive supervision and structured activities for clients. They usually include medical supports and are often operated under external licensing or standards. These programs are not required core services. This type of residential program includes nursing home beds, intensive residential treatment, substance abuse recovery programs, and supervised family living/long-term structured foster care. Tri County contracts with Lakeview Acres for five beds. Tri County provides in-kind reimbursement in the form of medication, psychiatric services, and emergency backup to all of the residents of Lakeview Acres. Lakeview Acres is owned and operated by the Harris County MHMR Authority and is located in Walker County. This is a highly structured residential treatment program for persons requiring continuous long-term monitoring and intensive supervision from staff. During FY 1989, the five beds at Lakeview Acres are expected to serve nine clients for a total of 1,296 client days. Tri County's cost per client day for these beds for FY 1989 is listed at zero (Tri County MHMR Services, 1988b, p. 33).

Intermediate Residential Programs

Intermediate residential programs offer moderate supervision and moderately structured activities for clients. On-site staff supervision 24-hours a day is the norm. These programs sometimes have a medical component and sometimes are not licensed or certified. Intermediate residential programs are often transitional in nature and may also include respite programs outside the client's own home. Tri County does not allocate a large amount of funds for housing for its mental health clients. Of all the possible types of intermediate residential programs, only respite care services are offered.

Supervised Family Living/Brief Respite Foster Care. These programs are designed to offer support and relief to the family or usual caretaker through 24-hour supervision of the client outside of his or her own home on a noncrisis basis when the client is not exhibiting a psychiatric crisis that presents a possible danger to self or others. Tri County does not have any programs of this type.

Residential Respite during Periods of Client Stress. According to the TDMHMR mental health services definition, this respite program allows the client to reside temporarily in a more structured residential environment than he or she has been accustomed to during periods of stress that could lead to a psychiatric crisis. While this program is an optional residential component, Tri County is developing a program for adults who are in service groups II, III, or IV who are experiencing periods of acute stress and needing respite. There are no beds for this now as it is still being developed. During FY 1989 it is estimated that this program will serve ten people for a total of 94 client days. The estimated cost per client day for this program is $83.13 (Tri County MHMR Services, 1988b, p. 33).

Tri-County does not provide many intermediate residential services. For example, personal care homes, therapeutic group homes, halfway houses, and substance abuse homes are not available through Tri County.

Semi-Independent Residential Programs

Semi-independent residential programs are defined by TDMHMR as programs that offer limited supervision and structure to clients (TDMHMR, 1987a). These programs include, but are not limited to, semi-independent or supervised apartments, boarding houses, quarterway homes, Fairweather Lodges, and co-op apartments. In general, there are no on-duty or live-in staff residing in semi-independent residential programs. For FY 1989, Tri County had projected that under this category it would serve 33 clients, for a total of 5,443 client days, at a cost per client day of $42.00 (Tri County MHMR Services, 1988b, p. 33). However, these estimates were made when it was anticipated that a new Fairweather Lodge would begin during this fiscal year; therefore fewer clients may actually be served during this fiscal year.

Tri County does not offer many semi-independent programs. Quarterway homes, which can usually be found at most areas that offer semi-independent residential programs, are not available at Tri County.

Fairweather Lodge. Tri County's contract for FY 1989 suggests that it has 12 beds in Fairweather Lodge programs. Tri County had originally intended to set up a second lodge in FY 1989, but lack of funding prevented this action. Currently there is one Fairweather Lodge in Tri County's service area. The lodge, located in Conroe, houses six people who have learned to live and work together. Tri County funds two staff persons for the lodge (Mitchell, 1989b). The lodge supports itself in all other ways. The six clients combine their salaries and spending money, and, in effect, share the "wealth." They all are employed at the same location. Tri County contract data suggest that only clients in service groups IV and V are referred to the lodge (Tri County MHMR Services, 1988b, p. 18). However, limited funds restrict the number of people who can participate.

Clients in the Fairweather Lodge program are taught skills for independent living in an environment that fosters the wellness of each person. It is a member-run cooperative that serves as a strong support group encouraging each client to maximize his or her own strengths. The training for Fairweather Lodge is through Tri County's San Jacinto House. The lodge is one of the work programs available at San Jacinto House (to be discussed in more detail later).

Board and Care Homes. There are currently no board and care homes in the Tri County service area. Board and care homes can be either informal or organized facilities that provide room and board for a fee. The paid staff prepares meals as needed and ensures the maintenance of the physical plant. Tri County refers clients only to personal care homes licensed by the Department of Human Services.

Supervised Apartments. Life Enhancement is a moderately structured program with a psychosocial therapeutic training component. The semi-independent, in-home type of supportive program originally began as a residential program called Willis House. As of September 1988, the group home's census of eight people dwindled and clients were helped to locate homes elsewhere that would offer independent living situations. Two women were set up in an apartment together, and one man was placed in a nursing home (Tri County MHMR Services, 1989).

Under this program, clients locate and support their own residence, and then the Life Enhancement staff goes out and provides varying degrees of supervision (Phillips, 1989c). Family support, activities of daily living, and socialization skills are among the services provided by the Life Enhancement program. This support program emphasizes independence, self-confidence, and self-determination. Tri County offers training support and access to social groups that aid the person in achieving personal, social, and vocational goals.

Independent Living. This is not a core program recognized by TDMHMR; however, Tri County case managers have assisted clients in finding inexpensive apartments or in accessing other resources for housing. Apartments are found and obtained at minimal rates; however, most case managers at Tri County report that there is a shortage of available housing for independent living in the area. Out of the 15 percent who apply, 1 percent of the total Tri County mental health population receives Housing and Urban Development (HUD) services (de Luna Gonzalez, 1989). There is a long waiting list for both HUD housing and inexpensive apartment locations.

There are only two HUD apartment complexes available in the three-county region. Sixty-five to seventy people are residing in the apartment complexes. Approximately 10 percent of the persons who are residing in the HUD apartment complexes are mental health clients (de Luna Gonzalez, 1989).

CLIENT AND FAMILY SUPPORT

Tri County projects that during FY 1989, 2,345 clients will receive client and family support services. The average cost per client for these services is $1,181.46 (Tri-County MHMR Services, 1988b, p. 33).

24-Hour Emergency Screening and Referral

This core service has three components: a crisis hot line, a crisis intervention team, and multidisciplinary assessment.

Crisis Hotline. The crisis hotline is a TDMHMR required core service. It is the primary mechanism through which the client population gains access to the services of the crisis intervention team. TDMHMR requires a hotline to be easily accessible to the public throughout each service area and to operate whenever the center is not open. Hotlines must have the backup of the crisis intervention team, which is on call on a 24-hour basis for consultation and for immediate face-to-face preliminary assessments of all clients who (1) are apparently experiencing a mental health crisis that could potentially endanger the safety of either the client or another person, or (2) may be experiencing hallucinations, delusions, disorientation, generalized confusion, or bizarre behaviors.

Tri County provides crisis screening during office hours through its intake and support units and 24 hours per day through its information and referral/crisis line. During office hours, screenings are done by therapists. Tri County receives approximately 85 calls per week (Phillips, 1989c). Crisis hotline calls are handled by trained staff who provide information about Tri County services and make crisis intervention referrals to the crisis team when needed. This core service targets all six of the service groups and serves anyone needing or requesting MHMR services (Tri County MHMR Services, 1988b, p. 20).

Crisis Intervention Team. This team is the 24-hour face-to-face crisis intervention component that provides the preliminary assessment of all clients who are apparently experiencing a mental health crisis with the potential for (1) life-threatening behavior or (2) an acute mental crisis involving bizarre behavior, hallucinations, generalized confusion, or disorientation.

Tri County's crisis intervention team is comprised of a screening therapist and nursing staff with psychiatric backup. There is a crisis intervention team for each catchment area. Psychiatric or administrative contacts are made by the crisis intervention team. This team is available on a 24-hour basis through the crisis telephone line (Phillips, 1989c). In FY 1989, this service is provided to all persons in the five service groups who are experiencing mental health crises (Tri County MHMR Services, 1988b, p. 20).

Multidisciplinary Assessment. Any client who is confirmed by the crisis team to be evidencing life-threatening or acutely dysfunctional behavior must then be provided with a multidisciplinary assessment. This assessment must occur within 24 hours of the intervention by the crisis team. The term "multidisciplinary" is defined as a physician (preferably a psychiatric) assessment and one or more psychological, nursing, or social service assessments. At Tri County this assessment is performed by a team consisting of nursing staff, a social worker, or a certified alcohol and drug abuse counselor, and a physician (Phillips, 1989c). The multidisciplinary assessment service is targeted to priority service groups I, II, III, and IV and serves persons in mental health crises (Tri County MHMR Services, 1988b, p. 20).

Tri County's multidisciplinary team is mandatory and is accessed through Intake and Support (I & S) units and through the Crisis Resolution Unit (CRU). After hours, a screener receives calls and goes to the location of the call. The screener evaluates the patient, consults with the doctor or nurse, and then makes recommendations. Recommendations for admission are followed immediately. Clients recommended to the CRU are accompanied by law enforcement or family.

The multidisciplinary team evaluates and assesses the entering client and performs diagnostics. At night clients receive the initial assessment at the CRU. During office hours, both the I&S units and the CRU assess and evaluate clients. All patients then receive service planning which is based on functional need rather than diagnostic category. Diagnostics are never used as the sole criterion for placement in Tri County's community adjustment programs. The multidisciplinary team refers clients to other services at the intake units.

Community and Hospital Activities

Caseworker Assignment. TDMHMR describes this as an assigned professional staff person who is known to the client within the agency and who serves as a point of contact and an advocate for the client in obtaining the services he or she needs within the agency. Tri County assigns each client a client program coordinator (CPC) to help the client gain access to the appropriate community and Tri County services.

Hospital Liaison. The hospital liaison is responsible for tracking clients as they enter the state hospital and then prepare to return to the community. The goal is to develop a joint treatment plan process between the center and the state facility and to facilitate a timely return of the client to community services. These services are time-limited and short-term in nature. Tri County provides this program to ensure continuity of services so that persons hospitalized will receive timely and appropriate aftercare services. The hospital liaison acts as the CPC sometimes in conjunction with their previously assigned caseworker during the hospital stay and helps to develop aftercare placement resources.

Currently there is one hospital liaison in Tri County who serves both mentally retarded and mentally ill patients (Taylor, 1989). The liaison serves up to 30 clients at a time. The average number of service contacts is between eight to ten visits. The criterion is a mental health or substance abuse admission to the state hospital. When a client from the Tri County area enters a state facility anywhere in Texas, the liaison is immediately contacted. If the client is in Rusk State Hospital or a state hospital near the Tri County area, the caseworker will visit the client once a month. The state facilities work with the liaison as a caseworker to coordinate plans, and to provide guidance and assistance to the client (Taylor, 1989). The caseworker immediately contacts case managers to begin planning for the client's discharge.

The termination criterion for hospital liaison assignment hinges on whether the client is discharged from the state hospital to a different catchment area or is transferred to a Tri County CPC. State facilities coordinate with the Tri County caseworker to ensure that the client has been to Tri County for services. At Tri County, the client is then screened and evaluated for programs that are available and that will help the client perform effectively in the community (Phillips, 1989c). The hospital liaison links clients to necessary services. If referred to a caseworker at an I&S unit, or to a case manager, the client will receive help in obtaining public support from those sources. This leads to greater efficiency and effectiveness.

Residential placement for Tri County clients discharged from state hospitals are sometimes located by caseworkers through the hospital liaison program. In attempting to provide guidance to the client, a caseworker may decide to send a staff member to a residential facility in Houston to ensure that the residence is appropriate for the individual. Due to the lack of housing in the Tri County area for mentally ill persons, clients may be referred to personal care homes in the Houston area.

Family Support Services

Family Support Programs. These programs provide support and counseling to a client's family members by sponsoring activities such as advocacy meetings and self-help groups for family members. All of these activities improve coping and problem-solving skills for the family and the client, strengthen constructive bonding within the family, and provide the opportunity for sharing of emotional support among families.

Family education at Tri County is one of the main areas of emphasis. There are many difficulties at times in involving the family in the treatment and recovery of clients. For example, many times the client requests that the family be excluded from participation, in which case the client's wishes are respected. The community education/family education program, offered in Liberty, Walker, and Montgomery counties, includes topics of interest to the clients themselves, such as insight into their mental illness. There is the opportunity for those with problems to use their experience to help others with similar problems. Tri County offers meetings three times a week in various locations to attempt to accommodate those throughout its service area.

In-Home Respite. These services include home health aid, homemaker, and supervision services for a mentally disabled individual in his or her natural or surrogate family home during the day. The respite care allows the primary caretaker to be absent for short periods of time to conduct necessary and normal personal tasks or for longer periods of time, such as overnight or weekends, in order to provide a period of relief.

Tri County has not offered respite services in the past, although staff members feel that it is an important service. Their philosophy is that respite should be used in conjunction with other programs and does not necessarily have to be offered on a periodic basis, as is traditionally the case with the developmentally disabled. They feel respite is useful for crisis situations, but the theory is that through intervention and the use of other programs, one can prevent the situation from deteriorating to a crisis level. The crisis unit at Tri County serves some of the functions of respite care, according to Tri County staff. Programs such as psychosocial rehabilitation also serve to reduce the need for respite. They do have short-term board and care for crisis situations, but not in the traditional respite sense. The program is not designed to be used for crisis intervention, but it can be used to accommodate clients overnight if necessary.

Medication-Related Services

TDMHMR requires mental health agencies to provide clients of each service area medication-related services, of which there are five components.

Medication Clinics. Tri County medication clinics provide periodic reviews of psychiatric status and updates on maintenance or revision of psychotropic medication treatment by physicians. Tri County provides medication services at the I&S units. In addition, clients receive medication services at the Conroe psychosocial location called San Jacinto House, where case management services are also located.

Laboratory Monitoring and Physical Examinations. Laboratory monitoring and physical examinations, core components of medication-related services, allow routine monitoring of the physiological status of the client. These tests are necessary for the provision of appropriate psychotropic medications. Laboratory tests are performed at the medication clinic. All lab work is contracted out to a private center in Houston, the National Health Laboratory (Audis, 1989).

Clients pay for lab monitoring and physical examinations at a set rate. If they cannot afford that rate, rates are then negotiated and based on the clients' ability to pay (Audis, 1989). If a client has no funds or sources for funding, Tri County provides monitoring assistance free of charge.

Medication Education and Mental Health Maintenance, Education, and Counseling. Tri County's nurse provides clients with medication education which includes instruction to the client about the side effects of psychotropic medications at the time of his/her appointment. Education on mental illness/mental retardation is also provided. This type of education helps clients develop specific coping strategies to use during times of stress (Mitchell, 1989b). These two types of education are provided also through psychosocial programs in San Jacinto House.

Provision of Medications. Although Tri County facilitates access to psychotropic medications, it tries to encourage clients to use their own personal resources (Riolo, 1989). If the intake unit determines that the client requires medications but has no source of funds, Tri County will provide medications free of charge. Generally, medications are provided on a sliding scale like other services. If clients are able, they may take their prescriptions to a retail pharmacy (Young, 1989b).

Psychosocial Rehabilitation Programs

Tri County's psychosocial rehabilitation model has two goals: (1) to improve services for the chronically mentally ill population and (2) to serve the larger overall community (Mitchell, 1989b). In developing a treatment plan for each client, Tri County focuses on issues such as what causes each person distress; what causes each individual to separate from the community; and what prevents each individual from working and living effectively in the community.

Tri County currently provides services that allow the clients to live in the least restrictive environment and to live independently in the community. Not enough adult mental health clients partake in psychosocial programming (Mitchell, 1989b). Approximately 10 percent of the clients participate in the psychosocial services that Tri County offers and promotes. To enhance client awareness of the programs available, Tri County changed the location of medication services to San Jacinto House, where clients can more easily participate in and familiarize themselves with the services available (Mitchell, 1989b).

San Jacinto House has recently moved to a new location, which is conveniently located in the same building with case management and medication offices. This provides a better location for education, which is stressed at San Jacinto House. GED classes, mental illness education, and socialization classes all aim at improving the lives of the members. A new psychosocial program is ready to open in Liberty County. Defined psychosocial programs at Tri County are the following:

1. Social Support activities--these include activities that ensure the development of a normalized social network in the community.

2. Independent Living Skills--which includes activities that increase the ability of clients to independently accomplish tasks demanded by the general community.

3. Vocational Skills Development--these include services which provide the chronically mentally ill client an opportunity to develop and use work-related skills. Two types of programs are prevocational training and vocational training.

4. Stations in Industry--offers an alternative between sheltered and competitive employment; clients work under the supervision of training staff to carry out production goals.

5. Transitional Employment--trained employment located in normal places of business.

Social Support Activities and Independent Living Skills. TDMHMR requires mental health authorities to provide social support activities for their clients. These activities enable the client to develop a social network which provides the client with a source of companionship and normalized social activity.

San Jacinto House, located in Conroe, is a Tri County program loosely based on the Fountain House model, which supports clients in vocational training and psychosocial skills. Open primarily from 8:00 a.m. to 5:00 p.m. five days a week and two evenings until 7:00 p.m., San Jacinto House facilitates effective social networking. If a program runs late, the house will stay open until the program is complete. San Jacinto House soon plans to open on weekends but currently only does so occasionally for special events.

San Jacinto House has a static capacity of 80 clients (Mitchell, 1989b). The goal of the house is to develop social support activities designed to meet client requests. The members of San Jacinto House meet three times a week to express their interests, request changes, and offer input for services they are receiving. This low-pressure, informal approach allows them to learn at their own pace and encourages a high level of participation.

San Jacinto House provides a natural support system. Psychosocial services include social support activities, independent living skills, and prevocational and vocational skills training. Activities include member-organized outings, social clubs, independent member meetings, client-generated newsletters, and other activities. The service groups targeted by San Jacinto House are groups II, IV, and V (Tri County MHMR Services, 1988b, p. 21).

Transportation is a problem in Liberty County. Without a van and without state dollars for transportation services, many people are not receiving services. Walker County still offers no psychosocial programs.

Independent living skills, also a core service required by TDMHMR, increases the ability of clients to independently accomplish tasks imposed by the community. Clients acquire skills such as managing money, purchasing and preparing food, utilizing public transportation in the community, and more.

Vocational Skills Development. These services consist of an array of vocationally-related services which provide the chronic client an opportunity to develop and use work-related skills. The vocational components of psychosocial rehabilitation programming must include, but are not limited to, prevocational training and vocational training. Although Tri County's vocational programs are relatively new, they have a high rate of successful completion of the programs.

Prevocational training is provided at San Jacinto House. Loosely based on the Fairweather model, clients form vocational groups that meet for four to six weeks (Tri County MHMR Services, 1989). The client's skills, abilities, work tolerance, and training needs are assessed through many formal and informal tests. A rehabilitation teacher allows the members to develop their own rehabilitation program. All members are taught to prepare their own resumes and to develop interview skills. The staff videotapes members learning to prepare for an interview. After being taught interviewing skills, they then watch the "before" and "after" tapes to see their progress.

Vocational training, one of TDMHMR's required core services, is designed to enhance the vocational skills of clients in a particular vocational area. Clients are given the opportunity to choose their own work programs from among the following: job readiness training; supportive employment with a job coach; Fairweather Lodge; work program (for transitional work which is paid); sheltered workshop; and community education and client education programs.

All members who complete the program are guaranteed jobs upon completion of the program. The Texas Rehabilitation Commission (TRC) contracts for work programs, and the Private Industry Council (PIC) provides Job Training Partnership Act (JTPA) funding for some vocational services (Mitchell, 1989b). San Jacinto House acquires contracts for clients to work in a supervised setting, and clients, in turn, get paid on a piece rate (based on what they produce).

Job readiness training prepares mentally ill and mentally retarded individuals for future employment. Clients receive approximately 25 hours of intensive training to enhance essential and practical skills and behaviors that lead to obtaining a job. TRC contracts for work programs and helps to organize the curriculum for the skills received.

Stations in Industry is a noncore service provided at Tri County. The service is a method of delivering vocational programs. Competitive employment is provided, and work is used as a training mechanism. A client is helped in acquiring a job located in a business office. A vocational trainer is stationed at the business to supervise the client. The employer pays Tri County for the work done, and, in turn, Tri County pays the client and the supervisor. The program is funded through vocational funds or through contracts with the private businesses (Young, 1989b).

Transitional employment is a program that employs individuals in normal places of business, from large corporations to small local shops. Clients usually work at an entry-level position. No adjustment or lowering of regular work standards is made by employers. At San Jacinto House, clients have formed a janitorial work crew to clean buildings. One individual stocks vending machines and picks up money. These programs are training for possible future placement in Fairweather Lodges. Clients receive minimum-wage salaries working at transitional employment positions.

The NETS (Networking Effective Transition System) program is not a core service. It is part of a joint program that has been funded for one year only. TRC funded eight mental health and mental retardation centers within the state to participate in this program (Mitchell, 1989b). The Texas Education Agency is encouraging students in high school who have emotional disturbance to prepare for the transition into adult life while they are still in school. This program gives them job skills and is similar to the job readiness training program.

Case Management

Case management is a core service required by TDMHMR and provided by Tri County. Case management is a system in which an individual performs activities in the service of the client and is accountable for the client's progress. The case manager is responsible for ensuring that the client has access to and receives any and all resources and services that may help in his or her optimal functioning. All activities planned for the client are individually designed with the goal of assessing, identifying, linking, coordinating, and monitoring all services and resources required by clients in order to maintain their continued success in the community.

Case management personnel at Tri County provide services for priority populations I, II, III, and IV (Tri County MHMR Services, 1988b, p. 23). In the average community mental health center in Texas, case managers serve just under 9.68 percent of the total mental health clientele (TDMHMR, 1989, p. 132). In Tri County, this figure is a bit higher, approximately 15 percent (Taylor, 1989). For FY 1989, Tri County has estimated that it will provide case management services to 115 MH clients, mostly those from service groups I and III (Tri County MHMR Services, 1988b, p. 33). The projected cost of case management services per client per year is $2,948.51 (Tri County MHMR Services, 1988b, p. 33). Characteristics of the priority population include dependency upon external public support systems, multiple hospitalizations, commitments for reasons of dangerousness, and long-term hospitalization. These clients, if not treated in the community, are likely to become candidates for hospitalization, rehospitalization, or institutional placement. Fixed, in-office appointments are the primary method of contact.

Case managers are available to their clients 24 hours per day. Tri County case management has service locations in all three counties with a home base in Montgomery County (Young, 1989b). Case managers help link clients to services available such as food stamps, protective services at the Department of Human Services, adult education, legal problems, and HUD housing. Case managers also help assess clients with support, semiannual reviews, and Individual Program Planning (IPP) goals. To prepare an IPP, the needs of the client must be identified and a four- to six-month needs assessment of the individual must be designed (George, 1989).

The duration of case management for mental health patients in Tri County is as long as needed for severely mentally ill clients; however, the average length for most clients is four months (Audis, 1989). Tri County employs seven case managers. Each case manager serves both mentally ill clients and mentally retarded clients. The case managers represent four full-time-equivalent (FTE) positions for mental health clients and three full-time-equivalent positions for mental retardation.

Caseloads per case manager at Tri County are between 14 and 20, with 18 as the average. TDMHMR imposes a maximum client load of 25 slots for each case manager. Tri County has its own maximum load of 22 clients, allowing 3 slots per case manager to be available for emergency cases. However, so far the 22-client maximum has not been reached (Riolo, 1989).

The case management waiting list, with clients ranked in order of need, has a four- to five-month wait. Emergency cases receive special services and never need to wait prior to receiving case management services (Riolo, 1989). Immediate discharge planning is the goal of the caseworkers here. Clients are usually maintained as follow-up patients. There is no difference in the manner in which case managers treat short-term mentally ill clients as compared with long-term mentally ill clients. The only difference is the length of follow-up.

Other Necessary Support Services

Income Support. Upon entry into the Tri County Mental Health System, eligibility for income support is always assessed. Determining the financial capacities of admitted clients is a priority. Clients are always helped in obtaining federal support. Tri County could not provide information on how many of its clients are receiving public support (Riolo, 1989).

Substance Abuse Outpatient Services. Tri County has provided substance abuse services since April 2, 1984, when it began to receive TCADA funding. Tri County has tried to prevent clients from "falling through the cracks" as a result of TDMHMR and TCADA not wanting to serve the person since they see the cause of the problem as most appropriately dealt with by the other agency.

Tri County offers substance abuse outpatient services to clients of all five service groups. However, clients who are not in the priority population must pay for these services on a sliding fee scale. These services are provided at the LifeSync offices and are designed for people who have had detoxification treatment or those who are not in need of detoxification prior to treatment. It can involve either group therapy or individual therapy and is tailored to each individual's needs. It also involves referrals to Alcoholics Anonymous, Al-Anon, and other groups, and it attempts to involve the family in the therapy.

These services are readily available to all, not just the priority population. All of the 12 detoxification beds in the CRU are used for substance abuse patients, some of whom are in the priority population. These services are funded by TCADA, as there is no TDMHMR support.

In-Home and Family Support--House Bill 1154. House Bill 1154 requires the community mental health center to provide necessary support services for MH clients for in-home and family support. During FY 1988, TDMHMR required Tri County to expend $44,000 of its general revenue obligation for HB 1154 compliance. However, only $15,173 was expended. As a result, the remainder from the previous year has been added to the FY 1989 obligation of $117,000, resulting in a total of $145,827 for HB 1154 compliance (Tri County MHMR Services, 1988b, p. 35).

The in-home and family support program became operational in Tri County in August of 1988. Tables 3.6 and 3.7 summarize Tri County's HB 1154 funding for FY 1988 and the first quarter of FY 1989. The tables provide information on how many individuals applied for HB 1154 assistance and how many applications were approved. In addition, they detail the different types of services that were requested and the number of each type approved. Clinical and health services consisted mainly of dental care. Transportation services included vehicle repairs, liability insurance, and wrecker service. The Unique Services category refers to rent and utility assistance, clothing, furniture, and emergency food. HB 1154 funds are used to fill the gap while a client waits to receive other state or federal assistance or when other types of assistance have been expended (Phillips, 1989a).

Discrepancy in Service Provision

While Tri County makes every effort to provide its services throughout the three counties, some of its services are available only in Montgomery County.

In Huntsville a case manager and a job coach serve Walker County. Medication services, screening, and family support services (general counseling and education) are also available in Walker County.

Table 3.6. Tri County MHMR Services
HB 1154 In-Home and Family Support
FY 1988

	Applied	Approved	Denied	Actual Funding Provided
Client Applications	46.00	10.00	36.00	
Services				
Clinical and Health	35.00	6.00	29.00	$9,575.00
Attendant Care	1.00	0.00	1.00	
Transportation	29.00	4.00	25.00	$1,667.75
Unique Services	38.00	23.00	15.00	$4,260.37
Architectural	5.00	0.00	5.00	
Total	108.00	33.00	75.00	$15,503.12
Total Funding				$15,503.12
Total Clients Served				10.00
Total Family Members Served				NA
Average Cost Per Individual Served *				$1,550.31
Average Cost Per Service				$469.79

Source: Phillips, 1989a.

* Individual served includes both clients and family members.

Table 3.7. Tri County MHMR
HB 1154 In-Home and Family Support
FY 1989

	Applied	Approved	Denied
Client Applications	39	39	0
Services			
Clinical and Health	48	42	6
Transportation	64	56	8
Unique Services	61	49	12
Total	173	147	26

Total Funding	$31,270.83
Total Clients Served	105
Total Family Members Served	46
Average Cost Per Individual Served *	$207.09
Average Cost Per Service	$212.73

Source: Phillips, 1989a.

Liberty County has a community support program in the town of Liberty. The new program in Liberty County is being developed similar to San Jacinto House in Conroe, which provides clients with vocational training as well as socialization and independent living skills. Case managers are located in both Liberty and New Caney. Medication services, intake units, and general family support services can also be found in Liberty County.

Tri County cannot reach all individuals in need of services because of the few resources available among the three counties. The philosophy of Tri County stresses the importance of education in training clients to become adjusted, productive citizens in the community. GED classes, mental illness education, and socialization classes all aim at improving the lives of members. Without transportation, however, many clients do not have access to services.

FINANCING

The first part of the discussion below reviews Tri County's budget from FY 1984 to FY 1988. That is followed by a more detailed examination of the center's expenditures on MH services during FY 1988.

Fiscal Years 1984-1988

Table 3.8 presents Tri County's sources of revenue from FY 1984 to FY 1989. During its first full year of operation, the center's budget was approximately $1.6 million. The total budget grew nearly 500 percent over the next five years, for a total budget in FY 1988 of $9.3 million. The source of revenues that increased most significantly during that time period was local funds, due in large part to Tri County contracts with the Department of Highways and Public Transportation. Another large component of the local funds category is patient fees and insurance, which grew by 657.5 percent over the five years. In addition, the center increased its level of reimbursement under Medicare by 481 percent and under Medicaid by 657.5 percent. The center has never received city tax funds; the percentage of county tax funds in the center's budget increased approximately 124 percent from FY 1984 to FY 1988.

During the five-year period, the local funds category as a proportion of the total revenues grew significantly, while the state funds category decreased in similar proportion. Federal funds comprised 4.6 percent of total revenues in FY 1984, and by FY 1988 this had dropped slightly to 3.5 percent.

Tri County's expenditures grew 543.5 percent over the five years, with personnel salaries growing at a comparable rate and personnel benefits growing at nearly twice that rate (Table 3.9). Expenditures on other operating expenses, including utilities, postage, telephone, and insurance, grew by 1385.5 percent. Capital outlay and funds spent on services provided by consultants or other agency contracts grew the least over the period, each only about 179 percent.

Fiscal Year 1988

Revenues. TDMHMR provided 40.4 percent of Tri County's total funding in FY 1988 (Table 3.10). These funds were from general revenue appropriations, MH staff-to-patient earnings, MR staff-to-client earnings, and state facility contracts. The majority of these funds, 24.1 percent, came from general revenue appropriations. In addition, Tri County earned funds through the $35.50 program (MH staff-to-patient) and the $55.60 program (MR staff-to-client), which together amounted to over 15 percent of the center's total budget in FY 1988. (Tri County's MH staff-to-patient earnings are discussed further in the final section of this paper.) The "other state funds" category constituted less than 1 percent

Table 3.8. Tri County MHMR Actual Revenues by Source FY 1984 - FY 1988

Source of Revenue	FY 1984	FY 1985	FY 1986	FY 1987	FY 1988	% Change 1984-1988
Local Funds:						
City Tax Funds	0	0	0	0	0	
County Tax Funds	159,692	217,860	247,044	271,677	357,494	123.9%
Other Local Tax Funds	24,000		6,810	1,189	0	-100.0%
Patient Fees and Ins.	148,554	255,730	327,021	756,845	1,110,960	647.8%
Misc. Income Contributions	187,538	487,494	299,007	334,703	314,424	67.7%
Medicare	2,521	4,643	6,250	23,142	14,648	481.0%
Medicaid	3,987	10,314	14,051	28,274	30,201	657.5%
TCADA					571,752	
DHS Title 4-B			21,290	0		
ICF-MR Contract				468,824	527,657	
ICS-MR Contract					260,942	
TRC	1,604	13,642	3,634	42,152	65,619	3991.0%
Tex. Highway Dept.			369,210	780,805	1,962,040	
Subtotal Local Funds	527,896	989,683	1,294,317	2,707,611	5,215,737	888.0%
Local Funds as % of Total	33.9%	35.2%	38.3%	44.6%	56.1%	
State Funds:						
General Revenue	875,415	820,238	820,238	1,853,513	2,245,403	156.5%
Staff to Patient MH			561,788	549,895	761,236	
Staff to Client MR			347,597	596,691	672,148	
Other State Funds	83,740	893,659	111,441	80,300	80,300	-4.1%
Subtotal State Funds	959,155	1,713,897	1,841,064	3,080,399	3,759,087	291.9%
State Funds as % of Total	61.5%	61.0%	54.5%	50.7%	40.4%	
Federal Funds						
MH Block Grant	0		138,628	137,582	137,582	
Other Federal Funds	71,604	105,273	105,905	147,775	192,199	168.4%
Subtotal Federal Funds	71,604	105,273	244,533	285,357	329,781	360.6%
Fed. Funds as % of Total	4.6%	3.7%	7.2%	4.7%	3.5%	
Total Revenues	$1,558,655	$2,808,853	$3,379,914	$6,073,367	$9,304,605	497.0%

Source: Hereford, Lynch, & Company, 1984; Hereford, Lynch & Company, 1985; Reynolds, Davis, White & Company, 1986; Reynolds, Davis, White & Company, 1987; Davis, 1988.

Table 3.9. Tri County MHMR
Actual Expenditures
FY 1984 - 1988

Expenditure Category	FY 1984	FY 1985	FY 1986	FY 1987	FY 1988	% Change 1984-1988
Personnel						
Salaries	689,013	1,333,536	2,018,860	3,189,813	4,484,606	550.9%
Benefits	72,860	177,629	266,235	436,288	841,755	1055.3%
Travel	30,190	51,200	62,175	103,571	191,332	533.8%
Consummable Supplies	112,835	243,828	255,210	430,502	452,253	300.8%
Capital Outlay	74,027	133,714	69,979	146,992	206,539	179.0%
Building	137,709	113,168	231,882	493,938	435,605	216.3%
Consultants/Contracts	150,268	141,588	263,753	305,712	419,699	179.3%
Other Operating Expenses	133,140	389,903	437,724	1,057,825	1,977,855	1385.5%
Total Expenditures	$1,400,042	$2,584,566	$3,605,818	$6,164,641	$9,009,644	543.5%

Source: Hereford, Lynch, & Company, 1984; Hereford, Lynch & Company, 1985; Reynolds, Davis, White & Company, 1986; Reynolds, Davis, White & Company, 1987; Davis, 1988.

Table 3.10. Tri County MHMR
Revenues and Expenditures by Source of Funds
FY 1987 and 1988

Revenues By Source	FY 1987	FY 1988	% Of Total
Local	$2,817,388	$5,215,737	56.1%
State			
General Revenue	$1,853,513	$2,245,403	24.1%
Staff-to-Patient MH	$541,946	$761,236	8.2%
Staff-to-Client MR	$593,753	$672,148	7.2%
Other State	$80,300	$80,300	0.9%
Federal			
MH Block Grant	$137,582	$137,582	1.5%
DHS - Liaison Worker	$140,159	$192,199	2.1%
TOTAL	$6,164,641	$9,304,605	100.0%

Expenditures By Source	FY 1987	FY 1988	1988 % Of Total
Local	$5,750,382	$4,920,776	54.6%
State			
General Revenue	$2,245,403	$2,245,403	24.9%
Staff-to-Patient MH	$759,322	$761,236	8.4%
Staff-to-Client MR	$767,724	$672,148	7.5%
Other State	$80,300	$80,300	0.9%
Federal			
MH Block Grant	$137,582	$137,582	1.5%
DHS Liaison Worker	$147,775	$192,199	2.1%
Total	$9,888,488	$9,009,644	100.0%

Source: Reynolds, Davis, White, & Company, 1987, pp. 21-22.
Davis, 1988, pp. 21-22.

of the center's total budget in FY 1988. These funds were received from Rusk State Hospital. Tri County had a contract with Rusk during FY 1988 in the amount of $80,300. Of this total, $69,316 was for MH residential services, and the remaining $10,984 was for MH management and support services (Tri County MHMR Services, 1987).

Federal funds for community centers are broken down into a mental health block grant and other federal funds. The MH block grant is distributed by TDMHMR. During FY 1988,Tri County received 3.6 percent of its total funding from federal funds; 1.5 percent of this came from the MH block grant, and 2.1 percent of the center's total funding came from the other federal category, DHS--Liaison Worker, funded by Medicaid administrative funds.

The category of revenues called local funds includes funding from a wide variety of sources that are not considered direct state or federal funding (Table 3.11). Local revenues provided 56.1 percent of Tri County's funding during FY 1988. Approximately 21 percent of that amount came from the Department of Highways and Public Transportation. These funds were earned by Tri County through a contract with this agency to provide litter pickup services on the highways. The next biggest share of the local category of revenues during FY 1988 was patient fees and insurance. Tri County serves nonpriority population clients on a fee-for-service basis, thus obtaining a valuable source of income for the center's services. This is evident in that 11.9 percent of Tri County's total revenues came from this source. County tax funds from Walker, Montgomery, and Liberty contributed 3.8 percent to Tri County's total revenues for FY 1988. As noted above, Tri County receives no city tax funds.

The Texas Commission on Alcohol and Drug Abuse provides funding to the center for its Crisis Resolution Unit and its outpatient substance abuse services. Although it is a state agency, these funds are considered local because Tri County obtains them through an annual contract with TCADA based on reimbursement for actual services. The same is the case with Tri County's funding from the Texas Rehabilitation Commission. During FY 1988 Tri County's Medicaid and Medicare reimbursements amounted to less than 0.5 percent of total center funds.

Expenditures. Although Tri County's total budget grew nearly 500 percent over the last five years, the mental health portion of the budget grew by only 341.2 percent during the same period (Table 3.12). For FY 1988, the budget was broken out into MH and MR program categories; they are funded equally by the center (Table 3.13).

Well over half of Tri County's expenditures during FY 1988, 64.2 percent, were for employee salaries and benefits (Table 3.14). The center employed 247.4 FTEs during that fiscal year. The following is a description of how Tri County expended its mental health dollars during FY 1988.

MH Residential Services. For FY 1988, $1,407,432 was budgeted for MH residential services; $1,216,803 was actually expended (Table 3.15). Tri County served 633 clients, with an average cost per client day of $89.62. Both of these workload measures were greater than planned, but client days were lower than anticipated.

Tri County's structured crisis residential programs during FY 1988 were the Crisis Resolution Unit, Laurelwood Hospital, and the D.E.A.R. unit. (The D.E.A.R. unit is now the detoxification side of the CRU.) The budget for these programs was $1,191,299, but actual expenditures were $1,000,290, resulting in a difference of $191,009 (Table 3.16). It was estimated that these programs would serve 477 clients, for a total of 10,800 client days. In fact, 595 clients were served, for a total of 8,282 client days. Client length of stay in the

Table 3.11. Tri County MHMR
Local Revenues
FY 1987 and 1988

Local Revenues	FY 1987	FY 1988	1988 % Of Local Total	1988 % Of Grand Total
City Tax Funds	0	0	0.0%	0.0%
County Tax Funds	271,677	357,494	6.9%	3.8%
Other Local Tax Funds	1,189	0	0.0%	0.0%
PatiGeneral Revenue	756,845	1,110,960	21.3%	11.9%
Misc. Income/Contribs.	334,703	314,424	6.0%	3.4%
Medicare	23,142	14,648	0.3%	0.2%
Medicaid	28,274	30,201	0.6%	0.3%
ICF-MR Contract	468,824	527,657	10.1%	5.7%
ICS-MR Contract	0	260,942	5.0%	2.8%
TCADA	0	571,752	11.0%	6.1%
TRC	42,152	65,619	1.3%	0.7%
State Highway Dept.	780,805	1,962,040	37.6%	21.1%
Total Local	$2,707,611	$5,215,737	100.0%	56.1%
Total Revenues	$6,073,367	$9,304,605		

Source: Reynolds, Davis, White, & Company, 1987, pp. 21.
Davis, 1988, pp. 21.

Table 3.12. Tri County MHMR
Mental Health Expenditures by Revenue Source
FY 1984 - 1988

Source of Revenue	FY 1984	FY 1985	FY 1986	FY 1987	FY 1988	% Change 1984-1988
Local Funds	194,170	582,250	680,220	1,228,226	1,959,004	908.9%
State General Revenue	695,452	548,657	595,642	542,169	1,174,031	68.8%
Staff-to-Patient MH			480,322	460,654	761,236	
Other State Funds	42,368	597,768	56,476	73,876	80,300	89.5%
Federal MH Block Grant	0	0	118,033	116,945	137,582	
Other Federal Funds	0	0	13,170	0	0	
Total Expended Mental Health	$931,990	$1,728,675	$1,943,863	$2,421,870	$4,112,153	341.2%

Source: Hereford, Lynch, & Company, 1984; Hereford, Lynch, & Company, 1985; Reynolds, Davis, White, & Company, 1986; Reynolds, Davis, White, & Company, 1987; Davis, 1988.

Table 3.13. Tri County MHMR
Expenditures by Program Category
FY 1988

Program Category	Budgeted 1988	Expended 1988	Expended a % of Total
MH Programs			
Residential Services	$1,407,432	$1,216,803	13.5%
Client/Family Support	$2,929,886	$2,619,044	29.1%
Case Management	$167,295	$186,108	2.1%
Management and Support	$522,646	$482,436	5.4%
Sub-total Mental Health	$5,027,259	$4,504,391	50.0%
MR Programs			
Residential Services	$2,013,301	$1,792,203	19.9%
Client/Family Support	$2,263,773	$2,187,661	24.3%
Case Management	$109,735	$106,327	1.2%
Management and Support	$522,645	$419,062	4.7%
Sub-total Mental Retardation	$4,909,454	$4,505,253	50.0%
Total Expenditures	$9,936,713	$9,009,644	100.0%

Source: Davis, 1988, p. 24.

Table 3.14. Tri County MHMR
Expenditures by Object of Expense
FY 1987 - 1988

Object of Expense	FY 1987	FY 1988	88 Expenditures as % of Total
Personnel			
Salaries and Wages	3,189,813	4,484,606	49.8%
Benefits	436,288	841,755	9.3%
Consulants/Professional Fees	268,972	267,180	3.0%
Travel	103,571	191,332	2.1%
Consumable Supplies			
Drugs	88,106	85,577	0.9%
Food	106,698	139,734	1.6%
Other	235,698	226,942	2.5%
Furniture and Equipment			
Capital Expenditures	51,029	117,425	1.3%
Rental and Lease Payments	11,855	6,840	0.1%
Repairs and Maintenance	32,585	33,688	0.4%
Buildings			
Capital Expenditures	85,663	73,216	0.8%
Rental and Lease Payments	333,997	357,398	4.0%
Repairs and Maintenance	67,120	78,208	0.9%
Vehicles			
Capital Expenditures	10,300	15,898	0.2%
Rental and Lease Payments	116,895	22,989	0.3%
Repairs and Maintenance	20,313	145,840	1.6%
Contracts with Service Agencies	36,740	152,519	1.7%
Debt Service	92,821	295,398	3.3%
Other:			
Utilities, Postage, Telephone	245,886	289,343	3.2%
Audit Fees	10,250	9,500	0.1%
Insurance	57,049	74,570	0.8%
Client Earnings	424,407	808,433	9.0%
Dues and Subscriptions	10,173	18,193	0.2%
Miscellaneous	128,412	273,060	3.0%
Total Expenditures	$6,164,641	$9,009,644	100.0%

Source: Davis, 1988, p. 13.

Table 3.15. Tri County MHMR MH Residential Services Expenditures and Method of Finance FY 1988

Object of Expense	Budgeted 1988	Expended 1988	% of Tota
Exempt Salaries	$80,985	$77,321	6.35%
Classified Salaries	$746,274	$683,175	56.15%
Salary Increase	$0	$0	0.00%
Employee Benefits	$132,851	$118,364	9.73%
Travel for Staff/Board	$6,500	$2,780	0.23%
Consumable Supplies	$101,253	$78,523	6.45%
Capital Outlay	$25,000	$11,942	0.98%
Building Repair/Renovation	$15,453	$15,087	1.24%
Consultants/Contracts	$65,184	$37,448	3.08%
Other Operating Exp.	$233,932	$192,163	15.79%
TOTAL	$1,407,432	$1,216,803	100.00%

Method of Finance	Budgeted 1988	Actual 1988	% of Total
Local	$678,597	$475,599	39.09%
General Revenue	$244,139	$244,139	20.06%
Staff-to-Patient MH	$341,172	$342,557	28.15%
Staff-to-Client MR	$0	$0	0.00%
Other State	$69,316	$80,300	6.60%
Other Federal	$0	$0	0.00%
MH Block Grant	$74,208	$74,208	6.10%
Total	$1,407,432	$1,216,803	100.00%
Total FTE Positions	47.9	37.6	

Workload Measures	Planned 1988	Achieved 1988
Service Group I	161	148
Service Group II	141	136
Service Group III	67	81
Service Group IV	125	141
Service Group V	21	35
Service Group VI	0	0
Total MH Clients Served	515	541

Source: Tri County MHMR Services, 1988a, p. 3.

Table 3.16. Tri County MHMR MH Residential Services Workload Measures

Workload Measures	Planned 1988	Achieved 1988
Structured Crisis		
Capacity	41	41
Clients Served	477	595
Client Days	10,800	8,282
Cost per Client Day	$110.31	$120.78
Total Funds	$1,191,299	$1,000,290
Structured Noncrisis		
Capacity	5	5
Clients Served	6	8
Client Days	1,060	1,194
Cost per Client Day	$0.00	$0.00
Total Funds	$0.00	$0.00
Intermediate		
Capacity	14	14
Clients Served	25	15
Client Days	4,000	2,826
Cost per Client Day	$37.52	$51.44
Total Funds	$150,073	$145,358
Semi-Independent		
Capacity	6	6
Clients Served	7	15
Client Days	2,457	1,276
Cost per Client Day	$26.89	$55.76
Total Funds	$66,060	$71,155
Total Clients Served	515	633
Average Cost per Client Day	$76.84	$89.62

Source: Tri County MHMR Services, 1988a, pp. 3-6.

CRU, calculated by dividing total client days by clients served, seems to have been approximately 14 days, much lower than the 23 days expected. The average cost per client day for these programs during FY 1988 was $120.78.

During FY 1988, Tri County had five beds available under the structured noncrisis residential category. The beds were located at Lakeview Acres, a program run by Harris County MHMR Authority serving chronically mentally ill clients in New Waverly (Walker County). Tri County did not expend any funds for this program (Table 3.16). The beds are available through a reciprocal agreement with Harris County MHMR Authority. In return for the beds, Tri County provided clinical services to all the Lakeview Acres clients (Tri County MHMR Services, 1988a, p. 4). This program served eight clients, for a total of 1,194 client days during FY 1988.

During FY 1988 Tri County operated Willis House, an intermediate residential program with a capacity of 14 clients. The budget was originally $150,073 for Willis House; $145,358 was in fact expended (Table 3.16). Fewer clients were served than expected, entailing fewer client days, accounting for the difference between the budgeted and actual expenditures. Fifteen clients were served for a total of 2,826 client days and a cost per client day of $51.44. The cost per client day was expected to be $37.52. The lower number of client days drove up the cost of delivering this program. This program is no longer in operation.

Tri County operates a Fairweather Lodge, which falls under the semiresidential category. In FY 1988, $66,060 was budgeted for this program, $5,095 less than what was actually expended (Table 3.16). The actual cost per client day for this program was $55.76, more than twice the expected cost of $26.89. This increase may be attributed to greater attrition of residents than anticipated. Tri County planned to serve 7 clients with this program, for a total of 2,457 client days. However, 15 clients were served, totaling 1,276 client days.

MH Client and Family Support. The client and family support category includes all of the TDMHMR required core services except for case management. It is funded by local funds, state general revenue, and state MH staff-to-patient funds (Table 3.17). For FY 1988, $2,929,886 was budgeted for this category, and $2,619,044 was expended. Tri County served 2,259 clients from the six service groups, 639 fewer than planned. The average cost per client served was $1,159.38.

MH Case Management. Mental health case management services are funded by local funds, state general revenue, and state MH staff-to-patient funds (Table 3.18). During FY 1988, $186,108 was expended for these services, approximately $19,000 more than was budgeted. This can be attributed in part to the fact that case management services were delivered to 17 more clients than planned; 162 clients were served for a cost per client of $1,148.81.

ISSUES FOR ANALYSIS

"Private Enterprise" Model

Tri County MHMR has a unique structure and philosophy behind its services. While providing services to the TDMHMR priority population, it has expanded its services for nonpriority population clients on a full fee-for-service basis at the LifeSync offices (formerly Tri County Associates).

LifeSync has main offices in Conroe and Kingwood. There are satellite offices in Liberty, the Woodlands, and Huntsville. Service to New Caney and Liberty is out of the Kingwood office. Until recently, the staff of Tri County Associates performed all of the

Table 3.17. Tri County MHMR MH Client and Family Support Expenditures and Method of Finance FY 1988

Object of Expense	Budgeted 1988	Expended 1988	% of Total
Exempt Salaries	$76,971	$74,630	2.85%
Classified Salaries	$1,031,315	$902,782	34.47%
Salary Increase	$0	$0	0.00%
Employee Benefits	$202,745	$212,819	8.13%
Travel for Staff/Board	$51,555	$46,440	1.77%
Consumable Supplies	$190,273	$145,430	5.55%
Capital Outlay	$94,007	$83,639	3.19%
Building Repair/Renovation	$14,301	$15,502	0.59%
Consultants/Contracts	$223,597	$201,351	7.69%
Other Operating Exp.	$1,045,122	$936,451	35.76%
Total	$2,929,886	$2,619,044	100.00%

Method of Finance	Budgeted 1988	Acutal 1988	% of Total
Local	$1,976,752	$1,648,885	62.96%
General Revenue	$710,236	$710,236	27.12%
Staff-to-Patient MH	$242,898	$259,923	9.92%
Staff-to-Client MR	$0	$0	0.00%
Other State	$0	$0	0.00%
Other Federal	$0	$0	0.00%
MH Block Grant	$0	$0	0.00%
Total	$2,929,886	$2,619,044	100.00%
Total FTE Positions	69.86	43.95	

Workload Measures	Planned 1988	Achieved 1988
Service Group I	570	419
Service Group II	568	272
Service Group III	314	212
Service Group IV	534	470
Service Group V	412	334
Service Group VI	500	552
Total MH Clients Served	2898	2259
Cost per Client Served	$1,011.00	$1,159.38

Source: Tri County MHMR Services, 1988a, p. 7.

Table 3.18. Tri County MHMR MH Case Management Expenditures and Method of Finance FY 1988

Object of Expense	Budgeted 1988	Expended 1988	% of Total
Exempt Salaries	$3,463	$3,361	1.81%
Classified Salaries	$100,104	$102,823	55.25%
Salary Increase	$0	$0	0.00%
Employee Benefits	$17,737	$18,401	9.89%
Travel for Staff/Board	$8,900	$9,200	4.94%
Consumable Supplies	$814	$1,174	0.63%
Capital Outlay	$3,800	$4,111	2.21%
Building Repair/Renovation	$408	$421	0.23%
Consultants/Contracts	$902	$1,083	0.58%
Other Operating Exp.	$31,167	$45,534	24.47%
Total	$167,295	$186,108	100.00%

Method of Finance	Budgeted 1988	Actual 1988	% of Total
Local	$0	$4,005	2.15%
General Revenue	$23,347	$23,347	12.54%
Staff-to-Patient MH	$143,948	$158,756	85.30%
Staff-to-Client MR	$0	$0	0.00%
Other State	$0	$0	0.00%
Other Federal	$0	$0	0.00%
MH Block Grant	$0	$0	0.00%
Total	$167,295	$186,108	100.00%
Total FTE Positions	5.8	5.1	

Workload Measures	Planned 1988	Achieved 1988
Service Group I	60	65
Service Group II	26	25
Service Group III	16	21
Service Group IV	28	40
Service Group V	5	11
Service Group VI	0	0
Total MH Clients Served	135	162
Cost per Client Served	$1,239.22	$1,148.81

Source: Tri County MHMR Services, 1988a, p. 8.

client screening; state funds were allocated to the Associates. As of April 3, however, Tri County Associates became LifeSync. As a result of this change, most of the screening tasks have been assumed by the intake and support units, located in the two regions. LifeSync will continue to perform some screening, counseling, and crisis services for nonpriority population clients upon referral from the intake and support units (Young, 1989d).

While the current goal is for LifeSync to become self-supporting, eventually it is hoped that it will produce excess revenues to be used in enhancing services (Young, 1989d).

Rehabilitation Philosophy

Tri County structures programs around rehabilitation due to the fact that it focuses not on clients' problems but on the productivity of their lives. Many rehabilitation models focus only on skills development. Tri County's model searches for a much broader kind of development. Individuals require different kinds of support at different times in their lives. Tri County focuses on each person as a different individual for more effective treatment. Tri County's goals include the improvement of services for chronically mentally ill people. The staff want services to reflect a rehabilitation approach or focus. This is due to their philosophy, which strongly suggests that chronic mental health patients should not be institutionalized for any indefinite period of time but should be treated and helped to be functional in the community.

Results at Tri County indicate that traditional therapy treatments alone do not prove very successful among chronic mental health clients (Mitchell, 1989b). However, work adjustment training has been proven to be therapeutic by improving client's social lives. Working helps seriously mentally ill persons to improve their self-esteem and purpose in their lives. Under a relatively new noncore program at Tri County, persons with mental health problems join mobile work crews. This is part of Tri County Industries, whereby clients are based out of sheltered workshops but actually enter the labor force performing skills in lawn maintenance, roadside park landscaping, and janitorial employment (Mitchell, 1989b).

The mobile work crews are an innovative way to generate community support for day treatment programs. State as well as county highway contracts help to support mental health clients in jobs. There are approximately 14 persons from Tri County currently working on state highways picking up trash and landscaping the roadside parks (Mitchell, 1989b). The highway contracts, however, are facing difficulties, and renegotiation is necessary (Mitchell, 1989b). There is not a perceived need for highway litter pickup as there was earlier in the decade when the slogan "Don't Mess with Texas" first appeared. Funds that were available are dwindling.

Tri County chooses to help clients have a fuller life by participating as fully as possible in the life of the community. Clients gain self-esteem through work and rehabilitation. Member-run cooperatives strengthen support groups and encourage clients to maximize their strengths. They are given high goals and no restrictions.

Single Portal of Entry

There is a state law in Texas for the designation of no more than six local mental health authorities as single portals of entry to the mental health system of care for their local service areas as a pilot or demonstration program. The goal is to streamline entry into the mental health system of care and to promote continuity of care by the establishment of a responsible authority.

In determining the pilot organizations to be single portals of entry, TDMHMR established a committee, comprised of TDMHMR representatives and people from outside the agency, to review applications from centers describing the types of services they offered. Tri County was one of three designated a single portal of entry starting in February of 1989. Tri County was chosen because its existing system of care is structured effectively to ensure continuity of care.

The purpose behind the idea of a single portal of entry is to create local accountability. Centers will be the gatekeepers to the mental health system, and courts will send people to them for screening and evaluation instead of to the state hospitals. Although Tri County is now officially considered a single portal of entry, this simply legislated by law what it had been consistently doing voluntarily in its service area (Tri County MHMR Services, 1989). Although few changes were required for Tri County with this new designation since it already fulfilled the requirements, Tri County staff feel it is important that this be implemented statewide and they are happy to be a pilot program. Critics have warned that there is a risk in the mental health authority being designated as the single portal of entry since it earns money by keeping a patient out of the hospital and consequently would have an incentive not to send the patient to the hospital even if it would be in the patient's best interest. The Tri County response is that there is no true incentive to keep a client out of the hospital to earn $35.50 per day when it costs $160 per day or more to treat a person in the community. Tri County feels that if TDMHMR is worried about this posing a problem, the key is for TDMHMR to provide more management and technical assistance to the programs (Tri County MHMR Services, 1989).

Technically, with this designation no one should be admitted to Rusk State Hospital without going through Tri County first. In reality, there are isolated cases where someone is admitted to Rusk State Hospital directly, but this happens rarely. By and large the single portal of entry serves the purpose of ensuring continuity of care so that each person receives the proper treatment in the proper setting.

East Texas Round Table

In recent years there has been a coordinated effort among centers and state facilities in the East Texas area to develop a comprehensive mental health and mental retardation delivery system. In December of 1979, the East Texas Round Table of Chief Executives was formed around the concept of "continuity of care" and "joint budget planning." This group was formed in a cooperative effort in East Texas to reduce the number of admissions to Rusk State Hospital. The group experienced a number of changes and complications based on its relationship to TDMHMR.

Initially, a large group of East Texas facilities was invited to participate, but it evolved into the chief executive officers of the Lufkin State School, Rusk State Hospital, Beaumont State Center for Human Development, Deep East Texas MHMR Center (Lufkin), East Texas MHMR Center (Tyler), Southeast Texas MHMR (Beaumont), and Sabine Valley. These were the key players who attempted to improve their systems of care for the mentally ill. When Tri County MHMR Services was formed in 1983, it too became a member because its new service area was contiguous with the three major state facilities involved.

Because of friction and lack of cooperation and accomplishments with the representatives of TDMHMR, the East Texas Round Table was disbanded temporarily. It is now about to resume its activities with the support of TDMHMR (Tri County MHMR Services, 1989). The members of the new Round Table will continue to invite the deputy commissioners of TDMHMR but will themselves be in control of its activities. They will set the agenda to deal with the problems in their region, and they feel that they will be better able to accomplish their goals by having this control.

The $35.50 Program

Tri County MHMR Services began operating during the first quarter of FY 1984. This was one year prior to the onset of the $35.50 program in the first quarter of FY 1985. The program was designed with a goal of encouraging community centers to reduce state hospital bed utilization by expanding their programs to serve more clients in the community. Tri County has been very successful since its establishment at decreasing its clients' use of state hospital bed days, from 5,165 in the fourth quarter of FY 1983 to approximately 750 in the first quarter of FY 1989. In fact, Tri County had made great reductions in bed day usage even before payments were made to the centers for doing so. At the beginning of FY 1988, the $35.50 program was revised with the addition of incentive payments and a new incentive baseline. The incentive payments were a higher bed day reimbursement amount for reductions of bed days below the incentive baseline and for centers with a very low bed day usage in relation to the population of their service area.

Tri County believes that it was in effect penalized for its successful bed day reduction efforts (Tri County MHMR Services, 1989). If the center had waited to reduce bed day usage until the beginning of the incentive program, its earnings over the life of the program would have been substantially higher because the center could have been earning up to $60 per bed day instead of $35.50 per bed day.*

The CMHMR Facilities Acquisition Program

At the end of 1988, the Texas Council of Community MHMR Centers closed a transaction to produce almost $38 million in bonds for 15 community centers. The bonds will be used to refinance approximately $20 million in existing loans at lower interest rates, and approximately $20 million will be used to acquire facilities and/or major equipment items (Texas Council of CMHMRCs, 1989, p. 1). Tri County is one of the centers included in this project. It will receive $3,955,000 of the total amount. Tri County has the following plans for the funds: acquire real property consisting of five buildings located in Conroe for use as clinics and administrative offices; renovate the clinics and offices located at Riverwood Court and River Pointe Drive in Conroe; refinance a 9,600-square-foot central administrative facility located in Conroe; refinance a 12,000-square-foot sheltered workshop located in Conroe; and refinance seven mental retardation group homes located in the Tri County service area.

CONCLUSIONS

Tri County MHMR Services has made substantial progress over the five years of its existence. Services have been expanded greatly, the number of staff has grown accordingly, and the budget has risen by a dramatic 500 percent.

Tri County has been very successful in deterring the majority of admissions to the state hospitals from its service area by developing programs that enable the maintenance of clients in the community. A prime example of such a program is the Crisis Resolution Unit. The availability of 18 beds for people experiencing mental health crises decreases the need to admit clients to the state hospital for resolution of such episodes. Another example is case management services, which are effective at coordinating the care of chronic and acute individuals. Unfortunately, case management services are extremely limited at Tri County, as they are across the state. It is likely that many more individuals could benefit from such services, reducing even more the necessity of state hospital care for meeting an individual's basic needs.

---

*See section IV of <u>Financing Care for the Chronically Mentally Ill in Texas, 1990.</u>

Tri County emphasizes the benefits of psychosocial and vocational programs for its clients as a way of increasing client self-worth and respect. Both Tri County's executive director and associate executive director have backgrounds working with the mentally retarded, a population for which vocational programs traditionally are successful. Once again, however, the psychosocial and vocational programs at Tri County have limited capacities. The Tri County staff has goals to establish psychosocial programs in all of Tri County's major communities (Young, 1989d). Increased funding will determine if and when this will occur.

Residential services are minimal in the Tri County service area. There is a need to improve structured residential services, and the Tri County staff would like to expand the Fairweather Lodge program in the future if funding permits (Young, 1989d).

Limited availability of services is aggravated by transportation difficulties in the Tri County service area. Some of the center's programs are available only in Conroe, the main city in Montgomery County. There is no system of public transportation in the Tri County area, and many of Tri County's clients do not have their own mode of transportation. Thus the center needs to, and is attempting to, expand its programs to other cities throughout its service area.

It should be clear from this report that Tri County is by no means able to solve all the problems of the Tri County service area. There are many gaps and shortcomings in services and availability, most of which are funding-related. Tri County has been more effective than many community centers at accessing various forms of local funds, including trying to maximize patients' fees and insurance. Nonetheless, the fact remains that the state continues to be a major source of funding for mental health services throughout the state, and until action is taken to increase the level of state funding for mental health care and to create a more rational financing system, even the most successful centers like Tri County will have to stretch too few dollars over too few programs to adequately serve persons in need.

References

Audis, Carol. 1989. Case Manager, Tri County Mental Health Mental Retardation Services, Conroe, Texas. Telephone interview by Carolina Martinez, March 29.

Davis, Kenneth C. 1988. Tri County Mental Health Mental Retardation Services, Audited Financial Statements. Huntsville, Texas.

de Luna Gonzalez, Rosa. 1989. Director of Program Operations, Tri County Mental Health Mental Retardation Services, Conroe, Texas. Telephone interview by Carolina Martinez, March 29.

George, Larry. 1989. Case Manager, Tri County Mental Health Mental Retardation Services, Conroe, Texas. Telephone interview by Carolina Martinez, March 23.

Hereford, Lynch, & Company. 1984. Tri County Mental Health Mental Retardation Services, Audited Financial Statements.

____________. 1985. Tri County Mental Health Mental Retardation Services, Audited Financial Statements.

Kingston, Mike, ed. 1988. Texas Almanac and State Industrial Guide. Dallas, Texas: Dallas Morning News.

Mitchell, Tom. 1989a. Director, Community Support Services, Tri County Mental Health Mental Retardation Services, Conroe, Texas. Telephone interview by Tim Tompkins, February 23.

____________. 1989b. Telephone interviews by Carolina Martinez, Conroe, Texas. March 23 and 24.

____________. 1989c. Telephone interview by Tim Tompkins, Conroe, Texas. March 27.

Phillips, Johnny. 1989a. Director, Community Assistance and Crisis Services, Tri County Mental Health Mental Retardation Services, Conroe, Texas. Internal memo dated March 16.

____________. 1989b. Telephone interviews by Tim Tompkins, Conroe, Texas. February-April.

____________. 1989c. Telephone interview by Carolina Martinez, Conroe, Texas. March 24.

Reynolds, Davis, White, & Company. 1986. Tri County Mental Health Mental Retardation Services, Audited Financial Statements. Huntsville, Texas.

____________. 1987. Tri County Mental Health Mental Retardation Services, Audited Financial Statements. Huntsville, Texas.

Riolo, Rona. 1989. Director, Case Management, Tri County Mental Health Mental Retardation Services, Conroe, Texas. Telephone interviews by Carolina Martinez, March 27 and 30.

Taylor, Adelle. 1989. Caseworker, Tri County Mental Health Mental Retardation Services, Conroe, Texas. Telephone interview by Carolina Martinez, March 31.

Texas Council of Community Mental Health and Mental Retardation Centers (Texas Council of CMHMRCs), Inc. 1989. Letter to Wayne Holtzman, Hogg Foundation, January 6, Austin, Texas.

Texas Department of Mental Health and Mental Retardation (TDMHMR). 1987a. Mental Health Service Definitions. Austin, Texas, May.

____________. 1987b. Texas Population Data by Texas Department of Mental Health and Mental Retardation Local Service Areas 1987-1993. Austin, Texas, May.

Thompson, Mary Ellen. 1989. Director, Consumer Support Services, Tri County Mental Health Mental Retardation Services, Conroe, Texas. Telephone interview by Joellen M. Harper, March 29.

Tri County Mental Health Mental Retardation Services. 1987. Contract for Services (FY 1988). Conroe, Texas, September.

____________. 1988a. Community MHMR Center Budget and Quarterly Report. Conroe, Texas, November 21.

____________. 1988b. Contract for Services (FY 1989). Conroe, Texas, September.

____________. 1989. Interviews with administrative and executive staff, Conroe, Texas. February 2 and 3.

Young, Dot. 1989. Associate Executive Director, Tri County Mental Health Mental Retardation Services, Conroe, Texas. Telephone interviews by Tim Tompkins, February-April.

____________. 1989b. Telephone interview by Carolina Martinez, Conroe, Texas, March 29.

____________. 1989c. Telephone interview by Joellen M. Harper, Conroe, Texas, April 20.

____________. 1989d. Telephone interview by Joellen M. Harper, Conroe, Texas, May 3.

Chapter 4. Concho Valley Center for Human Advancement

Hugh F. Crean, Norma Rodriguez, Rodolpho R. Vega

INTRODUCTION

The Texas Department of Mental Health and Mental Retardation's report entitled Future Directions 1988-1993 states:

> Currently 75 percent of the area of Texas is considered rural, and this 75 percent is occupied by 25 percent of the population of the state. To obtain appropriate psychiatric services, a rural Texan may have to travel as much as 100 to 150 miles. Rather than traveling such distances, mentally ill persons frequently delay treatment until the illness has progressed so far that hospitalization for long periods is required. While it is true that the majority of the population is urban, the one fourth of Texans in rural areas, including isolated populations such as those in West and South Texas, should have access to early treatment programs as well (TDMHMR,1988a, p. 12).

The Concho Valley Center for Human Advancement (CVCHA),* located in San Angelo, exemplifies many of these issues associated with rural mental health. For this reason, the CVCHA was selected as the subject for this case study. Among the overriding concerns and issues facing such a rural mental health center are

1. attitudes of a conservative community--the family and state institutions are often viewed as the responsible provider of care;
2. geographical inaccessibility--lack of outreach services to rural areas; and
3. stigma often attached to those with mental illness--conservative attitudes impact upon this as does the difficulty in maintaining confidentiality in small communities.

The mission of the Concho Valley Center for Human Advancement is ". . . to provide to service area residents with mental illness or mental retardation the opportunity consistent with the rights of the individuals served to develop and function as contributing members of the community" (CVCHA, 1987, p. 3).

DEMOGRAPHIC CHARACTERISTICS OF THE CONCHO VALLEY

The Concho Valley Center for Human Advancement is located in San Angelo, which is the seat of Tom Green County. San Angelo lies in the middle of the western portion of Texas and is equidistant from Austin on the east and New Mexico on the west. Situated at the juncture of the North Concho and combined South and Middle Concho rivers, this city has often been called the "Oasis of West Texas" (Sharpe and Weddle, 1982).

---

*In March 1989, the Concho Valley Center for Human Advancement changed its name to MHMR Services for the Concho Valley. This change occurred midway through this research project. All references and materials throughout this report are cited as the Concho Valley Center for Human Advancement (CVCHA).

The city of San Angelo strikes one as traditional and conservative with a small-town demeanor. There is a strong sense of community in San Angelo as well as within the neighboring counties, and one is impressed with the apparent friendliness among the people.

Seven counties constitute the CVCHA catchment area: Coke, Concho, Crockett, Irion, Reagan, Sterling, and Tom Green (Figure 4.1). Although the square mileage of the catchment area may seem rather large--9,369 square miles, the population density is only 13.3 persons per square mile (compared with an average density of 54.3 for the state as a whole). When Tom Green County is excluded, the other six counties cover 7,854 square miles with a 1989 population of 21,214, for a population density of only 2.7 persons per square mile. The total population of these seven counties in FY 1988 was 117,700 (CVCHA, 1988a). Table 4.1 shows the population distribution by county as well as other demographic information for the CVCHA catchment area.

Table 4.2 presents data on the ethnic breakdown of the Concho Valley as compared with the state of Texas. Of note, the Concho Valley has significantly fewer blacks than the rest of the state.

The per capita personal income for the city of San Angelo was $12,115 in 1984, while the per capita personal income for the state was $12,575. The average weekly wage for Tom Green and the surrounding counties was $311.29 in 1985 (Kingston and Crawford, 1987).

In FY 1988, CVCHA provided services to 624 clients with mental illness (CVCHA, 1988b). Of these, 37 percent were male and 63 percent were female. The ethnic background of the clients was predominantly white (69 percent), while Hispanics and Blacks comprised 24 percent and 7 percent respectively (CVCHA, 1988a). Approximately 95 percent of the population served was of low socioeconomic status. The age group most frequently served during FY 1988 was that between 22 and 44 years of age, which included 336 clients (54 percent), followed by the 45-64 age group, which comprised 191 cases (31 percent). Figure 4.2 summarizes the demographic characteristics of the 624 clients served during FY 1988.

Of the mental health clients served by CVCHA, most were assigned to service group IV (31 percent), followed by service group V (24 percent), and then service group I (19 percent). Of DSM III diagnoses, most of the clients served in FY 1988 were either in the categories "Undiagnosed" (15 percent) or "Other" (32 percent), making up 47 percent of the clients served. Significantly, 18 percent of the total clients served had a primary diagnosis of alcohol (15 percent) or drug-related (3 percent) disorders. Thus, strict primary mental health diagnoses comprised 35 percent of the clients served (schizophrenia and related disorders, 19 percent; depressive disorders, 12 percent; anxiety/somatoform/dissociative disorders, 2 percent; other nonorganic psychoses, 1 percent; and other organic disorders, 1 percent). It is unknown how many of those clients served were of the "dual diagnosis" type. Figure 4.3 graphically represents CVCHA's clients served according to service group and DSM III diagnosis.

Approximately 85 percent of clients served resided in Tom Green County (Tom Green County comprises 83.3 percent of the service area population). There are no other large clusters of clients from surrounding counties (TDMHMR, 1989). It is interesting to note that the CARE data indicate that 10 percent of the clients served come from outside CVCHA's catchment area while only 5 percent come from those counties other than Tom Green which are within CVCHA's catchment area.

Figure 4.1. Map of the State of Texas Highlighting the Concho Valley Center for Human Advancement's Catchment Area

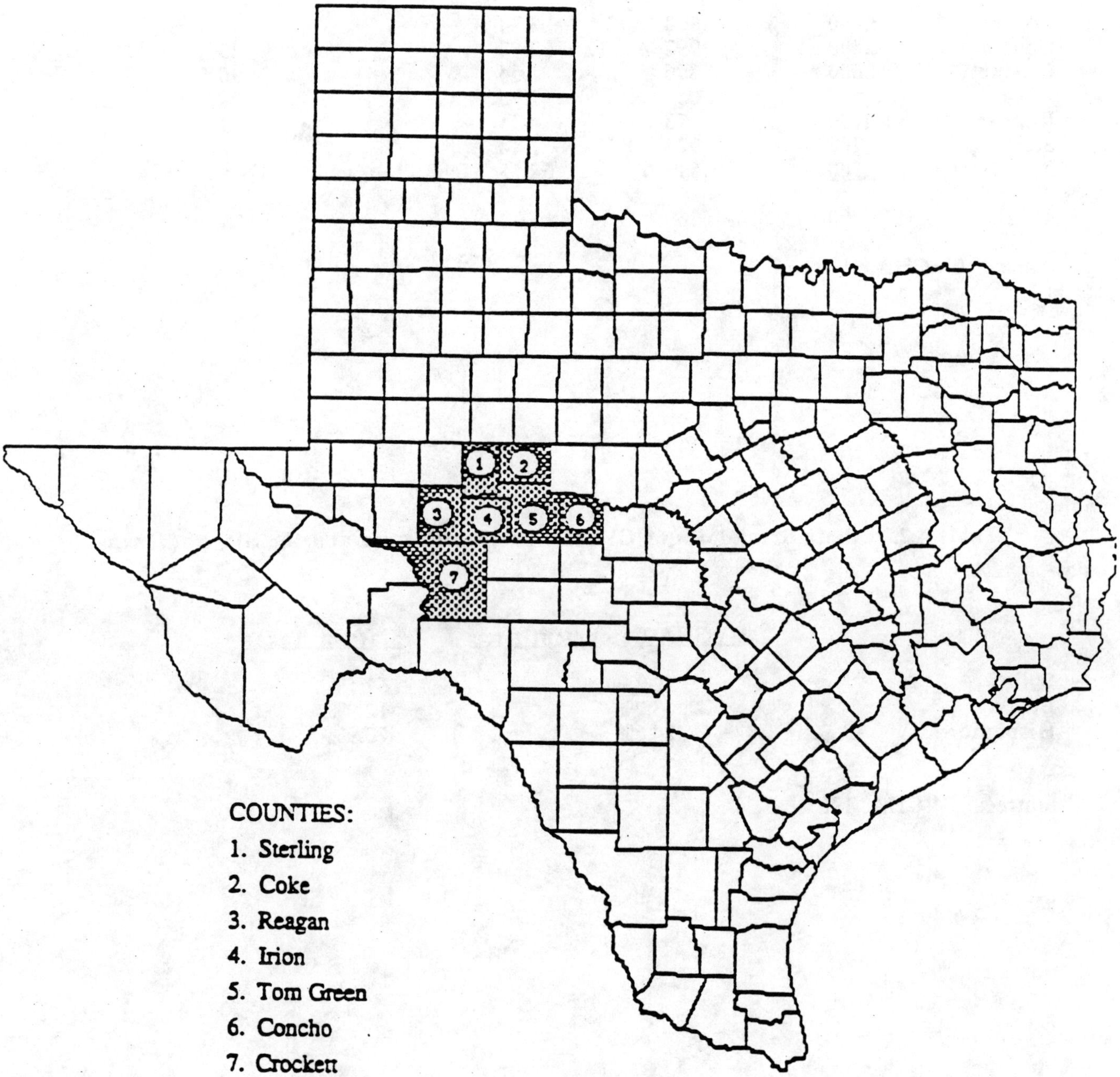

Source: Concho Valley Center for Human Advancement. "Demographic Overview of Service Area," San Angelo, 1988.

Table 4.1. Demographic Overview of CVCHA Catchment Area

County	Population	Square Miles	Population Density (people/sq. mile)	Distance to CVCHA (in miles)
Coke	3,400	908	3.74	47
Concho	2,800	992	2.82	45
Crockett	4,600	2,806	1.64	90
Irion	2,000	1,052	1.90	28
Reagan	5,100	1,173	4.35	71
Sterling	1,700	923	1.84	48
Tom Green	98,100	1,515	64.75	NA
Total	117,700	9,369	13.33	NA

Source: CVCHA, 1988a.

Table 4.2. Ethnic Breakdown of CVCHA Catchment Area and the State of Texas

	CVCHA Catchment Area	State of Texas
White	72.2%	67.1%
Black	3.2%	12.0%
Hispanic	24.6%	20.9%

Source: CVCHA, 1987.

Figure 4.2. Demographic Characteristics of CVCHA's Clients Served Fiscal Year 1988

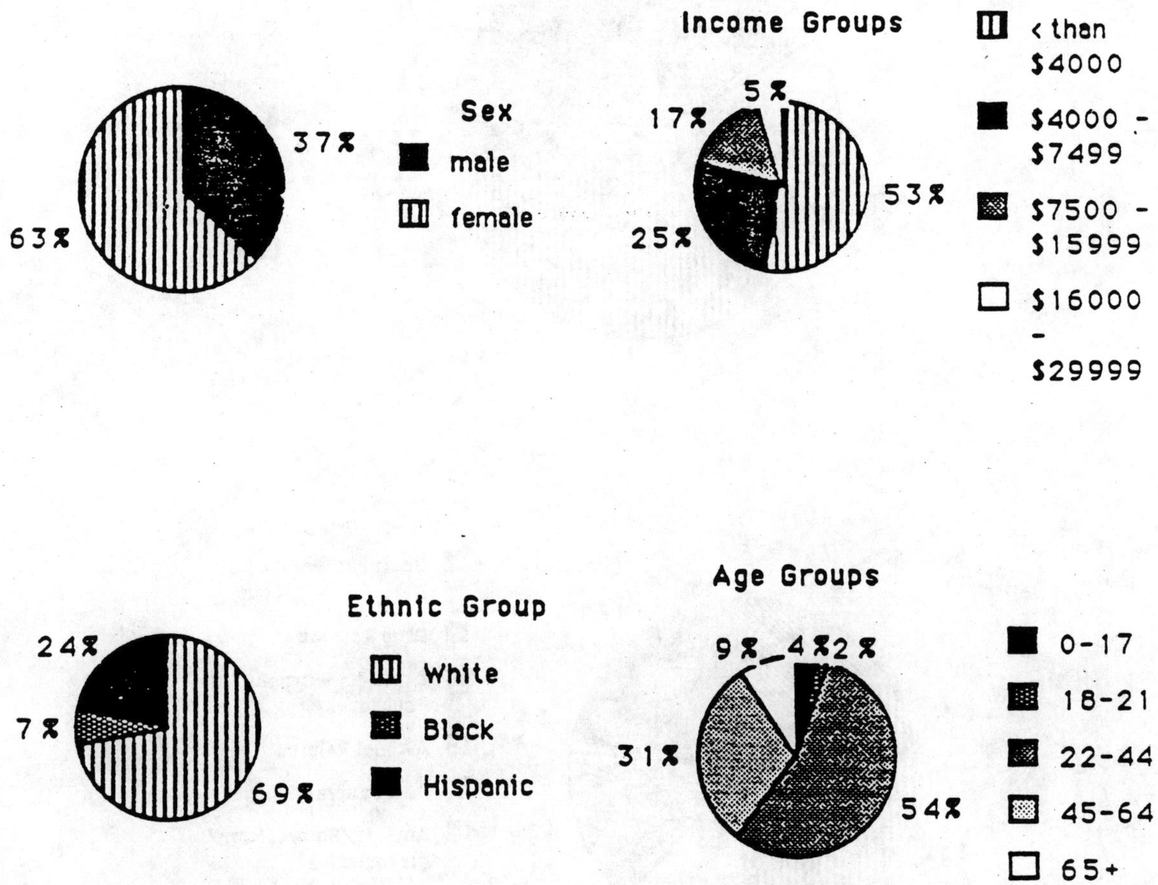

Source: Concho Valley Center for Human Advancement, <u>Characteristics of Clients Served: Center Totals</u>. San Angelo, 1988b. (Unpublished report)

Note: Total number of clients served = 624 (FY 1988)

Figure 4.3. CVCHA Clients (N = 624) Broken Down According to Service Groups and DSM III Diagnosis

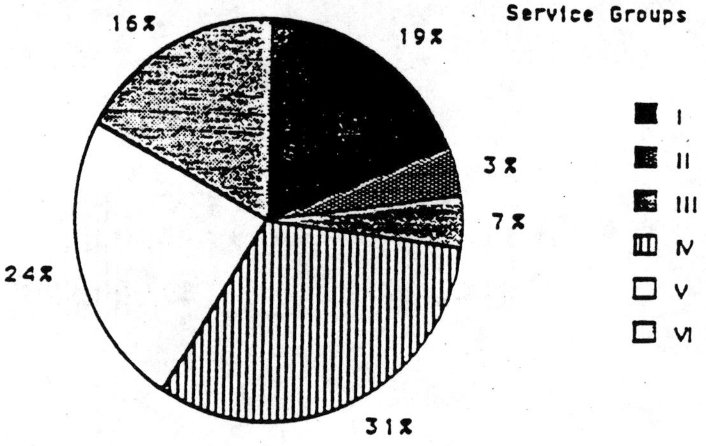

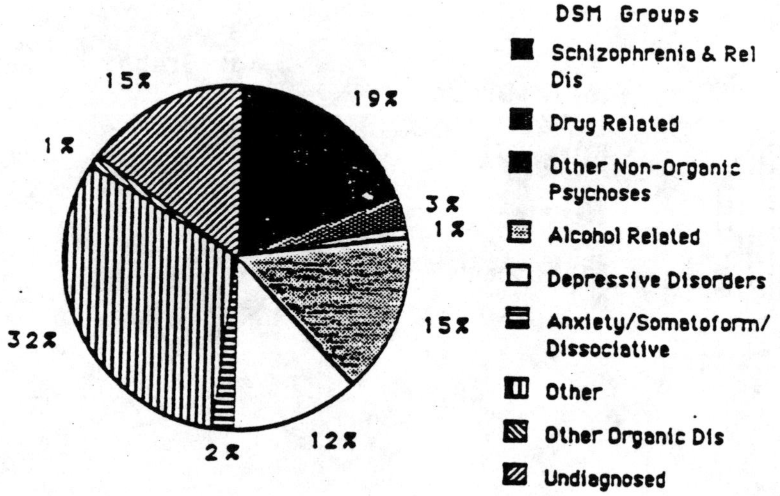

Source: Concho Valley Center for Human Advancement, Characteristics of Clients Served: Center Totals, San Angelo, 1988b. (Unpublished Report)

Note: Total number of clients served = 624 (FY 1988)

LEGAL STRUCTURE

According to Texas Laws Relating to TDMHMR, " . . . local agencies which may establish and operate community centers are a county, a city, a hospital district, a school district, or any organizational combination of two (2) or more of these . . . [and] the board of trustees shall consist of not less than five (5) nor more than nine (9) members" (TDMHMR, 1986, p. 7).

The Concho Valley Center for Human Advancement was established in 1966, but it did not officially open its doors until September 1967. The center provided its first actual services in March 1969 (Young, 1988). At the time that this center was established, the 1965 state law (House Bill 3) was used to organize the structure of the center. Many amendments have been added pertaining to the establishment and organization of community centers, but because the CVCHA was established prior to the enactment of these laws, the center was not forced to meet such requirements (Young, 1989). For instance, a university can no longer establish a community center and there is no longer a requirement of nine board members.

The sponsoring agencies for CVCHA include the City of San Angelo, Tom Green County, San Angelo State University, and San Angelo Independent School District. The relationship between CVCHA and the sponsoring agencies and the nonsponsoring counties will be discussed in a later section.

A board selection committee has been established which selects possible representatives for the board of trustees should a vacancy occur. Recommendations are provided by the county and city commissioners and by school and university officials. At this point, the board selection committee submits names of the persons whom they would like to have considered for a position on the board to all of the sponsoring agency's representatives. The sponsoring agencies then decide whom they wish to appoint for the position(s) (Young, 1989).

Presently, there are nine board members. Board members must be registered voters and residents of the catchment area (currently all of the board members are from Tom Green County). Appointments are made for two years, and they expire every other year on October 31. Board members can be reappointed, and there is no limit to the number of terms they may serve. They convene on the third Thursday of each month, and their responsibilities include the establishment of policy and direction, and the monitoring and reviewing of the center's activities (Young, 1989).

ENTRANCE INTO THE CVCHA SYSTEM

Individuals enter the CVCHA system in various ways. They may be self-referred or referred by the local sheriff's department, the local police department, county judges, city-county jail staff, local physicians (predominantly local emergency room physicians), or family members by either calling the center via the crisis hotline or by a person walking into the outpatient clinic at 244 N. Magdalen Street. If the crisis occurs at a local emergency room or the county jail, the on-call professional staff person will report to the scene of the crisis. Crises usually consist of suicide attempts, major episodes of mental illness, or severe depression (Young, 1988). The center's crisis intervention services will assure that those individuals undergoing a crisis become stabilized. Clients who reside in CVCHA's catchment area and who are sent to Big Spring State Hospital (BSSH) are automatically referred to the center upon discharge.

All individuals entering the system are screened to determine whether they fit in service group definitions I through IV. This is accomplished through an assessment of the presenting problem, mental status assessment, and other history information gathered by the staff person. Every morning at 8:15, the professional staff (those with an M.S. degree or above) meet to review any new cases and/or crises calls from the previous 24-hour period. In this meeting, the individual's eligibility for services is determined. If the individual is not eligible for services, he or she is then referred to another, more appropriate agency. Those eligible for services are admitted as new cases. Their cases are discussed at the full-staff or treatment team meetings, which occur at least bi-weekly, but may occur more frequently. Typically, these staffings occur as needed immediately following the 8:15 morning meetings, as professionals from various treatment teams are usually present at this time. Prospective clients and their needs are discussed at this meeting before the clients are assessed by the psychiatrist. All the information obtained from the initial screening, the morning meeting, the treatment team, and the psychiatrist's observations become part of the multidisciplinary assessment. Based on the conclusions of this assessment, a treatment plan is established. This treatment plan should be developed within 30 days of the client's initial contact with the center or, if the client is a BSSH discharge, within 21 days. Regarding case management, all clients in service groups I through IV are screened for this service by the professional staff. The admission criteria for case management will be discussed in a later section.

Should medications be prescribed to the client, they can be obtained at the city pharmacy, with which the center has a contract, on a sliding scale basis. While the center does charge a minimum fee of $2.00 per prescription, prescriptions are not denied clients due to an inability to pay. Supervision and monitoring of the medications is done at the Outpatient Clinic at Oasis House, which is located at 244 N. Magdalen Street. Oasis House is the site for the Community Support Program. If the client requires a laboratory examination and/or physical examination, he or she will be referred to the city health department. Clients are referred for these services by the Center physician and are also billed on sliding scale basis.

The treatment team may also refer the patient for psychosocial and/or residential services. Such services are provided at the Oasis House and will be discussed in greater detail in a later section.

What follows is a discussion of each of the services provided by CVCHA arranged by budget categories as outlined by TDMHMR (TDMHMR, 1987). In addition, pertinent financial information related to each of the services will be furnished.

RESIDENTIAL SERVICES

The residential programs offered at CVCHA consist of a semi-independent residential apartment living program as well as inpatient contracted beds which are specifically used for crisis stabilization. Thus, there are no structured noncrisis programs or intermediate residential programs.

The residential units are comprised of two small frame houses, a two-story brick house, and two garage apartments. All are located immediately adjacent to the center. The setting is designed for clients who require a minimal degree of supervision. In order to live in the apartments, the clients must either be referred from BSSH or must be at risk of returning to BSSH. In addition, clients must not have been violent for at least two years prior to their move-in date (CVCHA, 1988c; Blaydes, 1988).

At any given time, the apartment units are occupied by no more than four clients per unit (Jeffers, 1988). Currently, 15 clients reside at this residential setting. This is considered the maximum capacity for the apartment units, although the center has occasionally housed up to 16 individuals. Each client is required to meet with a staff person at least twice a week in order to obtain supervision and assistance in the upkeep of his or her apartment.

Once the clients move into the apartments, they must participate in the psychosocial program offered by the Oasis House. The program coordinates psychiatric medical services and medical evaluations as well as provides support to members in assisting in transportation services, community job placement, and program-based work crews (CVCHA, 1988c; Jeffers, 1988). In addition to center-based residential services, clients are assisted in locating living arrangements in other apartment complexes.

A written financial agreement is drawn up between the client and the center. Essentially, the center's staff act in a conservator's role for those clients who have problems handling their money. This problem usually results in the clients' careless spending of any or all monthly benefits within the first few days of each month. Whenever the center acts as conservator, one-third of the clients' entitlements (eg., SSI, SSDI) are allocated to rent, one-third to groceries, and one-third to the clients' savings account. Money can only be withdrawn from this account for "legitimate reasons." Legitimate reasons may include such things as televisions, radios, and other personal amenities, but such purchases must first be discussed with the community support program director. Such clients are allocated $15.00 per week "spending money," and any money earned through outside employment is retained by the client (Jeffers, 1988). Table 4.3 provides summary data for the semi-independent apartment living program.

The other residential service provided by CVCHA consists of inpatient crisis stabilization beds contracted from River Crest Hospital, a privately owned hospital in San Angelo. The contract stipulates the use of one bed, but if more than one bed is needed and available, CVCHA is provided with it. Essentially, CVCHA is contracting with River Crest for $50,000 worth of psychiatric inpatient services which can be utilized as CVCHA management deems necessary. For example, if more than one crisis occurs, beds may be allocated to accommodate such needs.

The explicit purposes of this unit are to provide a setting for crisis stabilization and to reduce any unnecessary admissions to Big Spring State Hospital (Blaydes, 1989b). The contract with River Crest Hospital started in January 1988, and the center began serving clients in February 1988 (Blaydes, 1989). Prior to the contract with River Crest Hospital, the center had a contract with St. John's Hospital. When St. John's Hospital changed its service philosophy, it became increasingly more difficult for CVCHA to place clients in St. John's small psychiatric unit (Blaydes, 1988).

During FY 1988, 30 clients utilized the contracted inpatient bed service (CVCHA, 1988d). The contracted amount for the inpatient bed is $249.86 per day. However, once the contract services, staff salaries, professional consultations, transportation, and other overhead costs are included, the cost per day increases to $347.08 (CVCHA, 1988d). In FY 1988, the contracted funding for the inpatient bed was expended between the 7th and 8th month of its 12-month span (Blaydes, 1989b). Thus, for those individuals who underwent a crisis at the end of the year, the center's only residential alternative was to send the individual to BSSH. Unfortunately, no data presently exist to identify which clients who went to BSSH could or should have been serviced at River Crest had additional funds been available.

Since River Crest Hospital has neither the facilities nor the staff to handle violent patients, BSSH is the appropriate choice in such cases. However, some critics have asserted that males who are mentally ill often have difficulty getting into River Crest because of the misperception that all mentally ill males are violent (Shannon, 1989).

The average stay per client for the River Crest contracted inpatient bed in FY 1988 was 10.87 days (CVCHA, 1988d). It should be noted that CVCHA's guidelines recommend that a client who is expected to have a length of stay greater than 7 days be strongly considered for admission to BSSH (CVCHA, 1988c). Table 4.4 provides summary information for the inpatient crisis bed.

In FY 1988, 141 clients from the CVCHA service area were admitted to BSSH. Of these, 106 (75 percent) were admitted on a voluntary basis whereas 35 (25 percent) were involuntarily committed (TDMHMR, 1989). Table 4.5 illustrates trends in admissions to BSSH from CVCHA's catchment area by length of stay and admission type. Interestingly, since 1984, the percentage of clients referred on a voluntary basis has continually increased (from 62 percent in 1984 to 75 percent in 1988) whereas involuntary admissions have decreased (from 38 percent in 1984 to 25 percent in 1988). In 1988, the admission rate to Big Spring State Hospital from the Concho Valley catchment area was 133 per 100,000 population (Blaydes, 1989d).

Clients who exhibit either a substance abuse disorder or a substance-induced organic mental disorder will not be admitted to inpatient services as a CVCHA client. They will, however, be assessed and referred to the most appropriate treatment setting, which in most cases is either the local detoxification center or BSSH. As Table 4.6 indicates, a significant number of admissions to BSSH since FY 1984 continue to be for substance abuse disorders. Although admissions with a primary diagnosis of alcohol-related disorders have decreased by approximately 26 percent since 1984 while those with a drug-related disorder have increased by 12.5 percent, substance abuse disorders, on the whole, still comprise roughly 50 percent of CVCHA's admissions to BSSH.

During FY 1988, $215,020 was allocated for residential services; however, actual expenditures amounted to $240,428 (TDMHMR, 1988c), resulting in a difference of $25,408. Table 4.7 illustrates expenditures and sources of revenue for residential services during FY 1988.

Of significance in Table 4.7 is the amount of funding received under the line item "Other State." This $103,666 was used to fund the semi-independent apartment living program. Originally, this service was contracted to the center by BSSH and any state funds used for this service went through Big Spring. As of 1989, however, these funds will come directly to CVCHA through state general revenue funds in order to provide such services.

Also of significance is the amount of staff-to-patient money (from the R. A. J. vs. Jones settlement) budgeted and received. CVCHA reports being conservative in its budgetary estimates of R. A. J. incentive monies. For FY 1988 residential services, the center budgeted the amount of $13,995 as a line item. In FY 1988, it earned $48,777.** This additional amount of $34,782 enabled CVCHA to cover the residential services deficit as well as reallocate local funding of $9,374 into case management and management and support services (Blaydes, 1989a). For FY 1989, the center estimates earning anywhere from $40,000 to $80,000 from R. A. J. funding for which the amount of $15,000 was budgeted as a line item for FY 1989 (Blaydes, 1989b).

** Since R. A. J. funds are expected to fluctuate from year to year and an exact estimate of these funds is not possible, the budgeting of R. A. J. funding at a low level is a fairly common strategy among CMHCs. These additional funds are used at management's discretion in any of the mental health programs requiring additional funds.

Table 4.3. Summary Data for CVCHA Semi-Independent Apartment Living

	Planned FY 1988	Actual FY 1988
Capacity	15	15
Clients Served	27	35
Client Days	4,928	4,940
Cost per Client Day	$23.10	$25.76
Total Semi-Independent Funds	$113,828.00	$127,279.00
Total Residential Services Funds	$215,020.00	$240,428.00

Source: Texas Department of Mental Health and Mental Retardation, "Community MHMR Center Budget and Quarterly Report--Transmittal Form: Concho Valley Center for Human Advancement." Austin, 1988, p. 5.

Table 4.4. Summary Data for CVCHA Contracted Inpatient Crisis Bed

	Planned FY 1988	Actual FY 1988
Capacity	1	1
Clients Served	58	30
Client Days	405	326
Avg. Stay per Client (in Days)	7.0	10.9
Cost per Client Day	$249.86	$347.08
Total Inpatient Crisis Funds	$101,192.00	$113,149.00
Total Residential Services Funds	$215,020.00	$240,428.00

Source: Texas Department of Mental Health and Mental Retardation, "Community MHMR Center Budget and Quarterly Report--Transmittal Form: Concho Valley Center for Human Advancement." Austin, 1988, p. 5.

Table 4.5. Trends in Admissions to Big Spring State Hospital from CVCHA's Catchment Area by Length of Stay and Admission Type

	FY 1984	FY 1985	FY 1986	FY 1987	FY 1988
24 Hours or Less					
Voluntary	3 (1.74)	0 (0.00)	1 (0.83)	1 (0.67)	2 (1.42)
Involuntary	0 (0.00)	1 (0.78)	0 (0.00)	0 (0.00)	0 (0.00)
2 or 3 Days					
Voluntary	3 (1.74)	2 (1.56)	2 (1.65)	6 (4.03)	1 (0.71)
Involuntary	1 (0.58)	0 (0.00)	0 (0.00)	0 (0.00)	0 (0.00)
4 to 7 Days					
Voluntary	12 (6.98)	3 (2.34)	4 (3.31)	8 (5.37)	8 (5.67)
Involuntary	2 (1.16)	3 (2.34)	1 (0.83)	4 (2.68)	1 (0.71)
8 to 14 Days					
Voluntary	10 (5.81)	16 (12.50)	9 (7.44)	17 (11.41)	10 (7.09)
Involuntary	1 (0.58)	2 (1.56)	0 (0.00)	4 (2.68)	5 (3.55)
15 to 30 Days					
Voluntary	21 (12.21)	27 (21.09)	45 (37.19)	50 (33.56)	63 (44.68)
Involuntary	13 (7.56)	2 (1.56)	9 (7.44)	3 (2.01)	5 (3.55)
31 to 60 Days					
Voluntary	34 (19.77)	28 (21.88)	9 (7.44)	9 (6.04)	12 (8.51)
Involuntary	22 (12.79)	13 (10.16)	14 (11.57)	10 (6.71)	9 (6.38)
61 to 90 Days					
Voluntary	14 (8.14)	1 (0.78)	1 (0.83)	5 (3.36)	3 (2.13)
Involuntary	14 (8.14)	7 (5.47)	7 (5.79)	11 (7.38)	8 (5.67)
More Than 90 Days					
Voluntary	10 (5.81)	7 (5.47)	13 (10.74)	12 (8.05)	7 (4.96)
Involuntary	12 (6.98)	16 (12.50)	6 (4.96)	9 (6.04)	7 (4.96)
Total	172	128	121	149	141
Voluntary	107 (62.2)	84 (65.6)	84 (69.4)	108 (72.5)	106 (75.2)
Involuntary	65 (37.8)	44 (34.4)	37 (30.6)	41 (27.5)	35 (24.8)

Source: TDMHMR, 1989.

Note: Numbers in parentheses represent percentage of total admissions for that year.

Table 4.6. Trends in Admissions to Big Spring State Hospital from CVCHA's Catchment Area by Admitting Diagnosis and Year

	FY 1984	FY 1985	FY 1986	FY 1987	FY 1988
Seriously Mentally Ill	63 (36.6)	64 (50.0)	50 (41.3)	71 (47.7)	68 (47.9)
Alcohol-Related	94 (54.7)	46 (35.9)	44 (36.4)	52 (34.9)	41 (28.9)
Drug-Related	13 (8.6)	16 (12.5)	18 (14.9)	24 (16.1)	30 (21.1)
No Diagnosis	2 (1.2)	2 (1.6)	9 (7.4)	2 (1.3)	3 (2.1)
Total	172	128	121	149	142

Source: TDMHMR, 1989.

Note: Numbers in parentheses represent percentage of total admissions for that year.

Table 4.7. CVCHA Mental Health Residential Services Financial Statement (FY 1988)

Object of Expense	Budgeted FY 1988		Funds Expended FY 1988	
Total Salaries	$61,501	(28.6%)	$49,991	(20.8%)
Employee Benefits	11,152	(5.2%)	9,525	(4.0%)
Travel	1,260	(0.6%)	591	(0.2%)
Consumable Supplies	16,534	(7.7%)	14,496	(6.0%)
Capital Outlay	1,000	(0.5%)	754	(0.3%)
Building Rent and Repair	28,202	(13.1%)	35,849	(14.9%)
Consultants/Contracts	72,700	(33.8%)	95,752	(39.8%)
Other Operating Expenses	22,671	(10.5%)	33,470	(13.9%)
Total	$215,020		$240,428	

Method of Finance	Budgeted FY 1988		Funds Expended FY 1988	
Local	$24,140	(11.2%)	$14,766	(6.1%)
General Revenue	73,219	(34.1%)	73,219	(30.5%)
Staff-to-Patient (R. A. J.)	13,995	(6.5%)	48,777	(20.3%)
Other State	103,666	(48.2%)	103,666	(43.1%)
Other Federal	-0-		-0-	
MH Block Grant	-0-		-0-	
Total	$215,020		$240,428	

Full-time Equivalent (FTE) Positions; Residential = 3.25
Full-time Equivalent Mental Health Positions = 25.00

Source: Texas Department of Mental Health and Mental Retardation, "Community MHMR Center Budget and Quarterly Report--Transmittal Form: Concho Valley Center for Human Advancement," Austin, 1988, p. 4.

Case Management Services

Clients having a service group designation of I through IV and a diagnosis of a chronic mental disorder of at least two years' duration are eligible for case management services if they fall into one or more of the following categories: (1) the client has received inpatient psychiatric treatment on several occasions; (2) the client has received continuous inpatient psychiatric treatment for at least six months within the last year; (3) the client has a prescribed treatment and care plan that has not resolved the identified problems and the client is a high risk for inpatient psychiatric treatment; or (4) the client has received inpatient psychiatric treatment in a state hospital, having been involuntarily committed for reasons of danger to self or others within the past six months (CVCHA, 1988c).

All open cases are referred for case management services. An open case is defined as a client who has been diagnosed as having a major mental disorder and who has received services from the center more than twice (CVCHA, 1988c). Thus, open cases do not include clients who call in on the crisis hotline or people who are going through a crisis and come in for short-term services (i.e., seen up to 6 or 7 times). Clients felt to be appropriate for case management services are typically referred in several ways: (1) because of its size and relationships among co-workers, clients may be referred informally to case management staff as long as they are considered open cases; (2) they can wait until the scheduled staff meeting and then be recommended; or (3) they can be referred for case management services when initial screening is done (CVCHA, 1988c).

Once a client is referred for case management services and all the screening documentation is received, the case management supervisor determines the appropriateness of case management services within seven working days and notifies the client and other staff of the decision. If the client is eligible for case management services and a caseload opening exists, the client will be assigned a case manager. However, if a vacancy does not exist and the client is eligible for case management services, the client will be placed on a waiting list maintained by the case management supervisor. In the spring of 1989, there were 16 clients on this waiting list; the average length of wait is approximately one year (Blaydes, 1989b). The waiting list is reviewed quarterly by the case management supervisor, and as vacancies occur, clients are assigned to case managers by the supervisor according to intensity of need.

Upon acceptance into the case management unit, a treatment plan is completed within 30 days of admission. The treatment plan addresses problem areas identified in the case management assessment and provides appropriate intervention objectives and strategies. The planning includes the client and any significant others whom the client wishes to participate. Case management treatment plans are reviewed by the Interdisciplinary Team at least semi-annually (Blaydes, 1989b).

The frequency of contact between the client and his or her case manager is based on the extent of that particular client's needs. On the average, the two mental health case managers have face-to-face contacts with their clients at least twice each month. Clients can also contact the case manager or another staff member familiar with their case at any time of the day.

The case management unit is comprised of one full-time case management supervisor, two full-time mental health case managers, and two full-time mental retardation case managers. During FY 1988, 104 mental health clients received case management services at a cost of $920.70 per client (TDMHMR, 1988c). Table 4.8 illustrates the number of clients per service group receiving case management services in 1988.

Table 4.8. CVCHA Clients Receiving Mental Health Case Management Services

	Planned FY 1988	Actual FY 1988
Service Group I	30	52
Service Group II	20	3
Service Group III	0	5
Service Group IV	30	37
Service Group V	0	7
Service Group VI	0	0
Total	80	104
Cost per Client Served	$829.59	$920.70

Source: Texas Department of Mental Health and Mental Retardation, "Community MHMR Center Budget and Quarterly Report--Transmittal Form: Concho Valley Center for Human Advancement," Austin, 1988, p. 9.

Case management clients who do not accept or who withdraw from case management services continue to be active clients for at least three months. During this time, ongoing efforts are made to assist them in meeting their needs and in helping them to accept case management services. If, after three months, the client still refuses case management involvement, the case is closed for case management services and another center staff person is assigned as that client's caseworker. Case management services are also closed if the client dies or moves out of the CVCHA catchment area (Blaydes, 1989b).

Although only $66,367 was budgeted for mental health case management for FY 1988, $74,121 was actually spent, resulting in a difference of $7,754 (TDMHMR, 1988c). This overexpenditure was covered by funds that were reallocated from residential services through R. A. J. funding. Table 4.9 summarizes the financial data for case management services for 1988.

CLIENT AND FAMILY SUPPORT SERVICES

CVCHA provides the following core services under the Client and Family Support budget category: 24-hour emergency screening; multidisciplinary assessment; family support program; and medication-related services that comprise a medication clinic, laboratory clinic, laboratory monitoring, physical examinations, medication maintenance, education and counseling, and provision of medication(s) (CVCHA, 1988e). Another service under this budget category provided by the center is the psychosocial rehabilitation program consisting of social support activities, independent living skills, and vocational training programs. What follows is a brief description of these services based on observations made during on-site visits as well as information obtained from interviews with the mental health program director and the community support program director. Other pertinent information was obtained from the CVCHA's Service Plan (CVCHA, 1988f). Following that, the financial aspects of each of the client and family support services will be discussed.

Medication-Related Services

Medication-related services are provided at the center's outpatient clinic. The psychiatrist and the psychiatric nurse at this clinic usually have approximately 28 clients per day waiting for medication-related services. Both evaluate and assess the condition of each patient. In addition, the psychiatrist and the psychiatric nurse will inform the client about the medications and their possible side effects.

The clients obtain prescribed medications at the city pharmacy, where CVCHA budgets $45,600 a year to purchase medications and $12,700 to contract with the city pharmacy for dispensing medications (TDMHMR, 1988d). If needed, the patient undergoes a laboratory examination at the city medical laboratory, located in the same building as the city pharmacy. As stated previously, clients are charged two dollars per prescription. If unable to pay, clients are billed on a sliding-scale basis. Clients covered by Medicaid are allowed three free prescriptions per month, which can be used for either physical or psychiatric illnesses.

Supervision of medication takes place at the oupatient clinic as well as the Oasis House. Periodically, the physician will meet with the client in order to assess efficacy of the medication (Blaydes, 1989).

Table 4.9. CVCHA Case Management Financial Data

Object of Expense	Planned FY 1988		Actual FY 1988	
Total Salaries	$46,680	(70.3%)	$41,184	(55.6%)
Employee Benefits	8,402	(12.7%)	7,329	(9.9%)
Travel	1,000	(1.5%)	515	(0.7%)
Consumable Supplies	500	(0.8%)	797	(1.1%)
Capital Outlay	480	(0.7%)	1,528	(2.1%)
Building Rent and Repair	3,200	(4.8%)	16,508	(22.3%)
Consultants/Contracts	-0-	(0.0%)	13	(0.0%)
Other Operating Expenses	6,105	(9.2%)	6,247	(8.4%)
Total	$66,367		$74,121	

Method of Finance	Planned FY 1988		Actual FY 1988	
Local	$26,045	(39.2%)	$33,799	(45.6%)
General Revenues	40,322	(60.8%)	40,322	(54.4%)
Staff-to-Patient (R. A. J.)	-0-		-0-	
Other State	-0-		-0-	
Other Federal	-0-		-0-	
MH Block Grant	-0-		-0-	
Total	$66,367		$74,121	

Full-time Equivalent Positions; Case Management = 2.50
Full-time Equivalent Mental Health Positions =25.00

Source: Texas Department of Mental Health and Mental Retardation, "Community MHMR Center Budget and Quarterly Report--Transmittal Form: Concho Valley Center for Human Advancement," Austin, 1988, p. 9.

Crisis Intervention Services

Anyone experiencing a mental health crisis may phone or come into the center for crisis intervention assistance. Admission into ongoing mental health treatment services, however, is reserved for individuals who (1) exhibit symptoms of a major mental illness; (2) have a service group designation of I through IV; (3) are chronically mentally ill; (4) have a history of state facility admission due to a major illness or who are returning to the center's service area after having received treatment in a state facility for a major mental illness; (5) are mentally ill and, if not treated, are expected to continue suffering distress, leading to their inability to function independently; or (6) are not experiencing long-term mental illness but are going through a severe crisis (e.g., suicide) that cannot be significantly resolved within 30 days through either crisis intervention or referral to another community agency (CVCHA, 1988c).

The center maintains a telephone hotline service which is largely provided by volunteers who are trained in crisis intervention skills. These volunteers handle incoming crisis calls between 5:00 p.m. and 8:00 a.m. on the weekdays and 24 hours per day on weekends and on holidays.

Center clinical staff are also on call to assist volunteers with difficult cases. The center's on-call clinical staff, on a 24-hour, seven-day-a-week basis, attend to all mental illness and suicide crises at hospital emergency rooms as well as the city/county jail, and as previously mentioned, are available for any emergencies in which the volunteer requires further assistance. They also work with service area judges in reaching appropriate legal dispositions regarding mental health emergency cases. The center averages 60-65 crisis calls per month, not all of which are for mental illness problems. Calls regarding information as to other services available in the area as well as calls requesting information on problems of daily living are also impacting the center through the crisis hotline (Blaydes, 1989a).

Also mentioned previously, individuals exhibiting either a substance use disorder or a substance abuse mental disorder will not be admitted for ongoing center services. The center is not licensed to offer treatment for such disorders. These persons will, however, be assessed and referred to the most appropriate treatment setting, such as a state facility or a community resource. Individuals with a dual diagnosis of a major mental illness and substance abuse disorder will (if possible) be admitted to ongoing center services (Blaydes, 1989b).

The length of time a client receives services varies with the type of contact as well as the problems which are presented. Crisis situations involving someone who is not mentally ill may be resolved within 30 days through crisis intervention, referral, or both. Individuals exhibiting symptoms of mental illness may become active cases and receive center services for many years. Clients are discharged from center services when they (1) refuse to accept services; (2) progress to the point of no longer requiring services; (3) are referred to another, more appropriate primary service provider; (4) move to a location outside of the center's service area; or (5) die (CVCHA, 1988e).

Psychosocial Services

Psychosocial services, which are provided at the Oasis House, are considered one of the "brightest" areas of CVCHA (TDMHMR, 1988b). The overall goal of the program is to empower members to take responsibility for their own lives; thus independent living skills are stressed throughout all phases of the program. The caring and highly motivated staff at the Oasis House are very proud of having achieved a 100 percent rating compliance in TDMHMR's "Standards and Quality Assurance Report" (TDMHMR, 1988b).

The Oasis House began providing services for 12 to 15 clients in August 1982 (long before such services were mandated as a core service in 1987). At the outset of this program, the turnover of clients was quite high. This was largely due to the fact that not all the clients met the criterion of a major mental illness, and thus their conditions improved quite rapidly (Jeffers, 1988).

Currently, the Oasis House serves 60 clients--the maximum number possible because of building and staff limitations. All of these clients have a major mental illness and must be referred from outpatient services in order to be eligible for any Oasis House program (Jeffers, 1988).

A day in the Oasis House begins at 8:00 a.m. with the formation of work units. Clients choose one of the three work units in which they wish to participate. They can select from a clerical, maintenance, or cooking unit. By participating in these units, clients acquire independent living skills (Jeffers, 1988). Each unit performs its chores until midday, when lunch is served at a cost of 50 cents per client. The Oasis House is able to offer these reduced prices due to the generosity of the local food bank.

The afternoon activities include vocational training that consists of contracted employment, vocational evaluations, skills training, and workshop activities. In addition, Oasis House conducts other social support activities such as dances, social gatherings, and fun runs.

Continuity of Care

Often a crisis situation involves a decision regarding whether the state hospital is an appropriate disposition. Only professional staff are authorized to make decisions regarding admissions to state hospitals. Oftentimes such decisions are made at the 8:15 a.m. meeting. If it is decided that Big Spring State Hospital is the best alternative, then the caseworker, who in many instances is the "worker of the day," must make the arrangements with BSSH and any other agencies that may require such information, such as county judges (if commitment orders are required) and local sheriffs (Blaydes, 1989a).

In coming to such a decision, BSSH must be deemed to be the least restrictive environment available to treat such presenting problems. Reasons for considering it the least restrictive alternative as well as other pertinent demographic information must be documented. In addition, the initial screening assessment must be included. This documentation is then forwarded to BSSH. Phone contact also occurs in order to ensure that BSSH has all the available information before the client's arrival (Blaydes, 1989).

Once it has been decided that an individual has been cared for at BSSH, it becomes the role of the hospital liaison to ensure a smooth transition from the community into the hospital and then from the hospital back into the community. Thus, the primary focus of the hospital liaison's activities occurs at the juncture between the facility and center transition; services are typically based upon the person's length of stay and also upon establishing as stable a living situation as possiple upon discharge into the community.

CVCHA's hospital liaison goes to BSSH every two weeks and is responsible for all of the Concho Valley residents in BSSH, including subtance abuse commitments. While patients are in BSSH, the liaison works with the patient and the hospital staff in order to ensure continuity of treatment, i.e., to ensure that the hospital, the client, and CVCHA are all in agreement as to treatment goals and the methods and resources utilized for attaining such goals. The liaison is responsible for providing the hospital staff with any and all available community information impacting upon the particular client, such as available financial and social resources of the client, the client's living conditions, and resources that the community can provide that individual.

Upon readying a particular client for discharge, the hospital liaison, along with CVCHA's treatment team, must develop and document an aftercare plan. Hospital staff are responsible for documenting a community support plan. These documents are designed to overlap as much as possible, with the explicit goal being to ensure agreement in follow-up care among the client, the hospital, and the center (Blaydes, 1989a).

Once the patient reenters the community, the hospital liaison then becomes responsible for ensuring that follow-up care actually takes place. According to TDMHMR standards, the center is expected to make contact with each discharged patient within ten days after being discharged (TDMHMR, 1988b). Most of CVCHA's clients are scheduled to meet with the center staff within two to three days after discharge. For those who miss this initial appointment, the hospital liaison then becomes responsible for making contact with these clients. This contact is done primarily through phone contacts and mailings. Occasionally, the liaison will make a home visit, although this is rare and only occurs for those living in Tom Green County. A more active outreach for those clients residing in outlying areas is a need that CVCHA would like to see further developed.

Family Support

CVCHA provides in-home and family support services to clients and their families through funding provided by the HB 1154 program. Under this program, the client or family may be eligible to obtain up to $3,600 a year to purchase the following services:

1. health services such as medical, surgical, therapeutic, and diagnostic services;

2. counseling or training programs which assist the family in providing care for a person with a mental disability;

3. attendant care, home health aid services, homemaker services, and chore services that provide assistance with training, routine body functions, dressing, preparation and consumption of food, and ambulation;

4. transportation for the person with a mental disability;

5. transportation and room and board incurred by the family and the person during the person's evaluation for services or treatment that has been preapproved by the center;

6. original or unique services consistent with the intent of the program and negotiated between the person or family and center (e.g., short-term rental assistance);

7. architectural modifications to the home and/or purchase or lease of special equipment or supplies that improve or facilitate the care, treatment, therapy, general living conditions, or access of the person with a mental disability (CVCHA, 1988g).

During FY 1988, the center spent $12,409 on family support services (TDMHMR, 1988c). Of this amount, $9,000 was allocated toward HB 1154 compliance, and $3,409 was targeted to develop an educational component for the families of the mentally ill. Eleven clients were served in FY 1988 through HB 1154; the predominant service was housing assistance (Blaydes, 1989d).

Financial Data

During FY 1988, a total of $675,191 was spent on all of the services provided under the Mental Health Client and Family Support budget category (TDMHMR, 1988c). Although more clients were served during FY 1988 than initially planned, the center spent $25,561 below the budgeted amount of $700,752 for Client and Family Support Services. This amount of $25,561 was reallocated into other budget categories such as Case Management and Residential Services (Blaydes, 1989d). Table 4.10 illustrates the number of clients served under the Client and Family Support category by service group.

Table 4.11 presents financial information on client and family support services according to type of service offered.

Table 4.12 presents the planned and actual expenses of the client and family support services as well as the method of financing these expenses.

OTHER NONCORE SERVICES

Jail Evaluations

This service arose out of the concern of increased rates of suicide in the local jails as well as the growing number of mentally ill individuals entering the criminal justice system. Currently, CVCHA provides screening, crisis intervention services, psychological assessments, and medication maintenance services on a limited basis to inmates. CVCHA would also like to be able to provide instructional seminars on suicide prevention and mental health issues to jail and other criminal justice personnel.

Specific funds are not allocated for this service. The center sees this service as largely preventative in nature and is trying to reach these people before significant manifestations of mental illness are seen.

Sexual Abuse Treatment Services

This service is primarily funded by the Texas Department of Human Services (TDHS), Child Protective Services Division, via Title IV-B funds. Therefore, the primary admission requirement is a referral from the local TDHS office.

Services are provided to any or all involved in the abusive act; the victim, the nonperpetrator adult, the perpetrator adult, and any other members of the victim's family. Services include assessment; treatment planning; psychological testing; individual, group, and family therapy; play therapy; and, if needed, a babysitter for a mothers' group.

During FY 1988, sexual abuse services were provided to 68 clients. This figure includes family members as well as the victims (Blaydes, 1989d). Length of service varies from 6 to 18 months. The budgeted amount for sexual abuse services for FY 1988 was $48,000. The actual amount received was $33,598.

Rape Crisis Services

The objectives of CVCHA's rape crisis services are to decrease sexual assault via increased reporting, public education of rape awareness and prevention, and prosecution and conviction of the crime of sexual assault. Other service objectives include seeing that the victims and families of rape/sexual assault return to their normal lifestyles as soon as possible, preventing sexual assault by training children and adolescents to recognize and deal with potentially dangerous situations, and by preparing adults in a child's community--both teachers and parents--to detect and care for child victims of sexual assault.

Table 4.10. CVCHA Clients Served under Client and Family Support Services

	Planned FY 1988	Actual FY 1988
Service Group I	140	117
Service Group II	48	25
Service Group III	62	23
Service Group IV	140	194
Service Group V	150	148
Service Group VI	60	104
Total	600	611
Cost per Client Served	$1,167.92	$1,105.06

Source: Texas Department of Mental Health and Mental Retardation, "Community MHMR Center Budget and Quarterly Report--Transmittal Form: Concho Valley Center for Human Advancement," Austin, 1988, p. 8.

Table 4.11 CVCHA Client and Family Support Budget by Type of Service Provided

Client and Family Support	FY 1988
24-hour Emergency Screening and Assessment	$169,568
Community and State Hospital Liaison	112,534
Family Support Services	
Family Support Programs	3,409
H. B. 1154 Compliance	9,000
Subtotal	12,409
Medication-Related Services	265,278
Psychosocial Rehabilitation Programs	140,963
Total	$700,752

Source: Texas Department of Mental Health and Mental Retardation, "Community MHMR Center Budget and Quarterly Report--Transmittal Form: Concho Valley Center for Human Advancement," Attachment II. B., "Mental Health Services to be Provided," Austin, 1988.

Table 4.12. CVCHA Client and Family Support Budget Category Financial Information

Object of Expense	Planned FY 1988		Actual FY 1988	
Total Salaries	$390,376	(55.7%)	$382,549	(56.7%)
Employee Benefits	70,744	(10.1%)	70,528	(10.4%)
Travel	6,339	(0.9%)	7,414	(1.1%)
Consumable Supplies	53,732	(7.7%)	69,242	(10.3%)
Capital Outlay	3,300	(0.5%)	2,684	(0.4%)
Building Rent and Repair	23,700	(3.4%)	18,662	(2.8%)
Consultants/Contracts	91,746	(13.1%)	51,337	(7.6%)
Other Operating Expenses	60,815	(8.7%)	72,775	(10.8%)
Total	$700,752		$675,191	

Method of Finance	Planned FY 1988		Actual FY 1988	
Local	$196,153	(28.0%)	$183,427	(27.2%)
General Revenue	421,856	(60.2%)	421,856	(62.5%)
Staff-to-Patient (R. A. J.)	-0-		-0-	
Other State	13,990	(2.0%)	13,990	(2.1%)
Other Federal	48,000	(6.8%)	35,165	(5.2%)
MH Block Grant	20,753	(3.0%)	20,753	(3.1%)
Total	$700,752		$675,191	

Full-time Equivalent Positions; Client and Family Support = 21.75
Full-time Equivalent Mental Health Positions = 25.00

Source: Texas Department of Mental Health and Mental Retardation, "Community MHMR Center Budget and Quarterly Report--Transmittal Form: Concho Valley Center for Human Advancement, Austin, 1988, p. 8.

The first avenue of communication concerning a case is the 24-hour hotline. Immediate crisis counseling includes information regarding available medical aid and procedures involving the report of rape to law enforcement agencies. The call may come from the victim, family, friends, the hospital, the police department, or the sheriff's office. The hotline is also used to provide referrals, assistance, and information to a caller. Services are provided primarily through volunteers. Volunteers are available to accompany the victim to the hospital and/or law enforcement agency. Long-term services by volunteers include assisting the victim and the family through the final disposition of the case or referrals to mental health professionals should severe psychological problems arise. The crisis coordinator is responsible for the volunteers' training, although other community professionals are also utilized as instructors.

During FY 1988, CVCHA's rape crisis services were provided to 83 clients. This figure also includes family members as well as the victims (Blaydes, 1989d). These services were funded by five different mechanisms: the Texas Department of Health contracted with CVCHA for $9,100; the United Way provided $15,700.04 in donations; the City of San Angelo provided $4,850; the Children's Trust Fund provided $4,850; and miscellaneous donations amounted to $60.00.

A COMMUNITY PERSPECTIVE: CONCHO VALLEY ALLIANCE FOR THE MENTALLY ILL

Dr. Charles Shannon, president of the Concho Valley Alliance for the Mentally Ill (CVAMI), provided a community perspective of CVCHA's services and programs (Shannon, 1989). Dr. Shannon characterized the staff of the CVCHA as being "extremely helpful" with the affairs of CVAMI. For example, the center assists CVAMI with its mailouts and printing materials. He describes the members of the board as sensitive, concerned, and well informed about the mental health needs of the community. Dr. Shannon also stated that the center is very helpful with smoothing the admission process of its mentally ill clients to Big Spring State Hospital.

CVAMI consists of 32 members. Its primary goal is to raise community awareness of mental health issues in the San Angelo area. In a recent editorial in the local newspaper, for example, CVAMI indicated that 25 percent of the persons needing psychiatric treatment in San Angelo must go out of the area to receive such treatment. Furthermore, according to the editorial, there is a lack of mental health services for children and adolescents; despite such paucity of services, the city council is planning to reduce funding to the CVCHA (Shannon, 1988). In explaining this situation, Dr. Shannon remarked that the city of San Angelo is very conservative. For its residents, $60,000 is "a lot of money to be given away to the mentally ill or retarded."[***] Moreover, community leaders in San Angelo, according to Dr. Shannon, believe that the family, not the community, should be responsible for the care of the mentally ill. These are the types of community attitudes which CVAMI, along with CVCHA, is trying to change. In addition, the organization is assisting the center in writing a HUD grant that would provide funds for additional housing for the mentally ill. CVAMI is also involved in organizing church groups to clean and repair the apartment complexes managed by the Oasis House. Dr. Shannon would also like to involve San Angelo State University, of which he is a faculty member, in raising community awareness about mental health issues in the San Angelo area.

Critical of CVCHA, Dr. Shannon indicated that CVCHA needs an outreach program for the rural counties of its catchment area as well as respite services for the families of the mentally ill. Further, he stated that the Oasis House should have additional psychosocial

---

[***] $60,000 is the total contribution from the city of San Angelo; thus, $30,000 is designated for mental health and $30,000 is designated for mental retardation.

programming, geared more toward highly functioning mentally ill patients. CVAMI is presently concerned that CVCHA only has programs geared for the low-functioning mentally ill, and in some instances those who function at a higher level are either left without services or are placed in programs which are not geared toward their levels.

The relationship between CVCHA and CVAMI is somewhat unique. It is often an amiable relationship whereby each agency understands and respects the other's role. It is understood by many CVAMI members that CVCHA is working under many constraints; it is also understood by CVCHA staff that often the role of CVAMI members is to be critical of existing services and to advocate for the rights of the mentally ill and their families. In many other instances, CVAMI and CVCHA have been able to unite and work together such as in educating the surrounding areas as to mental health issues and needs.

BUDGET STRUCTURE OF CVCHA's MENTAL HEALTH SERVICES

The Concho Valley Center for Human Advancement operated with a total budget of $2,675,797 for FY 1989 (TDMHMR, 1988c). Of this total budget, mental health services utilized $1,102,922 (approximately 41 percent),[****] which represents an increase of approximately $90,000 from FY 1988 for mental health services. A complete summary of incoming revenues broken down by budget categories is shown in Table 4.13.

As can be seen in Table 4.13, general revenue, which flows through TDMHMR, is the most significant block of revenue (51 percent of total revenue). TDMHMR requires that such state funds must be matched by local funds in the amount equal to a certain percentage of the total general revenue funds allocated. In the case of the CVCHA, local funds must match in the amount equal to 18 percent of the total general revenue funds (TDMHMR, 1988d). This amount of local match funds is not to exceed $175,580 (TDMHMR, 1988d). Thus, of the $332,481 of local revenue, $175,580 is applied as "Local Matching Funds" while the rest is categorized as "Other Local" and "Other State" (Blaydes, 1989c). Taxes from the City of San Angelo and from Tom Green County contribute approximately $30,000 each toward the local mental health matching funds (the city and county also allocate approximately $30,000 each for mental retardation services). Other local matching funds consist of funds from patient fees, Medicaid, Medicare, and other miscellaneous contributions.

The remaining two sponsoring agencies (San Angelo State University and San Angelo ISD) both contribute various in-kind services. For example, SASU makes available printing services, while San Angelo ISD has agreed to lease to CVCHA the three buildings at 244 Magdalen Street for the amount of $1.00 for a term of 50 years beginning January 5, 1976. The fair market value of these various agreements is unknown.

It is important to note that of the 117,700 people in the catchment area's population, 98,100 (83 percent) reside in Tom Green County (CVCHA, 1988a). Thus, most of CVCHA's resources are concentrated in the city of San Angelo and outlying areas within Tom Green County. In the remaining six counties, there are extremely limited resources for mental health services. If more funds are made available, CVCHA management has discussed the possibility of implementing some form of rural outreach program (Blaydes, 1989b).

The remaining six outlying counties are considered contract counties. In the past, residents of these counties who received services were billed on a sliding scale basis. If the individual receiving such services could not or did not make payment, the county was then billed for the services received. However, as of FY 1988, TDMHMR has committed to

---

[****] It is important to note that the mentally ill clients represent over 70 percent of the 856 unduplicated clients served at CVCHA (CVCHA, 1988b).

Table 4.13. CVCHA's Incoming Mental Health Revenue by Type of Services Offered (FY 1988)

Budgeted	RES	CFS	CM	M & S	Total	
Local	$ 24,140	$ 196,153	$ 26,045	$ 86,143	$332,481	(30.1%)
General Revenue	73,219	421,856	40,322	34,640	570,037	(51.7%)
Staff-to-Patient	13,995	-0-	-0-	-0-	13,995	(1.3%)
Other State	103,666	13,990	-0-	-0-	117,656	(10.7%)
Other Federal	-0-	48,000	-0-	-0-	48,000	(4.4%)
MH Block Grant	-0-	20,753	-0-	-0-	20,753	(1.9%)
Total	$215,020	$700,752	$66,367	$120,783	$1,102,922	
	(19.5%)	(63.5%)	(6.0%)	(11.0%)		

Actual Expenditures	RES	CFS	CM	M & S	Total	
Local	$ 14,766	$ 183,427	$ 33,799	$ 90,260	$332,481	(28.9%)
General Revenue	73,219	421,856	40,322	34,640	570,037	(51.1%)
Staff-to-Patient	48,777	-0-	40,322	34,640	48,777	(4.4%)
Other State	103,666	13,990	-0-	-0-	117,656	(10.6%)
Other Federal	-0-	35,165	-0-	-0-	35,165	(3.2%)
MH Block Grant	-0-	20,753	-0-	-0-	20,753	(1.9%)
Total	$240,428	$675,191	$74,121	$124,900	$1,102,922	
	(21.6%)	(60.6%)	(6.6%)	(11.2%)		

Difference: -11,718

Source: Texas Department of Mental Health and Mental Retardation, "Community MHMR Center Budget and Quarterly Report--Transmittal Form: Concho Valley Center for Human Advancement, Austin, 1988.

Note: RES = Residential Services Budget Category; CFS = Client and Family Support Services Budget Category; CM = Case Management Services Budget Category; M & S = Management and Support Budget Category.

working toward equalizing each CMHC's per capita base. In FY 1988, CVCHA was receiving only $7.18 per capita while some CMHCs were receiving close to $12.00 per capita, although $6.68 was the average per capita amount for FY 1988 among the 34 CMHCs in Texas (TDMHMR, 1988e). As TDMHMR has attempted to equalize those with the lower per capita rates with those having the higher rates, CVCHA has stopped billing these outlying counties because it feels it is receiving explicit funds to directly serve these counties (Blaydes, 1989).

These outlying counties are also not required by CVCHA to provide "local match funding." The CVCHA management feels that it is unfair to request these counties to provide funds when the center is unable to provide what it feels would be adequate services to such counties. Between $1,600 and $6,000 would be required from the outlying counties as the local match (depending upon the population of the county); however, the center states that much more than $6,000 is required to provide adequate services (Blaydes, 1989d). The issue remains as to which agency is responsible for initiating such change.

It is also important to note that CVCHA staff feel that the timing of the $35.50 program was such that it rewarded centers that were not already working to keep clients out of the state hospital. Since the baseline was established at a time when CVCHA was already keeping state hospital admissions low, it receives what it feels is very little money from the $35.50 incentive. Had the baseline been set several years earlier, then CVCHA could have received significantly more money by saving more bed days (Young, 1988).

The center receives revenue approximating $118,000 in miscellaneous income and contributions. CVCHA receives a United Way donation in the amount of $17,300 for Rape Crisis Services, and other donations amount to $300.

Expenditures of the mental health budget of $1,102,922 are presented in Table 4.14. As can be seen, total salaries constitute approximately 53 percent of the center's total expenses. Employee benefits represent approximately 9.5 percent of total expenses. There are 63 full-time-equivalent positions at CVCHA, of which 25 are in the mental health area (TDMHMR, 1988d).

The San Angelo Council on Alcohol and Drug Abuse (SACADA), funded by the Texas Commission on Alcohol and Drug Abuse (TCADA), United Way, and the City of San Angelo, provides drug and alcohol treatment to the city of San Angelo. Currently, CVCHA does not contract with the council for these services, but there are ongoing negotiations to provide screening for admission to BSSH and to provide follow-up care from state facilities. According to the center, $150,000 is needed to contract with the council, enabling it to maintain its current detoxification, halfway house, and outpatient counseling operations, which is in minimal compliance with TDMHMR standards (TDMHMR, 1988c). As can be seen in Table 4.6, many of the BSSH clients from the Concho Valley catchment area are suffering from substance abuse and alcohol-related disorders. This strongly supports the need for additional funding required for the San Angelo Council on Alcoholism.

As of August 1988, the total fund balance was $325,190 for governmental fund types. This balance is not unusually high (TDMHMR, 1988c). As a percentage of total expenditures ($325,190/$2,733,164 = 12%), the fund balance is only 12 percent. If CVCHA lost all of its funding, it could operate for only 43 days.

Table 4.14. CVCHA's Mental Health Service Expenditures by Type of Services Offered (FY 1988)

Budgeted	RES	CFS	CM	M & S		Total
Total Salaries	61,501	390,376	46,680	82,650	581,207	(65.9%)
Employee Benefits	11,152	70,744	8,402	14,877	105,175	(9.5%)
Travel	1,260	6,339	1,000	3,050	11,649	(1.1%)
Consumable Supplies	16,534	53,732	500	1,675	72,441	(6.6%)
Capital Outlay	1,000	3,300	480	2,582	7,362	(0.7%)
Building Repair/Rent	28,202	23,700	3,200	4,200	59,302	(5.4%)
Consultants/Contracts	72,700	91,746	-0-	900	165,346	(15.0%)
Other Operating Expenses	22,671	60,815	6,105	10,849	100,440	(9.1%)
Actual Expenditures						
Total Salaries	49,991	382,549	41,184	82,106	555,830	(49.9%)
Employee Benefits	9,525	70,528	7,329	13,212	100,594	(9.0%)
Travel	591	7,414	515	1,709	10,229	(0.9%)
Consumable Supplies	14,496	69,242	797	3,584	88,119	(7.9%)
Capital Outlay	754	2,684	1,528	4,449	9,415	(0.8%)
Building Repair/Rent	35,849	18,662	16,508	2,554	73,573	(6.6%)
Consultants/Contracts	95,752	51,337	13	910	148,012	(13.3%)
Other Operating Expenses	33,470	72,775	6,247	16,376	128,868	(11.6%)
Total	240,428	675,191	74,121	124,900	1,114,640	
	(21.6%)	(60.6%)	(6.6%)	(11.2%)		

Difference -11,718

Source: Texas Department of Mental Health and Mental Retardation, "Community MHMR Center Budget and Quarterly Report--Transmittal Form: Concho Valley Center for Human Advancement, Austin, 1988.

Note: RES = Residential Services Budget Category; CFS = Client and Family Support Services Budget Category; CM = Case Management Services Budget Category; M & S = Management and Support Budget Category.

CONCLUSIONS AND RECOMMENDATIONS

The Concho Valley Center for Human Advancement was selected as a case study in order to examine the issues concerning a small-scale rural community mental health center. The following discussion will focus on the strengths and weaknesses of CVCHA and will provide recommendations as deemed necessary.

Rural community mental health centers face issues that differ from those experienced by urban CMHCs. For instance, CVCHA, being a relatively small facility, allows for good working relations among mental health professionals as well as greater cooperation with community service agencies and state facilities. Since the center's staff is well acquainted, the referral of clients from one service to another is facilitated in a much smoother and expedient manner. For example, staff members often refer clients for case management services without the formalities that are likely to be required in a more urban setting. Nevertheless, all referrals are documented. Similarly, the center maintains very good relations with the community as exemplified in the support provided by and to organizations such as CVAMI.

On the other hand, a center with the third largest catchment area in the state and one that operates in a rural area larger than the state of Massachusetts has its share of problems. Chief among them is the need for an outreach program for the rural counties in its catchment area. Counties as far away as 90 miles lack any public transportation to the CVCHA. As stated in TDMHMR's report entitled Future Directions 1988-1993, individuals who must travel this far to obtain services may postpone treatment until the illness requires longer periods of hospitalization, thus increasing the financial costs of mental health care (TDMHMR, 1988a).

The center's management as well as community advocates are quite concerned about the lack of outreach programs to these rural areas (Blaydes, 1988; Shannon, 1989). Two solutions have been proposed, both of which require a level of funding that the center currently lacks. First, management proposes the implementation of a "circuit rider" concept--a rural outreach program that purports to work as follows. San Angelo would be the home base of the program. The center would lease office space in conveniently located communities throughout the catchment area. A CVCHA staff member would visit each office for two days a week, lodging at local hotels. Twice a month, a physician would make the rounds to provide medication-related services.

The second option would be to provide services from local physicians' offices. Because rural residents are more likely to seek mental health services at the local doctor's office and because it is less stigmatizing for them to do so, CVCHA has discussed the possibility of providing its services at such locations. Tentatively, a mental health representative from CVCHA would visit selected doctors' offices once or twice a week. In addition to providing direct services, CVCHA would provide educational programs on rural mental health issues and psychotropic medication issues for physicians within the catchment area.

CVCHA has also discussed the implementation of a WATS line to its outlying counties. This would enable clients from rural communities to access the center at no charge. As a by-product of this approach, clients would seek services at an earlier, preventive stage. However, the benefits of such a service may be limited without sufficient programming and/or transportation to adequately meet the on-going needs of such new-found residents.

Of further concern to human service agencies located in rural areas are the conservative attitudes typically found in these settings. The people of the Concho Valley still hold the family and mental health institutions responsible for the care and treatment of the mentally ill (Blaydes, 1988; Young, 1988; Shannon, 1989). Directly reflecting these attitudes is the fact that city leaders are now seriously considering withdrawing the local contribution of $60,000 for mental health and mental retardation services. In a city the size of San Angelo, $60,000 is considered a lot of money, which people feel could be better utilized elsewhere. Mental health and mental retardation are not considered high priorities, partly stemming from the attitudes mentioned above. Another reason cited for the withdrawing of the city's $60,000 contribution lies in the belief that since the center serves Tom Green County and other counties, there is no reason for a city plus a county contribution. Whether this viewpoint is valid or not, one can clearly see some of the difficulties in working in such an area where the mentally handicapped and their families are still very much stigmatized. A great deal of energy is spent in merely educating the people as to the needs and abilities of this population.

Conversely many residents also expect the center to be producing dramatic results and offering more services. At the same time, TDMHMR is putting numerous demands on Community Mental Health Centers. The CVCHA staff feel that there is a great deal of paperwork, budget detail, and other activities which are especially onerous in a small center with very limited administrative overhead. It is because of these exacting demands that the center only opens cases after six or seven contacts with the center. Thus, individuals requesting acute crisis intervention or assistance in dealing with problems of daily living are not registered as open cases. This results in an underestimation of the total clients served. CVCHM staff estimate approximately 500 additional clients have been served in such a manner (Blaydes, 1989c).

Although the CARE system data indicate that 997 cases are open, this figure is problematic for two reasons. First of all, as mentioned above, not all individuals who are served are reported. Second, closed cases are not always removed from the CARE system. While it is likely that the CARE system data are unreliable, it is probable that this figure is an underrepresentation of the actual number of clients served.

Even with limited resources, CVCHA was either at the state average or above the state average in compliance during the 1988 Standards and Quality Assurance Review in all review categories except three: screening, crisis hotline, and vocational services. These three areas are currently being addressed by the center (Blaydes, 1989c). CVCHA staff "are proud of their performance and want to do even better" (Blaydes, 1989c).

Another issue which relates more specifically to TDMHMR is that standards are prescribed, yet there appear to be few or no consequences for not meeting set standards and little direct incentive from TDMHMR to make the needed changes. Budget structures often seem unrelated to past performance measures. Similarly, there are no penalties for those areas in which standards have not been met. If standards are to be maintained, then incentives must be built in for the maintenance of such standards. It does not make sense to take away funds as a penalty when standards are not met (and what criteria are to be used: 100 percent compliance, 90 percent, 70 percent?). Because centers do not always have the resources to fully implement such standards in the first place, taking money away makes compliance that much more difficult (Blaydes, 1989c).

CVCHA's assessment of standards is as follows: "The standards are important measures--they become, at times, goals to reach towards when financial resources are limited--standards are expensive, but needed. One does the best possible to meet standards with few/limited resources" (Blaydes, 1989c).

Another problem related to CMHCs located in rural areas is the limitation in services provided to minority clients (TDMHMR, 1988b). The two counties in the Concho Valley with the greatest percentage of Hispanics (Crockett and Reagan) are the farthest away from the center, yet they lack public transportation services (CVCHA, 1988a).

All of the core services provided by the center are in need of further development, primarily because of insufficient funding. The center has been quite specific in outlining what it feels are additional needs to better serve the people of the Concho Valley. What follows is a specific cost-needs analysis as outlined by the center for each of the three main budget categories: residential services, client and family support services, and case management.

Residential Services

The center acknowledges that its residential core services are not fully developed (CVCHA, 1988h). To fully develop these services, CVCHA feels that three broad areas must be targeted for improvement: expansion of crisis stabilization services, provision of more residential alternatives to clients, and improvement of the semi-independent apartment living services. A proposed budget that includes all the necessary services required to fully develop such residential programs would amount to $828,623, or approximately 3.5 times the FY 1989 amount budgeted ($221,097). New proposed services include the following:

1. Contracted Inpatient Beds. Services for 52 more patients, at an average cost of $250 a day, would result in a budget of $150,000 for contracted inpatient beds. The center also needs a contract with another hospital for medical problems not covered in the psychiatric inpatient program and a contract with a psychiatrist for inpatient psychiatric coverage (CVCHA, 1988h).

2. Supervised Family Living/Long-Term Structured Foster Care. The center would like to contract with three homes for one bed each at a cost of $30 a day for the entire year. This service would cost $32,850 and would provide residential settings for long-term patients discharged from psychiatric hospitals (e.g., BSSH) who are in need of a transitional setting before moving on to a less supervised apartment situation (CVCHA, 1988h).

3. Supervised Family Living/Respite Foster Care. This is a much needed service that the center is lacking. The center would like to contract with three homes for one bed each at $20 a day, year round, amounting to a cost of $21,900 (CVCHA, 1988h).

4. Supervised Apartment Living/Extended, Intermediate, or Transitional Foster Care. This service would require 15 homes with one bed each at $25 a day, year round, resulting in an additional $136,875 (CVCHA, 1988h).

5. Faiweather Lodge/Group Home. In order to implement this service, the center would require $55,620 dollars for a nursing staff consisting of three nurses at a cost of $18,540 each as well as rent assistance ($740 a month) and building repairs ($150), for a yearly amount of $8,400 and $1,800 respectively (CVCHA, 1988h).

6. Supervised Apartments. This service would require an increased staff of one Caseworker I at $17,364 and the upgrade of two MH Specialist positions from $14,496 to Caseworker I at $17,364 (a total cost of $5,736); additional furnishings for the apartments and equipment for fire safety compliance for a total of $8,000; a van costing $18,500 for the residential programs; $200 a month in rental assistance to ten clients for an expenditure of $24,000; and $5,000 in repair funds for the apartment units (CVCHA, 1988h).

Residential services are quite limited. Of primary concern is that the funds budgeted for contracted inpatient beds have, in the past, been used within six months. According to center guidelines, after spending 7 days at River Crest Hospital, clients are supposed to be considered for admission to BSSH. In FY 1988, CVCHA clients spent an average of 10.87

days at River Crest at a cost of $347 per day. This greatly exceeded the budgeted amount of $250 per day. However, a concern of CVCHA staff, which impacts on cost-per-day figures, is that clients who are experiencing acute crisis situations and who are referred to BSSH are likely to stay for longer periods of time than if served at River Crest (Blaydes, 1989c).

Financial costs, however, are not the only criteria by which such decisions are made. Oftentimes, clients are not directed to BSSH for various reasons. First, BSSH is 86 miles away from San Angelo. The center would like to keep the clients close to their families, friends, and community as long as possible. Second is the issue of stigmatization, one of primary importance in a conservative community. Staff members of the center, as well as its clients, feel that once a person is referred to a state mental hospital, even for a period as brief as three days, that person may have to bear the stigma of "being crazy" for the rest of his or her life. Third, every time a client is referred to BSSH there is an economic ripple throughout the county. Often, two deputies are required to transport the client to and from the hospital, a task which depletes county services elsewhere. In addition, the county judge needs to be involved when the client is involuntarily committed. In sum, the center believes that BSSH is not the most appropriate environment when an additional two or three days is all that is required to stabilize or improve the well-being of the client, precluding the need for state hospital admission (Blaydes, 1989a).

The center also lacks alternative residential services. The only residential services available are the semi-independent apartments and the crisis stabilization bed. More than 15 residential beds are required to sufficiently serve this area and other alternatives are required. The population being served has a great diversity of skills and needs, and yet only one type of living arrangement is currently being offered through the mental health authority (the semi-independent apartments). In spite of this, the center does attempt to personalize and individualize this service. However, as previously pointed out, there is substantial demand for more residential services.

Client and Family Support

In FY 1989, the CVCHA appropriated $700,752 for client and family support services. The professional staff and program directors of CVCHA feel strongly that these services need to be further developed to adequately serve the Concho Valley. To achieve such goals, CVCHA projects expenditures with needed increases to total $1,125,104, an increase of $424,352 above the budgeted amount of $700,752 for FY 1989. This added sum is broken down as follows :

1. The following staff positions need to be added or upgraded:

    a. The Oasis House needs $8,604 to upgrade three MH Specialist positions to Caseworker I.

    b. The sum of $187,938 is needed for additional staff in order to develop a highly necessary regional circuit, formalized family support services, a free-standing crisis intervention team, adequate case assignment and counseling of priority clients, and an adequate staff for a medication clinic, medical records, and clerical support.

2. Travel allowances amounting to $10,000 are needed in order to provide regional services.

3. Capital outlay is required for the following:

   a. A van for the community support programs ($18,000).

   b. A car for regional services ($14,000).

   c. Additional furniture and phones for the staff ($27,000).

   d. Additional office space ($1,500 a month) and repairs ($18,000).

4. Additional contracts for psychiatric services as well as laboratory and physical examinations are required at an estimated cost of $50,000.

5. A regional WATS line (enabling those in outlaying counties to utilize the crisis hotline toll-free) at a cost of $7,300 (CVCHA 1988j).

The center's first-level priority is persons at risk of immediate institutional placement, followed by persons with a previous history of institutional admission as well as those persons requiring services to maintain a functional level in the community (CVCHA, 1987). Because of financial constraints, psychosocial services are thus targeted toward lower-functioning clients. More vocational services should be made available to higher-functioning clients.

Case Management

Although CVCHA has appropriated $73,760 for case management for FY 1989, an additional $153,349 is required to meet its projected needs. This increased cost includes the following (CVCHA, 1988i):

1. Three additional MH case managers at a cost of $21,204 each and a Clerk Typist II are required in order to meet the projected staffing needs of this service.

2. Capital outlay for a car purchase ($16,000) is necessary in order to provide case management services via a circuit rider as well as funds for furnishing a regional office ($10,500).

3. Travel expenses amounting to $4,000 are required in order to provide such regional services.

4. Rental expenses of $15,900 are required for additional regional office space.

Although case management caseloads are similar in number to those found in urban areas, the relationships between clients and case managers are qualitatively different. It appears that more personal relationships exist between clients and case managers than may be expected in many urban CMHCs.

Overall, the CVCHA staff are proud of their accomplishments, given their limited resources. On the most recent Standards and Quality Assurance Review, CVCHA was at or above the state average in compliance in all but three areas. The center achieved a 100 percent rating on its community support program, it has maintained good relationships with other agencies, and, perhaps most important, it has established warm and personal relationships with its clients. Other strong points include the unique relationship between CVCHA and CVAMI and the appropriate and efficient utilization of volunteers in various roles by the CVCHA.

One of the main concerns of the center is that the outlying counties are receiving marginal services at best. Also of concern is the limited range of residential services currently being provided to clients. Within this area, adequate funding for year-round crisis stabilization services is needed. Of further concern is the question of how aggressively the center pursues additional funding and grants.

The center staff are highly dedicated and motivated; they are warm and caring professionals who foster a positive mental health environment. Provision of adequate mental health services to the rural areas of the state of Texas is one of TDMHMR's priorities. While CVCHA and others have shown a genuine concern for such issues, a more proactive and systematic approach to better meeting such needs remains to be implemented.

References

Blaydes, S. 1988. Program Director, Concho Valley Center for Human Advancement, San Angelo, Texas. Interviewed by R. Vega et al., December 16.

____________. 1989a. Program Director, Concho Valley Center for Human Advancement, San Angelo, Texas. Interviewed by R. Vega et al., February 16.

____________. 1989b. Program Director, Concho Valley Center for Human Advancement, San Angelo, Texas. Telephone interview by H. Crean, March 24.

____________. 1989c. Program Director, Concho Valley Center for Human Advancement, San Angelo, Texas. Letter to R. Vega et al., April 21.

____________. 1989d. Program Director, Concho Valley Center for Human Advancement, San Angelo, Texas. Telephone interview by A. N. Rodriguez, May 11.

Concho Valley Center for Human Advancement (CVCHA). 1987. "Concho Valley Center for Human Advancement Long Range Plan." San Angelo, Texas.

____________. 1988a. "Demographic Overview of Service Area." San Angelo, Texas.

____________. 1988b. "Characteristics of Clients Served: Center Totals." San Angelo, Texas.

____________. 1988c. "Description of Services." San Angelo, Texas.

____________. 1988d. "Mental Health Programs Contracts and Consultants." San Angelo, Texas.

____________. 1988e. "Outline of Services." San Angelo, Texas.

____________. 1988f. "Service Plan." San Angelo, Texas.

____________. 1988g. "Services Provided Through the In-Home and Family Support Program." San Angelo, Texas.

____________. 1988h. "Residential and Projected Increases: 06/13/88." San Angelo, Texas.

____________. 1988i. "Case Management Budget Current and Projected Increases." San Angelo, Texas.

____________. 1988j. "Client and Family Support Current and Projected Core and Single Portal Increases." San Angelo, Texas.

Jeffers, C. 1988. Director, Community Support Program, Concho Valley Center for Human Advancement, San Angelo, Texas. Interviewed by R. Vega et al., December 16.

Kingston, M., and M. G. Crawford. 1987. <u>1988-1989 Texas Almanac</u>. Austin, Texas: Texas Monthly Press.

Shannon, C. 1989. President, Concho Valley Alliance for the Mentally Ill, San Angelo, Texas. Interviewed by H. Crean and R. Vega, February 16.

Shannon, J. 1988. Editorial. San Angelo Standard Times, December 13.

Sharpe, P., and R. S. Weddle. 1982. Texas: The Newest, the Biggest, the Most Complete Guide to All of Texas. Austin, Texas: Texas Monthly Press.

Texas Department of Mental Health and Mental Retardation (TDMHMR). 1986. Texas Laws Relating to Texas Department of Mental Health and Mental Retardation. 6th ed. Austin, Texas.

____________. 1987. "Mental Health Services Definitions Fiscal Year 1988." Austin, Texas.

____________. 1988a. "Future Directions 1988-1993." Austin, Texas.

____________. 1988b. "Standards and Quality Assurance (SQA) Report--Quality Assurance Review--Concho Valley Center for Human Advancement." Austin, Texas.

____________. 1988c. "Concho Valley Center for Human Advancement Budget and Quarterly Report." Austin, Texas.

____________. 1988d. "Contract for Services: Concho Valley Center for Human Advancement." Austin, Texas.

____________. 1988e. "Executive Fact Book--Third Quarter 1988." Austin, Texas.

____________. 1989. "Texas Department of Mental Health and Mental Retardation Client and Registration (CARE) Data, 1984-1988." Austin, Texas. (Computer printout.)

Young, J. 1988. Executive Director, Concho Valley Center for Human Advancement, San Angelo, Texas. Interviewed by N. Rodriguez et al., December 16.

____________. 1989. Executive Director, Concho Valley Center for Human Advancement, San Angelo, Texas. Interviewed by N. Rodriguez, February 16.

Chapter 5. San Antonio State Hospital Outreach

Pamela M. Diamond, Minh Ly Griffin, Nicholas L. Hoover

INTRODUCTION

Rural mental health care delivery in Texas presents many problems. While the community has become the locus of mental health care in this era of deinstitutionalization, in rural areas this "community" is often spread out over hundreds of square miles in and around many small towns and cities. Many of these areas are underserved medically as well as psychiatrically. As an example of this, in 1986, there were 10 rural counties in Texas with no physician, 43 counties with no hospital, 28 counties with no licensed nursing facility, 14 counties with no pharmacist, and 30 counties with no dentist . By 1989, the number of counties without hospitals had increased to 52 (TDMHMR, 1989a). Many of the counties lacking one of the above services also lack the others (Walker, Mountain, Barry, & Mayo, 1986).

The availability of mental health professional staff is limited as well. In Texas, in 1986, only 4 percent of the psychiatrists practiced in rural communities, and 186 counties in Texas have no psychiatrist. Only 9 percent of the Licensed Professional Counselors practice in rural areas, and in rural areas, there are 45,552 people for each licensed psychologist (Walker et al., 1986). Implementation of community based models of mental health care in rural areas, therefore, often requires substantial modifications in order to meet the needs of these dispersed communities. There are also serious limitations in the variety of professional staff available in the rural community to provide multidisciplinary services. Often the staff is forced to provide care in several adjoining counties, traveling from one small clinic to another and not really being available at any one location all of the time.

Hospitals which are adequately prepared to provide community-based crisis services are rare. Laboratory work, required for adequate monitoring of psychotropic drug reactions, may not be available locally. And clients must often travel great distances to avail themselves of needed services. Locating a mental health clinic centrally within a region covering several hundred square miles does not insure accessibility. All of these problems, and many not discussed here, add to the difficulty of providing adequate, cost-effective mental health services in the rural community. As stated in the June working draft of the Texas Department of Mental Health and Mental Retardation's "Future Directions 1988-1993," "Rural mental health services are, per unit of service, more expensive to provide than are urban services. Few of the rural counties and communities provide adequate local financial support for community services" (TDMHMR, 1989a, p. 30). This realization coincides with increasing evidence that "rural communities in Texas are in a state of crisis because of plummeting oil and gas prices, declining land values, and the loss of the institution of family farming. A report on Rural Mental Health in Texas indicates an increase in child abuse, substance abuse, and suicide among the youth population and their families" (TDMHMR 1989a, p. 31).

Most of the population of Texas is served by community mental health centers (CMHCs). However, much of the area of Texas is not. According to TDMHMR, 87.95 percent of the population is served by the 35 CMHCs, and many of these are in rural areas, but these centers cover only 51.48 percent of the area of Texas (TDMHMR, 1989b). This leaves 12.05 percent of the population spread out over the remaining 48.52 percent of Texas.

To provide mental health services in the rural areas of Texas not served by CMHCs, the state hospitals and state centers have developed a number of small outreach mental health clinics (MHCs), administered by the hospital or center and located within the rural communities. There are some very important differences between these state-administered outreach MHCs and the CMHCs. A major difference is that the clinics are directly operated by the state, and essentially their sole source of funding is from state funds which are channeled through the state hospital or state center of which they are a part. The local communities do not directly provide funding for these clinics; however, they often do provide in-kind contributions such as equipment, facilities, utility payments, and, in one case, even staff (Schnee, 1989).

In addition to the difference in primary funding source, and partially because of the rural nature of most of the outreach areas, some of the core services normally associated with CMHCs are not always available at the outreach MHCs. For example, community-based crisis residential services are not universally accessible in areas served by outreach MHCs. Case management services are provided directly from the hospital or center, and they are not under the control of the clinic staff. The funds for case management in the outreach area are also handled by the state hospital or center and not by those directly in charge of outreach services (Esparza, 1989a).

To provide a more in-depth look at the delivery of state-operated mental health services in the rural areas of Texas, this case study will examine the outreach area for which San Antonio State Hospital is the Mental Health Authority.

A DESCRIPTION OF THE AREA COVERED BY SAN ANTONIO STATE HOSPITAL OUTREACH SERVICES

Currently the San Antonio State Hospital (SASH) Outreach program covers a total of 16 counties in Texas. These counties, which are primarily rural, span the width of South Texas, from Val Verde to Aransas, and cover approximately 16,000 square miles. The total population of the area is estimated to be 455,414 (SASH, 1989a), which yields a population density of about 28 people per square mile. Although SASH is located in Bexar County, this county is not a part of the outreach area since it is served by the Bexar County Mental Health and Mental Retardation Center.

There are ten mental health clinics operated by SASH Outreach serving four local service areas as defined by TDMHMR. The map in Figure 5.1 shows the locations of the outreach counties served by SASH Outreach. There are two substance abuse clinics which are operated by SASH Outreach as well, and SASH also provides consultant services to a local mental health clinic in Zavala County.

To facilitate its acceptance in the local community, each outreach clinic establishes a Mental Health Advisory Council (MHAC) in the community that the clinic will be serving. These MHACs are primarily for "networking" and coordinating services within the community, and they serve a public relations function which facilitates communication between the MHCs and the community. They often provide a fund-raising base in the local community for the clinics as well, and at times even provide some funds for the clinic. Some of the more active MHACs have even participated in the hiring of clinic directors (Schnee, 1989). Members of the MHAC usually include a law enforcement official, a physician, and other community leaders (Esparza, 1989a).

Table 5.1 lists the SASH Outreach MHCs and their locations along with some additional information about their staffing patterns and numbers of clients served.

As shown in Table 5.1, these clinics are fairly small operations, generally staffed with three or four individuals, one of whom is usually clerical. Most of the clinics have at

Figure 5.1. Area Served by San Antonio State Hospital Outreach

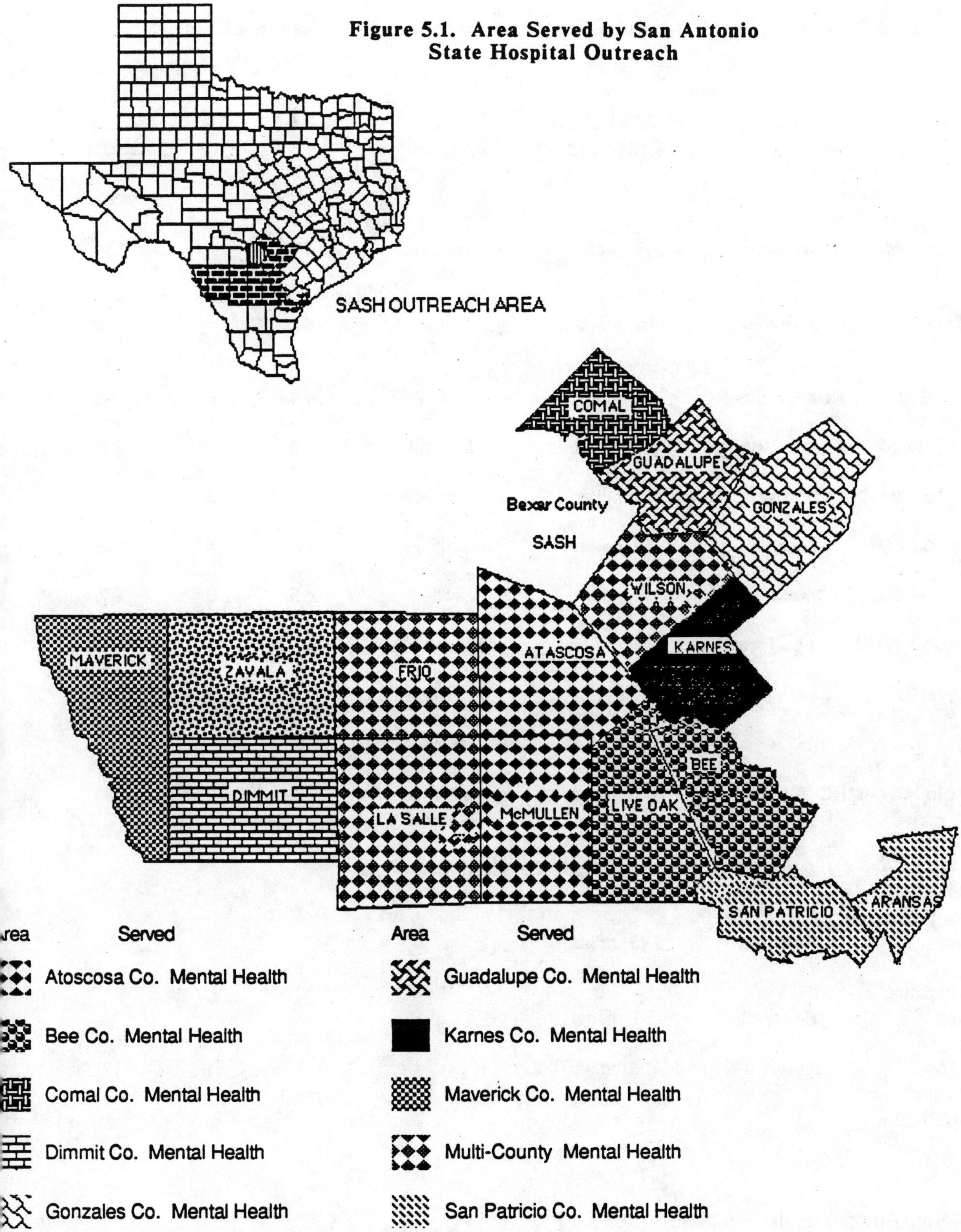

Source: San Antonio State Hospital, "Area Served By SASH Outreach." San Antonio, Texas. January 4, 1989.

Table 5.1. Locations and Clients Served by SASH Outreach Clincs

Clinic	Location*	Approximate Distance	Counties Served*	LSA*	Staff*	Active Clients**
Atascosa Co. MHC	Jourdanton	35 miles	Atascosa McMullen	47	4	118
Bee Co. MHC	Beeville	90 miles	Bee Live Oak	45	4	178
Comal Co. MHC	New Braunfels	32 miles	Comal	44	5	142
Dimmit Co. MHC	Carrizo Springs	105 miles	Dimmit	45	3	80
Gonzales Co. MHC	Gonzales	70 miles	Gonzales	48	3	118
Guadalupe Co. MHC	Seguin	40 miles	Guadalupe	44	5	158
Karnes Co. MHC	Kenedy	55 miles	Karnes	45	3	97
Maverick Co. MHC	Eagle Pass	130 miles	Maverick	45	4	199
Multi Co. MHC	San Antonio	n/a	Frio La Salle Wilson	45	5	130
San Patricio Co. MHC	Sinton	140 miles	San Patricio Aransas	45	5	161
Other Facilities Serving the Area						
Aransas Co. Substance Abuse Office	Rockport	145 miles				
Frio Co. Substance Abuse Office	Pearsall	50 miles				
Zavala Co. MHC (SASH provides consultant only)	Crystal City	105 miles				

*Source: San Antonio State Hospital, 1989b.
**Source: TDMHMR, Care System Data Base February 1989.

least one master's-level staff member, usually a social worker, and one licensed vocational nurse (LVN). Counties with larger populations, such as San Patricio, Comal, Guadalupe, and Maverick, have larger staffs of up to five full-time employees. In addition to the regular staff, SASH provides medical, psychiatric, and psychological consultants who see patients at the clinic two to four times per month to prescribe treatment and medication. Although only three are full-time, there are currently eight psychiatrists who work out of the outreach offices in San Antonio (Schnee, 1989).

There have recently been several newly created staff positions within the SASH outreach system. Five new master's-level positions have been added, and four have already been filled. Of the three new bachelor's-level positions, two are still open. However, four of the five new case manager positions have been filled, almost doubling the case management staff (Schnee, 1989). In general, more funds have been made available recently through the hospital to increase staff at the outreach clinics.

Table 5.1 also shows the number of clients currently served by the different clinics. These numbers were extracted from TDMHMR's CARE system database and represent active cases as of February 9, 1989. These numbers agree well with estimates of client load given by staff members of the clinics in interviews.

The ethnic mix of the counties covered by SASH Outreach varies a great deal, as shown in Table 5.2. Ten of the counties covered by SASH Outreach, however, are over 50 percent Hispanic, and there are few blacks in the entire region.

Figure 5.2 shows the ethnic distribution for the entire region combined. Compared with the ethnic distribution of Texas, this area has a higher percentage of Hispanics, and a lower percentage of blacks and Anglos.

Table 5.3 shows the ethnic breakdown of the clients assigned to SASH Outreach, broken down by diagnosis.*

---

*Diagnosis in this paper is based on the two-digit diagnostic code which is used in the CARE System Database. This code is computed from DSM III diagnoses and has been further consolidated into four categories for this discussion. The codes which define the four categories used in this paper are listed below.

01 Schizophrenia and related disorders
02 Depressive disorders
03 Other nonorganic psychoses
04 Alcohol-related
05 Drug-related
06 Other organic disorders
07 Autism/pervasive disorders
08 Other developmental disorders
09 Anxiety/somatoform/dissociative
10 Personality/factitious/impulse
11 Mental retardation
12 Adjustment/other nonpsychotic
13 No mental disorder
14 Undiagnosed

An individual with a diagnosis of 01, 02, or 03 is considered SMI (seriously mentally ill). If the diagnosis is 04 or 05, the individual is categorized as SA (substance abuse). Anyone coded as 13 or 14 is considered to have no diagnosis (NO DIAG), and anyone not already categorized is considered to be OTHER, which includes minor mental illness, developmental disorders, and organic illnesses (TDMHMR, 1989a).

Table 2.2. **Population and Ethnic Distribution of Counties Included in SASH Outreach Area**

Counties	Population	% White	% Black	% Hispanic
Aransas	20959	69%	1%	30%
Atascosa	33836	49%	0%	51%
Bee	31961	40%	2%	59%
Comal	53427	76%	1%	23%
Dimmit	14671	20%	0%	80%
Frio	18154	23%	0%	77%
Gonzales	18147	58%	8%	33%
Guadalupe	64389	68%	5%	28%
Karnes	14307	46%	2%	52%
La Salle	6331	24%	0%	76%
Live Oak	13819	69%	0%	31%
Maverick	57339	5%	0%	95%
McMullen	862	37%	0%	63%
San Patricio	71602	50%	1%	49%
Wilson	21792	62%	1%	38%
Zavala	13818	6%	0%	94%
Total	45,5414	43.76%	1.31%	54.93%

Source: Texas Department of Health, 1988.

Figure 5.2. Ethnic Distribution for All SASH Outreach Counties

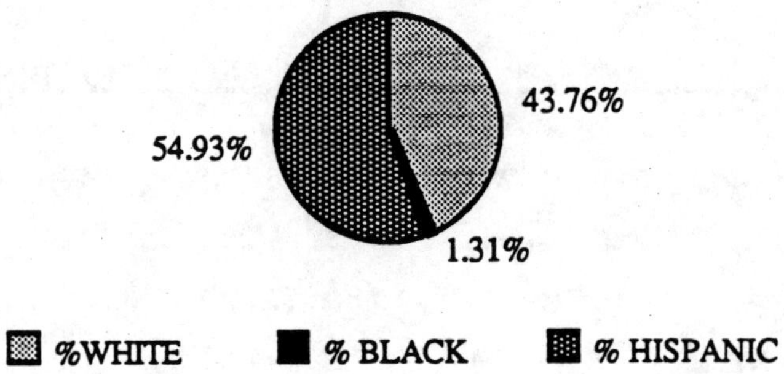

Source: Texas Department of Health, 1988.

Table 5.3. Open Community Cases Assigned to SASH Outreach Categorized by Service Group

ETHNICITY	TOTAL	%	SMI	%	SA	%	NO DIAG	%	OTHER	%
WHITE	663	(35%)	316	(37%)	96	(37%)	148	(29%)	103	(34%)
BLACK	100	(5%)	65	(8%)	5	(2%)	14	(3%)	16	(5%)
HISPANIC	1,145	(59%)	470	(55%)	160	(61%)	336	(66%)	179	(59%)
OTHER	20	(<1%)	6	(<1%)	2	(<1%)	8	(2%)	4	(1%)
TOTAL	1,928		857	(44%)	263	(14%)	506	(26%)	302	(16%)

SMI - Seriously Mentally Ill

SA - Substance Abuse

No Diag - No Diagnosis Assigned

Source: TDMHMR, CARE System Database, February 1989.

As shown in the Table 5.3, 44 percent of the clients assigned to SASH Outreach are considered seriously mentally ill (SMI). Hispanics are somewhat underrepresented in this category at 55 percent, even though they represent the largest number of clients overall, while blacks and whites are somewhat overrepresented. In the category NO DIAG, which includes undiagnosed cases as well as those with no mental disorder, Hispanics and Other (Asians, Native Americans, etc.) are overrepresented. This may indicate that clinicians find it more difficult to accurately diagnose individuals with a primary language other than English and from disparate cultures.

Table 5.4 shows the breakdown of SASH Outreach clients by service group and diagnosis. Fewer clients are represented in this table because not all active clients have been officially assigned to one of the service groups listed in this table.

As expected, the highest percentage of SMI clients are in service group I (53 percent). In fact, the SMI category accounts for the highest percentages in the first three service groups and is second only to NO DIAG in service group IV. In service group V, which contains everyone not assigned to the other service groups, NO DIAG is the most highly represented.

BUDGET AND FINANCIAL INFORMATION FOR SASH OUTREACH

As noted previously, 100 percent of the funding for outreach services comes directly from the budget of the state hospital. SASH Outreach is part of the Community Services Division at SASH, as is case management. For FY 1989, $2,862,133 is budgeted for SASH Outreach services. Of this amount, $584,741 (20.4 percent) is allotted for administration, and $933,769 (32.63 percent) is to be used for acute inpatient psychiatric care of children between the ages of five and eleven at the Southwest Neuropsychiatric Center (SASH, 1989a; Schnee, 1989). Professional services for the clinics are supported by a line item in the budget in the amount of $216,345 (Schnee, 1989). For FY 1989, $1,127,278 is specifically reserved for the clinics. The average yearly budget per clinic is $112,728. These budgets range from a high of $171,864 at the Multi-County MHC to a low of $74,362 at the Karnes County MHC (SASH, 1989).

Variations in budgets can be explained (to a certain extent) by the number of clients served by a clinic and by the number of square miles that it serves. The budget for SASH Community Services for FY 1989 is listed in Table 5.5.

While it is interesting to note the 34.38 percent increase in the budget, a direct comparison between the two years is difficult. During FY 1988 SASH Outreach operated other clinics which are now either a CMHC or are operated by other entities (e.g., Riceland). SASH also contracted with Bexar and Nueces county CMHCs for certain services which they did not provide during FY 1989 (Bayne 1989b).

Data on the individual offices are shown in Table 5.6. Since Zavala County has a verbal agreement with SASH Outreach for services, and is not officially part of the outreach clinic system, its budget breakdown has not been provided. It is virtually impossible to break down the funds by core services. Because of the small staff size within each clinic, there cannot be separate staff assigned to each core service. Each member of the staff must, instead, distribute his or her time among various duties that would be accomplished by different divisions or staff members at a community mental health center. This may be one of the reasons that the clinics, even with the sincere efforts of the staff, are often unable to fully provide both core and noncore services.

These tables generate some questions about the variation in funding for outreach MHCs. The figures showing the ratios of amount budgeted by the number of active clients range from a low of $554 at Atascosa County MHC to a high of $1,322 for the Multi-

Table 5.4. Open Community Cases Assigned To SASH Ooutreach Categorized By Service Group

	SMI		SA		NO DIAG		OTHER	
SERVICE GROUP I	209	(53%)	66	(16%)	74	(18%)	53	(13%)
SERVICE GROUP II	15	(38%)	11	(28%)	10	(26%)	3	(8%)
SERVICE GROUP III	11	(38%)	3	(10%)	9	(31%)	6	(21%)
SERVICE GROUP IV	48	(36%)	20	(15%)	53	(40%)	13	(9%)
SERVICE GROUP V	9	(24%)	3	(8%)	19	(52%)	6	(16%)

SMI - Seriously Mentally Ill

SA - Substance Abuse

No Diag - No Diagnosis Assigned

[Source: TDMHMR CARE System\ Database - active cases on 2-8-89]

Table 5.5. FY 1989 Budget for SASH Community Services

Operating Expense	Community Services
Exempt Salaries	$261,811
Classified Salaries	1,180,170
Longevity	14,840
Professional Svc.*	216,345
Drugs	124,660
Medical/Hospital Supplies	1,332
Maintenance Supplies	1,200
Other Supplies	36,361
Travel In-State	38,746
Maintenance and Repairs	8,100
Rental and Leasing	4,640
Purchased Services	1,425
Contracted Svc.**	933,769
Fees and Premiums	2,320
Other Expense	720
Capital Outlay	35,694
Total	**$2,862,133**
FY 1988 Expenditures	$2,129,941
Percentage Change FY 1988 to FY 1989	34.38%

Source: San Antonio State Hospital, "San Antonio State Hospital Monthly Operating Report," run date 7/12/89 as of 5/31/89.

* Professional Services is entirely for contract psychiatric services
** Contracted Services is for residential care services

Table 5.6. FY 1989 Amounts Budgeted for SASH Outreach Clinics

Outreach Mental Health Clinics

Operating Expense	Atascosa County	Bee County	Comal County	Dimmit County	Gonzales County	Guadalupe County	Karnes County	Maverick County	Multi-County	San Patricio County	TOTALS
Classified salaries	56,700	61,850	89,100	56,000	55,220	110,280	55,542	71,235	99,179	72,810	$727,916
Longevity		800	640	960	840	640	480	1,180	2,020	1,280	$8,840
Professional svc.	6,300	24,000	12,480	17,000	18,000	12,480	9,360	31,200	56,985	28,300	$216,105
Drugs	9,000	9,000	21,000	12,000	6,000	16,200	4,500	16,960	12,000	18,000	$124,660
Medical/Hospital	180	96	180	180		120	180		180	120	$1,236
supplies				600		3,000					
Other Supplies	1,634	3,550	600	1,500	2,770	600	2,500	2,587		3,500	$19,241
Travel In-State	4,800	900	4,100	900	900	480	360	800	900	480	$14,620
Maintenance and	600	480	360	480	480	600	480	600	120	480	$4,680
Repairs				360							$360
Fees and Premiums			480	360		480	600		480		$2,400
Rental and Leasing		780	180		600		360	800		900	$3,620
Total	$79,214	$101,456	$129,120	$90,340	$84,810	$144,880	$74,362	$125,362	$171,864	$125,870	$1,127,278
FY 1988 Budgeted	$55,824	$92,189	$109,330	$74,237	$75,666	$115,011	$51,802	$109,728	$132,028	$125,417	$941,232
Percentage Change FY 88-89	41.90%	10.05%	18.10%	21.69%	12.08%	25.97%	43.55%	14.25%	30.17%	0.36%	19.77%
Open Files 2/8/89	143	178	142	80	118	158	97	199	130	161	$1,406
Cost per Open File	$554	$570	$909	$1,129	$719	$917	$767	$630	$1,322	$782	$802
Sq miles served	2,381	1,937	555	1,307	1,068	713	753	1,287	3,457	1,573	$15,031
Cost per sq mile	$33	$52	$233	$69	$79	$203	$99	$97	$50	$80	$75.00
Staff	4	4	5	3	3	5	3	4	5	5	$41
1985 Population	29,500	36,800	46,200	11,900	18,800	54,600	13,400	34,200	38,900	79,300	363,600
Per Capita Cost	$2.69	$2.76	$2.79	$7.59	$4.51	$2.65	$5.55	$3.67	$4.42	$1.59	$3.10

Source: San Antonio State Hospital, "San Antonio State Hospital Monthly Operating Report, Fund 05, Community Services," run date 7/12/89 as of 5/31/89.

County MHC. There are many differences in these areas: for example, in the number of square miles served and the number and type of clients served. There are also fairly dramatic differences when examining the cost per capita between the different areas served. While there is a strong negative linear relationship between the cost per capita and population (r= -.809), there are some variations in costs that are unexplained by this relationship. For example, when comparing those clinics with approximately the same population, Bee, Maverick, and Multi-County, it can be seen that cost per capita varies from a high of $4.42 to a low of $2.76. Using a stepwise multiple regression analysis in which cost per capita was the criterion variable, and population, number of staff, number of open files, and number of square miles served were entered as predictors, only two of these predictor variables were found to significantly relate to cost. Population was the strongest predictor, as might be expected from the above strong correlation. However, when the variability related to population was removed, the only variable that added predictive information was number of open files (R^2 = .792). In other words, with population held constant, the number of open files explains much of the variability among the clinics in per capita cost, and none of the other variables which were looked at in this analysis add significantly to this prediction. Inferences should, however, be made with caution when using the data in Table 5.6, as there are many variables which may not have been considered in this analysis. However, they do illustrate that, from the data provided by SASH Outreach, there are differences in funding among the outreach clinics, and not all can be explained with the data available.

In interviews with clinic staff it was discovered that the clinics do not vigorously pursue payment from their clients; however, in most cases the clients are indigent and could not pay anyway. Karnes County MHC reported that only 2 out of its 88 clients were in the "100 percent pay" bracket of the sliding scale. Most of their clients pay little or nothing, and many are on public assistance programs of various sorts (Rossett, 1989a).

As mentioned earlier, an important difference between the CMHCs and the outreach clinics is in their funding sources. All of the funding for outreach clinics is from state funds channeled through the parent state hospital. The tax base in most of these communities was poor even before the downturn in the state economy. Many of these counties also suffer from unemployment rates which are much higher than the state average. For example, in 1988, the Texas unemployment rate ranged from 7 to 8 percent. Eight of the 16 counties covered by SASH Outreach, however, had unemployment rates well above this, ranging up to 29.1 percent in Maverick County (Suniga, 1989). Normally there are little or no funds that these communities can spare to provide mental health services. The only local match comes from in-kind support. For example, communities often provide free furniture, supplies, and office space to the clinics (Esparza, 1989a).

Since the chief budget arbitrator for the state hospital is its superintendent, the level of funding for outreach services has been, in the past, completely dependent on the priority placed on outreach by that superintendent. Since the primary focus of the superintendent was often the inpatient facility, outreach services did not always receive a high priority, especially when funds were tight. To eliminate some of the problems associated with this type of subjective funding allocation, a community-based funding formula has been put in place which creates a template for outreach funding which is now geared specifically to the region served by the clinics. This funding formula essentially determines the level of staffing and funds available for the outreach clinics irrespective of the superintendent's priorities (Schnee, 1989).

The funding formula idea, used for the outreach areas, takes into account the special needs of rural mental health care delivery. One system which has been developed is the "area teams" concept. An area team is composed of a specific number of mental health care professionals, a psychiatrist, social workers, LVNs, and clerical workers who are assigned to an area based on the population and the population per square mile. Each team is assigned to a specific location within the area so that it is placed as conveniently as possible for those living in the communities. Funding, in turn, is also based on the number of people per square mile and the population. Under this system, services can usually be expanded in rural areas. However, the Legislative Budget Board did not recommend allocating the full amount necessary to fund this type of system completely (Smith, 1989). This lack of funding for mandated outreach services was one of the reasons cited by David Pharis, court-appointed monitor for the R. A. J. vs. Jones lawsuit, for not agreeing to settle the lawsuit (Ward, 1989, p. B1). There should be some changes seen in funding as negotiations over the lawsuit continue.

The hiring of additional staff for the outreach clinics is not dependent on available funding alone. One major problem in rural health care delivery is the actual availability of professional staff. It is often very difficult to find professional staff, especially at the master's level, either residing in or willing to relocate to small towns. While more vacancies may appear for master's-level staff, it is common for these vacancies to be open for six months or more. Therefore, many of the SASH outreach clinics have open positions which they find difficult to fill. More often than not, the clinics must depend on paraprofessional employees who may not meet all of the qualifications for these positions. While these employees do not have the education desired by TDMHMR, they do posses the willingness to live in these communities and the desire to do the best job possible (Esparza, 1989a; Rossett, 1989a).

Since funding for the outreach clinics has at times been marginal at best, it was thought to be useful to look at each clinic individually to ascertain how each actually provides the mandated core services within its respective community and at what level of service. The next section provides an overview of each of the core services, with descriptions of how the different clinics interpret and implement them in their community. The information for this section was gathered from a series of phone interviews with clinic staff. A structured questionnaire was used to guide the interview (Appendix 5.A), and responses were gathered from eight clinics.

SASH OUTREACH MENTAL HEALTH SERVICES

The definitions of mandated core and other services, as developed by TDMHMR, are often interpreted rather idiosyncratically by the various outreach clinics. The services, as defined, do not take into consideration the unique situations found in rural communities. For example, "crisis intervention team" is often defined quite pragmatically in the outreach clinics--it consists of the entire clinic staff. This is but one example of the adjustments implemented by the individual mental health clinic directors as they adapt a given service definition to fit the requirements of their unique setting.

While the service definitions may result in different interpretations, the required services are generally being provided in some form by the clinics under SASH Outreach jurisdiction. Distance, however, serves as a permanent barrier which impedes service delivery in a variety of ways. The distance between the state hospital and the individual clinics in the rural communities can make a vital difference in a client's service program. For example, specific blood tests which are necessary before certain medications can be prescribed may not be available in the local communities. Although these tests can be obtained at SASH, the time required to deliver the samples, and the refrigerated conditions under which the samples must be maintained, often make it difficult or nearly impossible to do this routinely. These medications may be crucial for successful treatment. However, when the tests cannot be performed, the needed drug treatment may not be implemented. Furthermore, taking a patient to SASH to have the test performed can be very difficult for a rural clinic, as available staff dwindles down to the clerical employee (Rossett, 1989a).

A major service area which is adversely affected by distance is case management. Case management for the outreach clinics is provided by the SASH Community Services Division and not by the outreach clinics. Aside from being managed at the state hospital in San Antonio, case management is a shared program for the ten mental health clinics in the various counties. Typically, a case manager is shared between two mental health clinics and based in one of the counties served by the clinics. The distance between the outreach clinics can result in unnecessary delays in service provision when a case manager is needed at one clinic site while on call at another.

Despite the common problems brought about by insufficient resources, the various outreach clinics are delivering mental health services and programs. Conditions unique to rural communities are handled by clinic staffs with an aim to help the clients as best they can, given the resources available. The following sections present a survey of the SASH outreach clinics and discuss how the mental health core and noncore services are being delivered.

Crisis Stabilization Services

In analyzing crisis stabilization services offered by the SASH Outreach clinics, several vital features emerge. First, crisis stabilization for these rural service areas is mainly provided by the clinic staff--sometimes in conjunction with a local physician, a family doctor, or family members. Presently, there are clinics like San Patricio County MHC and Atascosa County MHC which are unable to provide any kind of 24-hour crisis stabilization services to their clients (Burk, 1989; Bruce, 1989). However, the common pattern evident with all the clinics is that each strives to do its best using local resources before resorting to the state hospital. Since these clinics serve small towns, they establish good relationships with other public organizations in their vicinity so that all agencies know how to contact the clinic staff in case of emergency.

A second consistent pattern among these clinics is the absence of mental health emergency beds in the community. Currently, none of the clinics surveyed contracts directly with a local hospital for emergency beds. There is a general consensus that such a service is needed, so there is an active effort by the various clinics to acquire emergency bed contracts with local hospitals. Several clinics (Gonzales County, Maverick County, and Multi-County) are in the process of negotiating with their local hospitals to contract emergency beds for the near future. The staff at the Comal County clinic also mentioned that one local hospital occasionally donates hospital beds for emergencies (Crabtree, 1989; Stockley, 1989; Parsons, 1989).

An important consideration, given the lack of contracted beds, is how the clinics handle emergency situations in which clients require immediate hospitalization. One approach is to use local facilities as much as possible, using the state hospital only when it cannot be avoided. Clinics in Atascosa County, Karnes County, and Maverick County try to do this (Bruce, 1989; Rossett, 1989b; Stockley, 1989). They typically send clients in emergencies to the local emergency room, where the clients are assessed by a physician. The physician then determines whether the client will stay the night or whether emergency commitment or protective custody is needed. These clinics do use the state hospital for crisis stabilization at times, but only when absolutely necessary. Otherwise, these clinics prefer to stabilize their clients locally. Dimmit County, Gonzales County, Multi-County, and San Patricio County clinics typically handle emergency situations requiring immediate hospitalization by transferring the client directly to the state hospital. Transportation is provided by a clinic staff member or a local law enforcement officer when commitment is necessary (Flores, 1989; Crabtree, 1989; Parsons, 1989; Burk, 1989).

Emergency Screening

Emergency screening for the SASH Outreach catchment area is not formal in the sense that it is staffed on a 24-hour, seven-days-a-week basis. These rural community clinics operate Monday through Friday from 8:00 a.m. to 5:00 p.m. However, clients can access mental health services during other hours with a telephone call to a staff member's home. Although staff members are officially not on duty at all times, they are available on call as the situation may dictate.

An important part of the required emergency screening services is a 24-hour crisis hot line. Half of the clinics surveyed have this coverage (Atascosa, Comal, Dimmit, and Multi-County). The other half responded that they do not have a 24-hour crisis hot line. A closer analysis of what is meant by a 24-hour crisis hot line, as understood and implemented by the clinics, demonstrates that this response is somewhat misleading. The towns in the SASH outreach service area are on the average small enough that community members are familiar with the clinic staff and are aware of the clinics as a mental health resource. Thus, all the clinics which responded to the survey provide some type of 24-hour crisis hot line to their clients if it is defined as the accessibility of clinic staff at any given time under emergency situations. For these clinics, a 24-hour crisis hot line service is fully covered when telephone numbers of the clinic and the clinic director (and sometimes home phone numbers of the entire staff) are made available to the community and to various other public entities, such as law enforcement agencies and hospitals. Good relationships among the community agencies aid this process as well.

A less common practice is the use of resources other than the director or individual clinic staff members for the 24-hour emergency hot line service. For example, Comal County MHC has a 24-hour crisis hot line which is manned after hours by volunteers. Karnes County MHC issues a calendar to the sheriff's department, the county courthouse, the local emergency room, and various other entities along with information as to the particular clinic staff member on call and that staff member's home telephone number (Rossett, 1989b). San Patricio County MHC is located in a very small community in Aransas. Its clients normally do not contact the clinic after hours, but when they do, they can call the police department, which will then contact the clinic director. Again, good rapport within the communities ensures that the clinic directors will be contacted when their services and expertise are needed (Burk, 1989).

A recent addition to the emergency services available to the outreach clinics is the availability of a WATS line through the state hospital which is manned 24 hours a day (Schnee, 1989). This service was established only this year, and from interviews with clinic staff, it is not yet well known or frequently used. As clinic staff become more aware of this service and make it known to their clients and communities, perhaps some of the gaps in 24-hour emergency coverage in these rural areas will be eliminated.

Another component of emergency screening is the crisis intervention team. As with other services, rural community clinics are not able to fully provide this service as formally defined as an assigned team on duty 24 hours per day, seven days per week. The SASH Outreach clinics make an effort to establish crisis intervention teams for their service areas through their only available resources--the clinic staff itself, working together with local hospital and medical personnel. If a client's initial contact for emergency services is made at the local general hospital emergency room, the clinic staff is generally notified by the local physician on duty at the time in order that they can participate in the process.

Maverick County MHC in Eagle Pass illustrates this process. In Maverick County, the crisis team is generally staffed by the clinic director, a contract general practitioner who is available eight hours per week, and a psychiatrist who visits the clinic four days a month.

Although there is no formal arrangement between the Maverick County MHC and the local hospital, the normal procedure, when the crisis team is not assembled and a client is in need of services, is to take the client to the general hospital emergency room. The hospital staff will assess the client's condition and contact the outreach clinic director. The clinic tries, whenever possible, to get the client into the emergency room long enough to assess his or her condition and to allow time to process his or her admission into the state hospital if needed. For that reason, the state hospital is not often used as an emergency screening facility by the Maverick County clinic because clients have usually been screened prior to their arrival at the state hospital (Stockley, 1989). Only one center, San Patricio County MHC, responded that it has no crisis intervention team. For this exception, the emergency screening is provided through the emergency room in a hospital which is about 15 miles away from the clinic in Sinton. San Patricio also often uses the state hospital as an emergency screening facility, even though it is located 140 miles from the center (Burk, 1989).

Other clinics also rely on the state hospital for emergency screening. The common practice is to transport the client to SASH with a commitment court order. This reliance on the state hospital brings up the problem of transportation. When a client needs to be transported to a state hospital for emergency screening, he or she is often transported by either law enforcement officers or by family. There are times when a staff member will transport the client, but such incidents are rare because the clinics are usually understaffed and cannot afford to have a staff member gone for much of the day. In Karnes County, the clinic's crisis intervention team consists of the director and the caseworker. Although this clinic tries to do emergency screening locally, when the state hospital must be used as an emergency screening facility, a staff member is often called upon to accompany the client and peace officer to SASH. Although this practice promotes good communication between the clinic and the state hospital regarding the client's condition, it often puts a strain on the clinic staff since the staff is so small and it takes several hours to travel the distance to and from the clinic to SASH. For that reason, it is not always possible for the staff person to accompany the client to the hospital, even though it might be preferable (Rossett, 1989b).

Multidisciplinary Assessment

In these rural outreach clinics, multidisciplinary assessment is not formally provided. The primary reason is that there are few psychiatrists in these rural communities. San Patricio County MHC provides an example of some of the difficulties encountered in the rural community. Since the psychiatrist for this clinic visits only twice monthly and the other primary clinician is available only two days every other week, the state hospital is often used for multidisciplinary assessment. The police department is usually used to provide transportation for these clients to the hospital (Burk, 1989). Maverick County handles multidisciplinary screening in a similar way, since there is no psychiatrist in that county. Comal County MHC handles this service differently. The county has one local private psychiatrist who works with the clinic to provide multidisciplinary assessment for clients requiring the service. In addition, the licensed vocational nurse (LVN) assists with multidisciplinary assessment (Battle-Ledford, 1989). In general, the clinics try to provide the needed services to their clients; but when there is a crisis or when resources are unavailable, the state hospital is used.

Family Support Services, Including Respite

Of the eight SASH Outreach clinics which responded to the telephone survey, none has any provision for respite care for the families of clients. At Atascosa County MHC, the Department of Human Services (DHS) is a provider of respite services; but these services are available only to individuals who are physically and mentally disabled (Burk, 1989). For Karnes County MHC, the only respite care facility is 30 miles away in Bee County.

This sole resource is a halfway house where the clinic has sent clients to stay for a maximum of 30 days. Maverick County MHC uses visiting nurses, but they are primarily for geriatric patients. Multi-County also uses visiting nurses, but they are unable to provide extensive care (Rossett, 1989b). Multi-County MHC also has some boarding homes and transitional living units, but it does not have respite care unless it uses SASH. Sometimes with local cooperation a patient can be admitted at the local hospital for an overnight stay (Parsons, 1989).

Although respite care in these rural mental health clinics does not really exist, the various clinics do offer other family support services. Only San Patricio County MHC has no family support services (Burk, 1989).

The family support services offered in the outreach areas take many forms; however, the most commonly offered services are support groups and medication education. Gonzales County MHC provides education on the nature of mental illness, medications, and other mental health issues (Crabtree, 1989). Similarly, Karnes County has medication classes which involve the family. Some of the other clinics have a more extensive family support services program. Atascosa County has a family support group which meets every other week for all the families of its clients. This outreach center also provides individual counseling in addition to formal education classes on mental health issues which are held annually (Rossett, 1989b). Comal County had a family support group which floundered. However, the barriers to hard-earned success have not deterred the clinic from its continued effort to institute family support services. Aside from its family support group, Comal County also has a medication class which meets monthly. Another aspect of Comal County's family support services is a member-led social club, which meets for daily activities (Battle-Ledford, 1989). Dimmit County's family support services include a family support group, family counseling, and medication education in which the family is included. The clinic director for Dimmit County also mentioned that part of the clinic's family support services program involved follow-up on the progress of the clients and their families (Flores, 1989). Maverick County has a support group that mainly targets clients requiring hospitalization or those who have been hospitalized. Education on the effects of medication is done primarily on an individual basis in Maverick County because of the bilingual nature of the community (Stockley, 1989). Multi-County has a family support group which gathers in Wilson County every two weeks. This outreach center also has a psychosocial group meeting every month. Furthermore, the clinic staff is available by telephone for the families of clients. Education programs at Multi-County on mental health concerns are also provided to the entire community (Parsons, 1989).

Case Management

There are two basic issues which are salient to the delivery of case management to SASH Outreach clients: distance and organizational structure. The result of these structural realities is a group of case managers who are shared among the many counties served by SASH Outreach but who are not a direct part of any one MHC organization. The SASH Outreach case managers must together cover approximately 16,000 square miles of territory. Until very recently there were only six individuals who split this huge territory (currently there are ten). These distances necessitate a sharing of case managers among the various counties and clinics, and render it almost impossible for adequate services to be promptly provided.

The organizational structure of case management services is determined by the TDMHMR policy which requires that the director of case management services be no more than two steps below either the executive director of the CMHC or the superintendent of the state hospital. In outreach services this means that case management is directed from the state hospital and the local clinics have no supervisory control over the activities of the case management staff. This policy was put in place to insure that case management remain independent, administratively, of other clinical services. The rationale behind this decision was to eliminate the possibility of case managers being required to fulfill clinical duties unrelated to case management in the clinics, thereby reducing their effectiveness and availability as case managers (Schnee, 1989). This arrangement is not always seen as optimal by clinic directors.

Atascosa County MHC shares a case manager with Wilson County, which is part of Multi-County MHC. Twenty-five of its clients receive formal case management services and there is a waiting list. Those who do not receive formal case management can obtain those services less formally from the clinic staff. The case manager lives in Atascosa County but is based at the Multi-County MHC office, which is in San Antonio. The clinic director finds that this arrangement allows for close enough supervision of the clients under case management; however, she spends much of her time driving to and from the various clinics (Bruce, 1989).

About ten of the Dimmit County MHC clients receive case management services. Based in Carrizo Springs, the case manager moves among the three counties in the service area (Maverick, Dimmit, and Zavala) to provide the needed case management. Unlike Atascosa County, this arrangement does not permit close enough supervision of the clients under case management. For Dimmit County, the main service gaps are caused by time and distance. The case management of the three counties is a considerable job for one person, but the added variable of distance increases the frustration experienced by both the case manager and the clinic staff (Flores, 1989).

Like the Dimmit clinic, the Maverick clinic also shares its case manager with two other counties. The case management services for this area are also based in Carrizo Springs. Approximately five clients of the clinic are receiving case management services. This structure of sharing a case manager is often confining and unrealistic, and it does nothing to enhance supervision of case-managed clients. For the Maverick clinic, the case manager visits only three days of the month. The clinic, however, cannot schedule case management crises to fit this arrangement (Stockley, 1989).

Karnes County MHC has similar problems. Approximately eight of its clients receive case management services, which are based at the Bee County clinic. This sharing of one case manager does not permit adequate case management supervision of the clients because Beeville is 32 miles away. If a crisis involving case management services occurs, the time and distance impose a barrier to quick access to the case manager. Consequently, the clinic staff is often forced to provide early intervention for these clients in the absence of the case manager (Rossett, 1989b).

The Multi-County clinic, which provides mental health services to Frio, LaSalle, and Wilson counties, has a number of clients on waiting lists for case management. The case management for Multi-County MHC is based at Atascosa County MHC. Not surprisingly, this arrangement is not efficient in allowing close enough supervision of clients under case management. The clinic director feels that each county should ideally have its own case manager. For this clinic, aside from the limited availability of case managers, there is the extra problem of distance to occupy case management time (Parsons, 1989).

San Patricio County MHC has 20 of its clients on case management. For this clinic, case management is based at Rockport, which is roughly 30 miles away in Aransas County. The case manager for this clinic consults/visits at least once a week. Evaluation of the case management services for the San Patricio County clinic is still rather difficult since the clinic only recently acquired its case manager (Burk, 1989).

The Comal County clinic has 30 clients on case management in addition to clients on a case management waiting list. Its case manager is based at the clinic. This arrangement allows for close enough supervision of the clients who receive case management. However, there are occasions when the clinic director needs direct supervision of the case manager. Since the case manager is under the supervision of the SASH supervisor, the clinic director has no direct authority. At times this arrangement is inefficient because SASH has to be contacted for any instructions pertaining to case management services (Battle-Ledford, 1989).

Since the telephone interviews with the individual clinics in March of 1989, several positive changes have taken place in the case management services operated by SASH Outreach. There are now ten case managers covering the outreach area instead of six. The four additional case managers have been assigned to San Patricio County, Maverick County, Frio and LaSalle counties, and Atascosa and Wilson counties (Brechtel, 1989). Even with this increase in staff, each case manager would be, on the average, responsible for approximately 1,600 square miles of territory. In spite of the fact that case managers are still responsible for extremely large areas, these additions to the staff will undoubtedly improve delivery of case management services in this area.

A case management program is rendered less successful and effective if issues concerning distance and availability of case managers are left unresolved. Case management is a dynamic component in a mental health service delivery program. The problems of distance and insufficient case managers can be ameliorated with more adequate resources. If the goal of mental health clinics is to expand services, then it is imperative to initiate parallel expansion of case management services and resources.

Another issue seen by some clinic directors as a problem in the delivery of case management services is management structure. While the recurrent source of concern facing the clinics regarding case management is distance, several clinics expressed dissatisfaction with the present program's administrative structure. Case management for these rural clinics is not under the management of the individual clinics. Rather, as stated earlier, case management is under the supervision of the SASH Outreach Services case management coordinator. This organizational structure means that the case managers are not actually part of the clinic staff (Esparza, 1989a). Some directors feel that this makes communication and delegation of responsibilities more difficult, and the director for Atascosa County MHC stated that she would like the case manager to function more as a part of the clinic and treatment team than as a separate entity (Bruce, 1989). Clearly, communication and a close working relationship between clinic staff and case managers are necessary for effective services to be provided. However, this does not necessarily require and given current policy, cannot require direct supervisory control of case managers by clinic directors. On the other hand, there is often a need for the case manager to be able to independently advocate for his or her client's needs within the clinic, and not be required by the clinic director to perform non-case management duties whenever staffing becomes tight.

Medication-Related Services

All eight of the clinics surveyed operate a medication clinic. With the exception of Multi-County MHC, all clinics have an LVN who dispenses medications. For the Multi-County clinic, the clinic director, who is an RN, dispenses the medications. The prescribed medications, which are dispensed at the clinics, are obtained either through local vendors or from SASH (Parsons, 1989).

Laboratory screening is essential to monitor the effects of certain types of psychotropic drugs. This laboratory screening requires that blood samples be drawn and analyzed at a laboratory facility. Since many of the tests are fairly complex, blood samples must often be sent to SASH for screening when local facilities cannot provide the services.

The Atascosa County and Dimmit County clinics send their blood samples either to SASH or to the local Texas Rural Health Initiative (RHI) Clinic. The Comal clinic mails its blood samples to SASH. It also uses the local hospital for blood testing when feasible. Furthermore, in the past, it has coordinated with the University of Texas Health Sciences Center at San Antonio and contracted for unusual laboratory work such as saliva testing when a client has particularly poor veins, which make it difficult to draw blood (Battle-Ledford, 1989). The Gonzales clinic does its laboratory screening at the local health agency (Crabtree, 1989). The Karnes clinic schedules clients to come in for drawing of blood samples on days when a consultant from San Antonio visits the clinic so that the blood samples can be taken directly to SASH (Rossett, 1989b). The Maverick clinic relies on SASH or the local hospital laboratory for medications monitoring (Stockley, 1989). The Multi-County clinic transports its blood samples to SASH (Parsons, 1989). San Patricio County MHC tries to get its clients to come in for laboratory screening whenever the doctor orders laboratory work to be done. However, since its community is small and consists largely of indigents, getting laboratory work completed can be a problem because it is not easy to work with indigents who have virtually no resources to pay for transportation to the clinic (Burk, 1989).

Given all of the variations and improvisation required to provide laboratory screening in these rural counties, it is not surprising that there are sometimes problems involved in the implementation of this service. Mental health services, therefore, can be incomplete or inefficient if the drugs used to treat the symptoms of specific mental illnesses cannot be used because of difficulties in monitoring the effects of the medications.

Another type of medication-related service is medication education. Basically all of the clinics provide this service in one form or another. In general, medication education is provided at the clinics at varying times over the year. Sometimes it is done individually, and other times in formal groups. Films, pamphlets, and videotapes are often used to enhance these educational programs. Families are often included in this process as well, and in many of the clinics this service overlaps with other family support services.

The Atascosa clinic has formal medication classes for each client at least once a year. It also has individual medication education classes. Other resources available to clients are handouts and films on the nature of medications (Bruce, 1989). At the Comal clinic the nurse answers questions which clients and their families have regarding medications. Every time a client is prescribed medication at this clinic, he or she receives an individual medication education session with the nurse and a booklet explaining the prescribed medication. Another method the clinic uses is to make available to clients a 20-minute videotape on medications provided by McNeil Pharmaceutical. The Comal clinic also has monthly medication education classes (Battle-Ledford, 1989).

At the Dimmit clinic, medication education is done on an individual basis and, when possible, reinforced with monthly group meetings (Flores, 1989). Similarly, the Gonzales clinic provides this service individually (Crabtree, 1989). The Karnes clinic has medication education for the family and for small groups. These groups are matched as to the types of medications prescribed for the members. The groups meet every two months to obtain information and instruction (Rossett, 1989b).

Maverick County MHC conducts medication education on an individual basis as needed when a client receives medication. The clients are also given a card with the state hospital pharmacy telephone number (Stockley, 1989). Multi-County provides medication education to individuals and to their families. When possible, this clinic also sets up monthly classes with groups (Parsons, 1989). At the San Patricio clinic, medication education is provided according to need--either individually or with the family present or even by telephone (Burk, 1989).

Another related service of the clinics is the provision of education on mental health issues and coping strategies. The sole exception is San Patricio County MHC, which has no programs of this type (Burk, 1989). The Comal clinic does not have a formal program for mental health concerns; however, it does have a social club and social support groups for clients. For the other clinics, mental health maintenance is typically done in both group settings and through individual counseling (Battle-Ledford, 1989).

Another component of medication-related services available from the clinics is the actual provision of medications to the clients. It is common for the clients to be unable to pay for this medication; therefore, the clinics charge their clients for medications on a sliding scale according to ability to pay. Typically, a client can afford to pay only a fraction of the medication's cost (Bruce, 1989; Flores, 1989; Crabtree, 1989; Rossett, 1989b; Stockley, 1989; Parson, 1989).

Psychosocial Rehabilitation Services

As is the case with other mental health services, psychosocial rehabilitation services for the rural community are limited. Extreme examples of this fact are the Karnes and San Patricio clinics. These clinics have no social support activities or day treatment programs (Rossett, 1989b; Burk, 1989). The other clinics are more fortunate in this service area.

The Comal clinic has a more extensive program. It has a cooking class that meets twice a month. There are also daily activities and a social club room. This room is open Monday through Friday and has a TV, VCR, and games available for the clients to use. The social club publishes a monthly club newsletter, and the members have an organizational meeting twice a month to plan the newsletter. In addition, the clinic has also established a program of weekly video rentals on Fridays (Battle-Ledford, 1989).

Atascosa County MHC has a coffee club which meets every other week or once a month. Aside from this social club, there are no other social gatherings or day treatment (Bruce, 1989). At Dimmit County MHC social support activities consist of a family group and an EA (Emotional Anonymous) group. Clients also have organized social clubs (Flores, 1989). The Gonzales clinic has a recreational group. Part of its social activity is a monthly birthday celebration (Crabtree, 1989). The Maverick clinic has social support activities that fluctuate from one group to the next. Currently, it has a social support group composed of long-term stabilized clients with a diagnosis of schizophrenia. It also has a social club for clients who occasionally have social gatherings (Stockley, 1989). The support activities for the Multi-County clinic is through a family support group that meets every two weeks in Wilson County. Another activity is a once-a-month discussion with the purpose of providing information to improve living skills and overall quality of life. A social activity usually follows the discussion (Parsons, 1989).

Another component of psychosocial rehabilitation services is vocational and/or prevocational training. At these clinics, this service is typically provided through referrals to the Texas Rehabilitation Commission (TRC). At the Comal clinic, this service is skeletal at best. Every Wednesday, the TRC liaison comes to the clinic to talk with clients who want to link up with TRC. A job coach paid by TRC visits the clients in the afternoon at the clinic. Under agreement between Comal County MHC and TRC, the clinic gives TRC the necessary support services and space in return for services offered by TRC (Battle-Ledford, 1989). Only the Atascosa clinic has prevocational training (Bruce, 1989).

Karnes County MHC works closely with TRC. The clinic staff makes recommendations to TRC, which then assesses these clients for vocational or prevocational training. This clinic has also enrolled four of its clients at a junior college to acquire some training (Rossett, 1989b). At Dimmit County MHC, there is no formal vocational or prevocational training. The case manager is relied upon to make certain that linkage to outside resources is available to the clients (Flores, 1989). The Gonzales clinic offers this service through its liaison with a TRC counselor (Crabtree, 1989). Maverick County MHC does not offer this service, but it tries to ensure that whatever resources available are fully utilized. For example, it will refer its clients to TRC, TEC, and DHS (Stockley, 1989). Like the other clinics, the Multi-County and the San Patricio clinics will make referrals to TRC for their clients to obtain vocational or prevocational training (Parsons, 1989; Burk, 1989).

Housing

Although the mandated core services do not cover residential services, the need for housing services is becoming increasingly apparent. In many cases, service delivery by the clinics is incomplete and ineffective without some type of housing being available for the clients. The outreach counties, however, are often not able to provide much in the way of residential services.

Rural areas typically do not have great demand for residential services. Yet a need does exist. This need will continue to grow and will be more aggravated if not attended to soon. Unfortunately, this need can be met only partially, given the limited resources available to the clinics. It is not unusual for the average outreach clinic to offer no residential services whatsoever. If a clinic does provide residential services, it is more than likely through nursing homes or board and care homes. Other traditional forms of housing services (including halfway houses, personal care homes, group homes, supervised apartments, and Fairweather Lodges) are nonexistent. Since the local service areas served through SASH Outreach mental health clinics are rural, the clients normally have no resources other than their own families and homes.

Although it is usual to find that residential services are unavailable in the rural areas for clients who need housing, a survey of the different clinics does uncover notable deviations. For Maverick County MHC, in emergency situations where housing is crucial for the client and/or the client's family, the staff invests energy and time to access whatever local housing resources are available. This clinic relies on two churches in town or places a client in a local motel or a shelter when necessary. At present, a local motel in the vicinity of the clinic is in the process of negotiations with SASH to contract residential services for this outreach center. The Maverick clinic is also unlike other clinics in that it has about 35 clients in public housing and about 15 clients in rent-subsidized apartments. These figures differ from the other clinics, which have on the average about 5 clients utilizing some type of residential services (Stockley, 1989).

The Comal County, Gonzales County, and Karnes County MHCs have low-income housing available to them. Clients who require residential services at the Comal clinic work with the clinic case manager to get Housing and Urban Development (HUD) Section 8 housing or some other form of subsidized housing. The usual procedure is to help these clients fill out the required forms. For clients at the Gonzales clinic, residential services are provided in the form of nursing homes, board and care homes, and low-income housing in the community. Currently, five of the Gonzales clinic clients are in a nursing home and two clients are in a board and care home (Crabtree, 1989). At the Karnes clinic, residential services are limited to HUD Section 8 housing. There is a board and care home, but it is located in Beeville; which is about 15 miles away (Rossett, 1989b).

Despite the limited availability of residential services, clinics continue to do whatever is possible to secure some level of housing for the clients who need it. An illustration of their extra effort and willingness to meet the needs of their clients is found at Atascosa County MHC. For this center, resources for residential services are limited to nursing homes. Even this resource demands added action before it can be utilized because at times the staff has to scramble to get funds for beds. But the rising need facing the clinic is the number of young clients who require residential services and who are inappropriate for nursing home care. In these cases, the clinic tries to find other types of placements (Bruce, 1989).

Although plagued with limited resources and inadequate facilities, the outreach clinics are trying to meet the core services requirements. A revealing discovery from the survey and an on-site visit to Karnes County MHC emphasizes the desire by the clinic staff to serve the clients to their utmost capacity. These individuals truly want to work for the benefit of the clients. Unfortunately, an adequate level of service delivery cannot always be met, despite their willingness and effort.

INPATIENT USE PATTERNS FOR CLIENTS FROM THE OUTREACH COUNTIES

Given that the outreach clinics cannot always provide the needed core services in the communities and often use the state hospital to fill these gaps, one might expect that the state hospital use patterns for these counties would differ from those of communities which have the services of a CMHC. Table 5.7 shows the admission rates for the first quarter of 1989 from both the SASH Outreach counties (grouped into their LSAs) and the admission rates from the neighboring LSAs which are served by either CMHCs or state centers. From this table it can be seen that the admission rates from the outreach counties are quite a bit higher than those from the other areas surrounding SASH (with the exception of Bexar County), which are served by alternate facilities. Overall, the actual number of admissions per year from these counties is small. However, the counties with the highest number of admissions in 1988 were San Patricio, with 154 admissions, and Guadalupe, with 122. Five of the counties had 20 or fewer admissions during the entire year (TDMHMR, 1988).

Figure 5.3 shows admissions from the 16 SASH Outreach counties to inpatient facilities (SASH and others) over the past five years. The San Antonio State Hospital was the most frequently used inpatient facility, with only a few other admissions to miscellaneous state centers and some to Kerrville State Hospital. Over the five-year period, there were no consistent trends noted in hospitalization use, except for a very slight upward trend from Wilson, Guadalupe, and San Patricio counties and a slight downward trend in seven other counties.

When admissions per 1,000 population were calculated for 1988, only four of the counties, McMullen, Aransas, San Patricio, and Bee, had admission rates of over 2.0 per 1,000, and McMullen, which had a total of 3.0 admissions in 1988, had the highest rate. Dimmit, which had a rate of 1.09 per 1,000, was the lowest of the counties in 1988.

Figure 5.4 shows the percentage of admissions to inpatient facilities that were voluntary, compared with those that were involuntary. During 1988, Wilson, Maverick, LaSalle, Guadalupe, Frio, Karnes, Dimmit, and Atascosa counties had more voluntary admissions than involuntary. This was a reverse of the pattern seen from 1985 until 1987 in most of these counties. The other counties had more involuntary admissions during all five years, with the exception of Live Oak and Comal, which had the reverse trend in 1984. These patterns may represent differences in philosophy among the county judges, variations in community resources over time, changes in the state hospital policies regarding voluntary admissions of substance abuse clients, and/or other problems idiosyncratic to the specific county.

Table 5.7. Admissions to San Antonio State Hospital During the First Quarter of Fiscal Year 1989

LOCAL SERVICE AREA	POPULATION / 1989	NUMBER OF ADMISSIONS	ADMISSION RATE PER 100,000
SASH OUTREACH			
44 Guadalupe and Comal	105,617	32	31.30
45 Maverick, Aransas, San Patricio, Bee, Frio, McMullen, Dimmit, Zavala, Live Oak, and Karnes	230,470	69	29.94
47 Wilson and Atascosa	48,960	16	32.68
48 Gonzales	20,319	7	34.45
NON SASH OUTREACH			
4 Bexar County MHMR	1,169,911	413	35.30
14 Gulf Bend MHMR Center	172,963	21	12.14
22 Nueces Co. MHMR	321,599	40	12.44
30 Tropical Texas Center	667,003	8	1.20
59 Laredo State Center	185,548	8	4.31
60 Rio Grande State Center	104,614	4	3.82

Source: Gonzales, 1989

Figure 5.3. Admissions to SASH and Other Inpatient Facilities from All SASH Outreach Counties

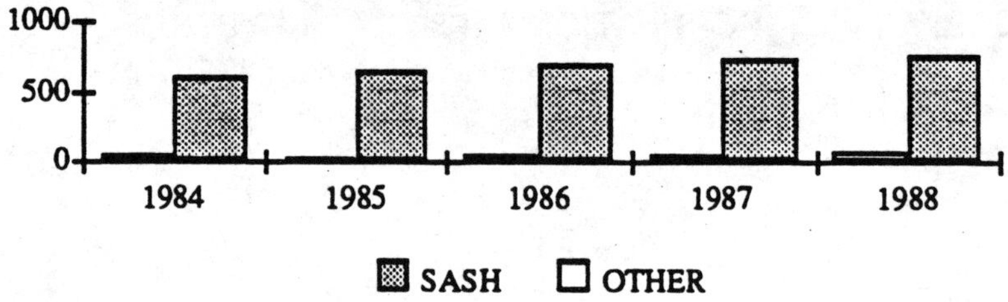

Admissions from Aransas County

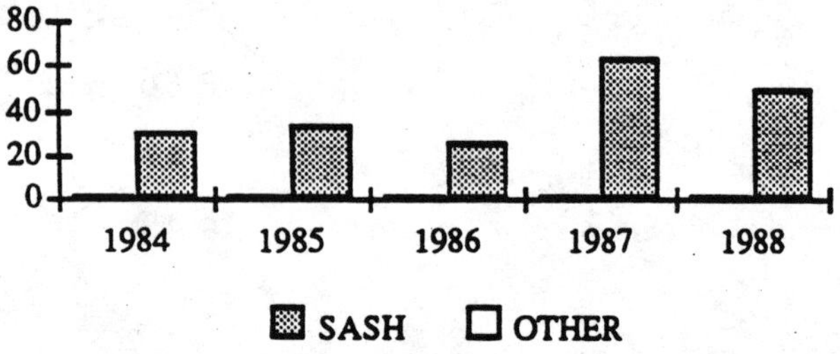

Admissions from Atascosa County

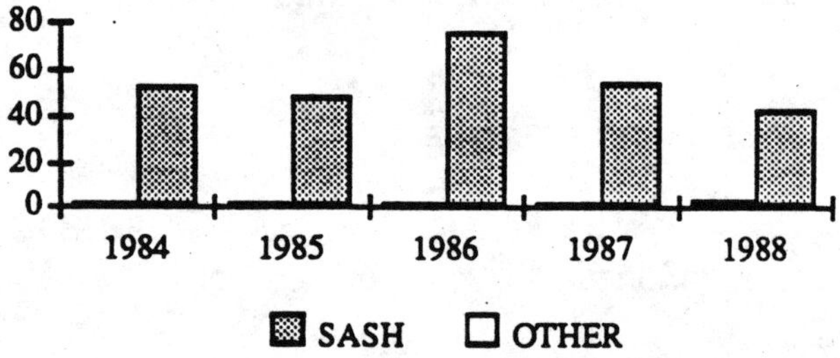

Admissions from Bee County

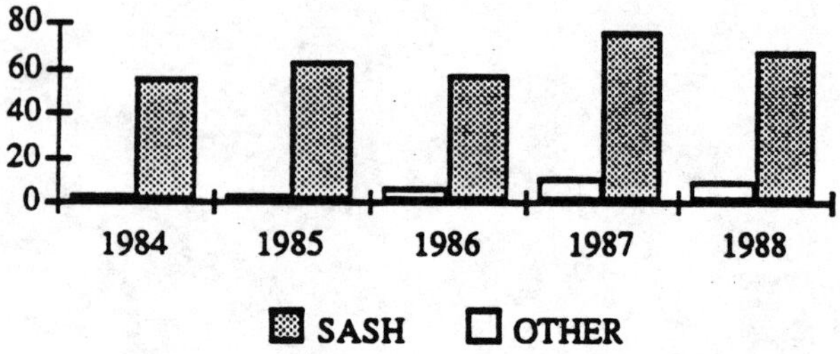

Admissions from Comal County

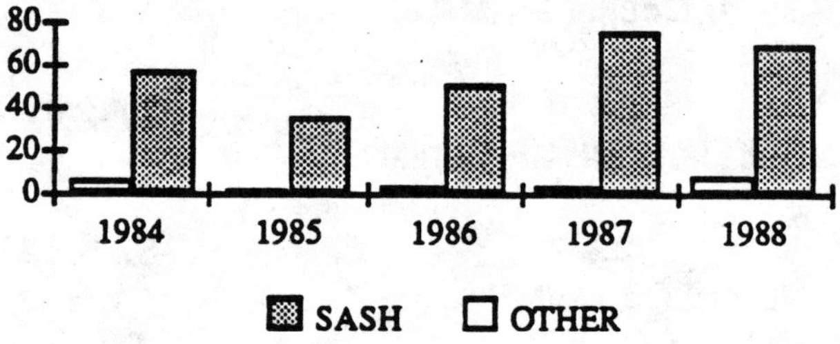

Admissions from Dimmit County

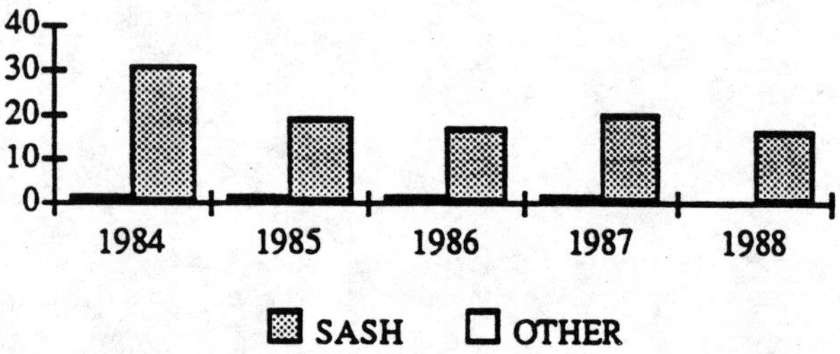

Admissions from Frio County

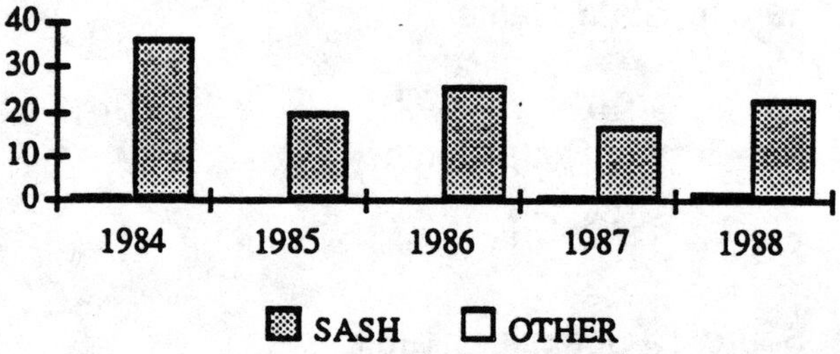

Figure 5.3 cont.

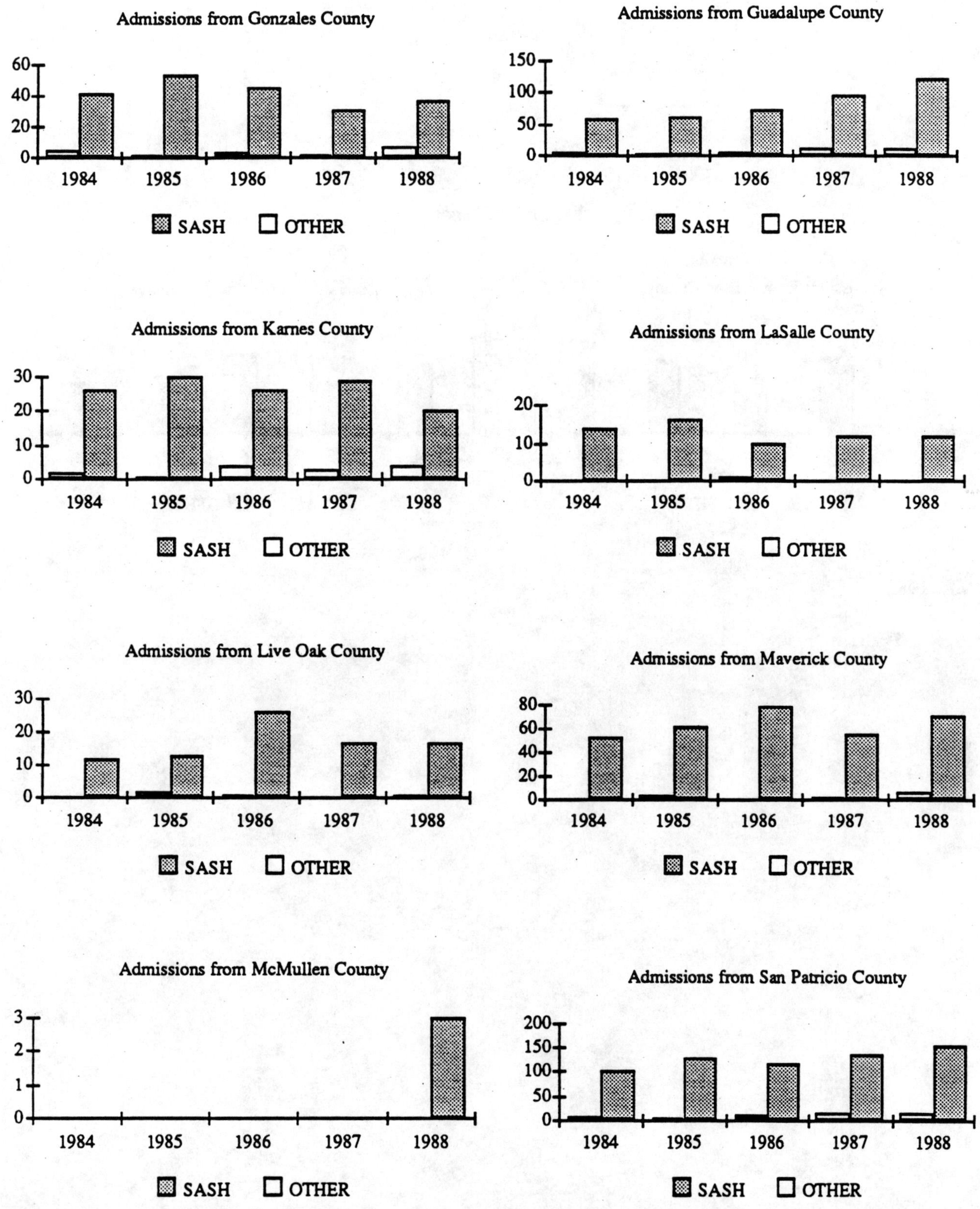

Figure 5.3 cont.

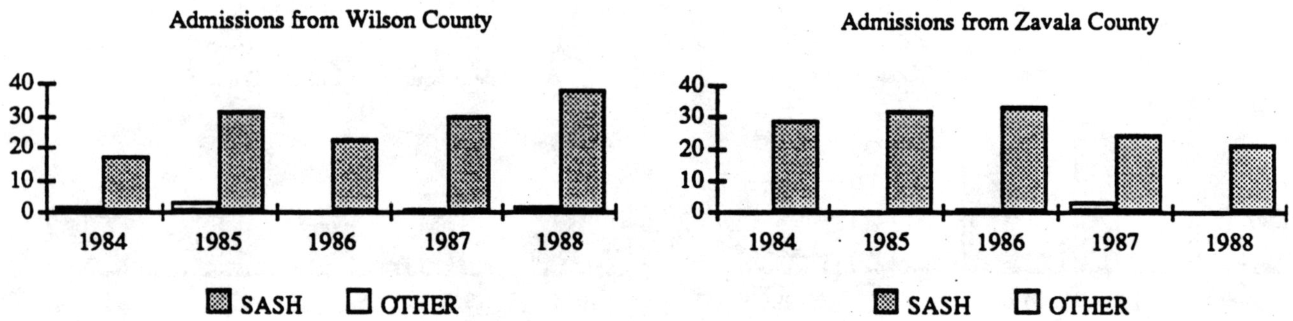

TDMHMR, 1988.

Figure 5.4. Percentages of Voluntary and Involuntary Inpatient Admissions by County

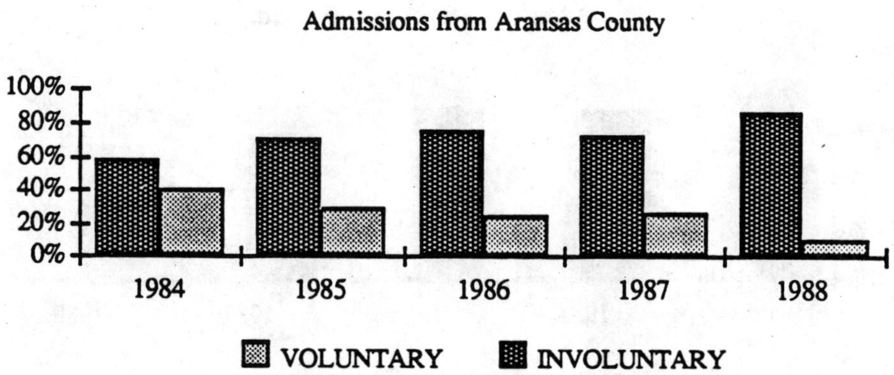

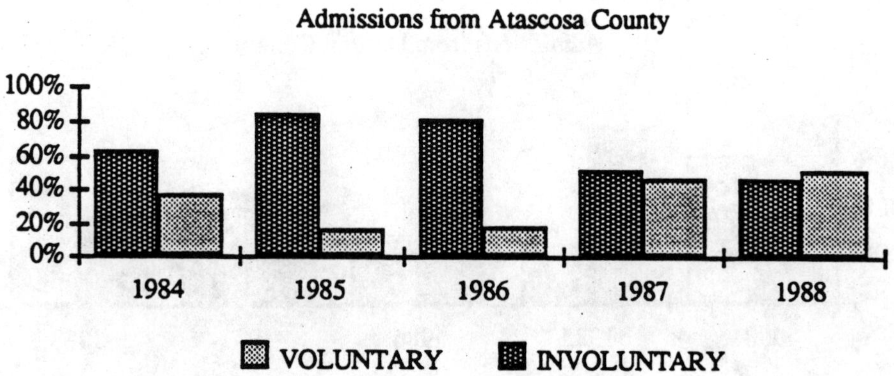

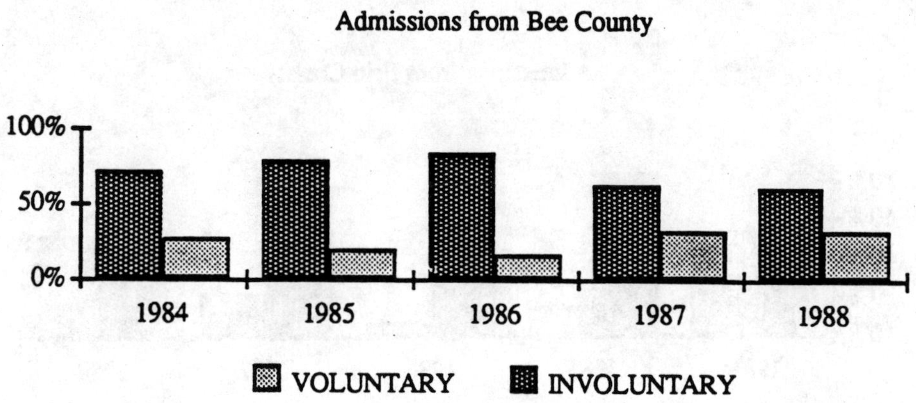

Figure 5.4 cont.

Admissions from Comal County

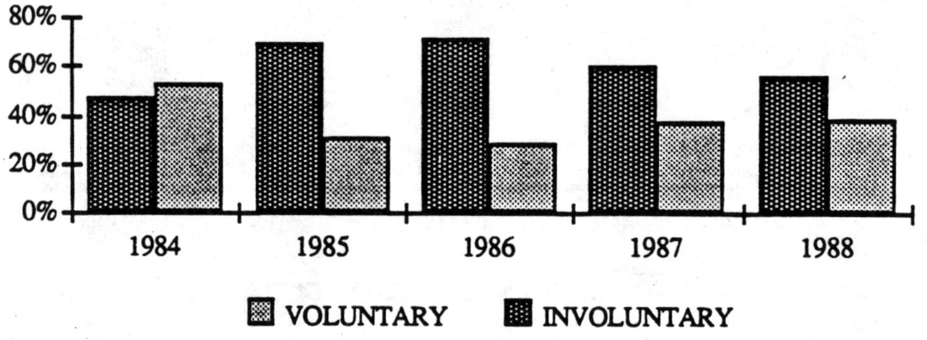

Admissions from Dimmit County

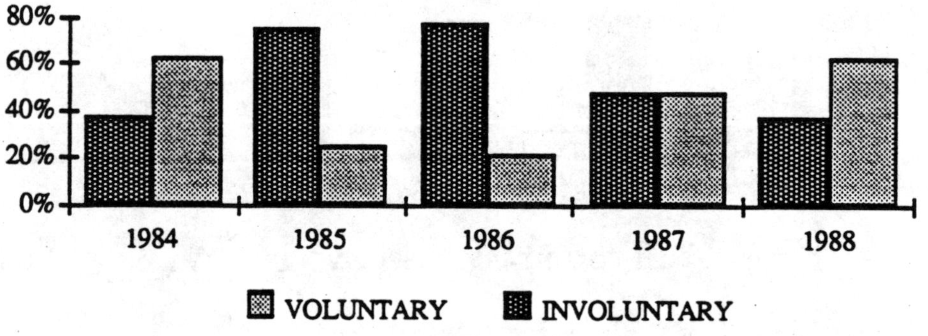

Admissions from Frio County

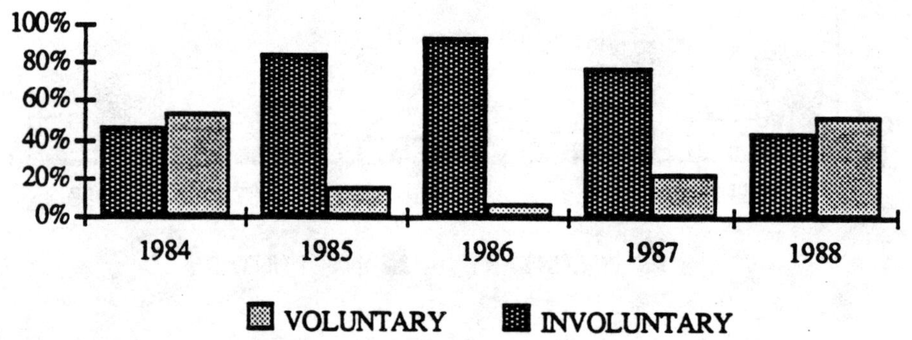

Figure 5.4 cont.

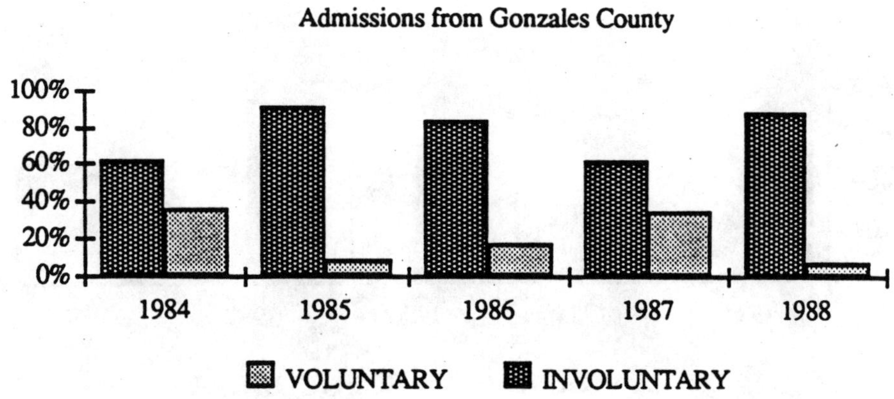

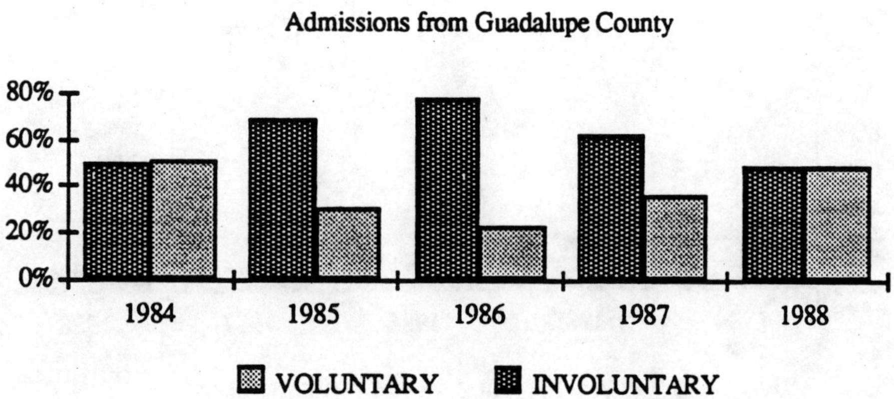

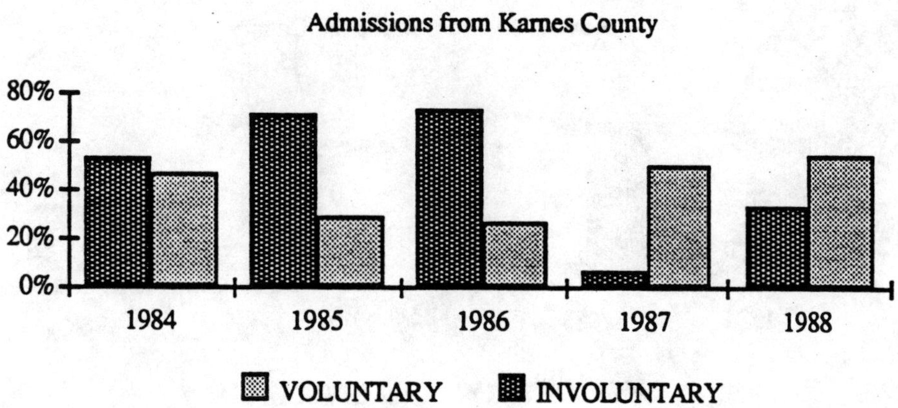

Figure 5.4 cont.

Admissions from LaSalle County

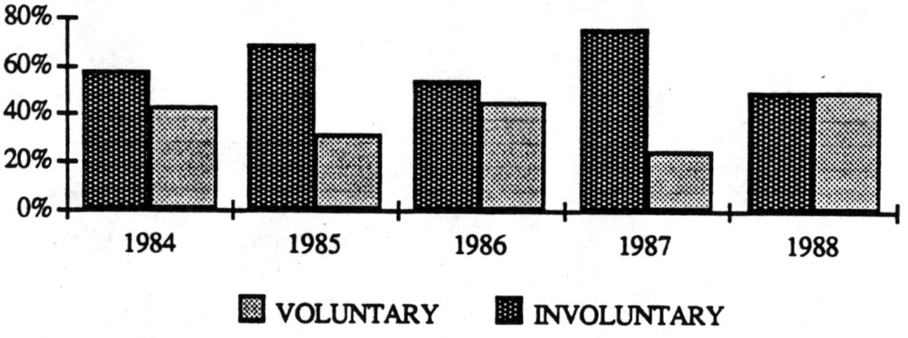

Admissions from Live Oak County

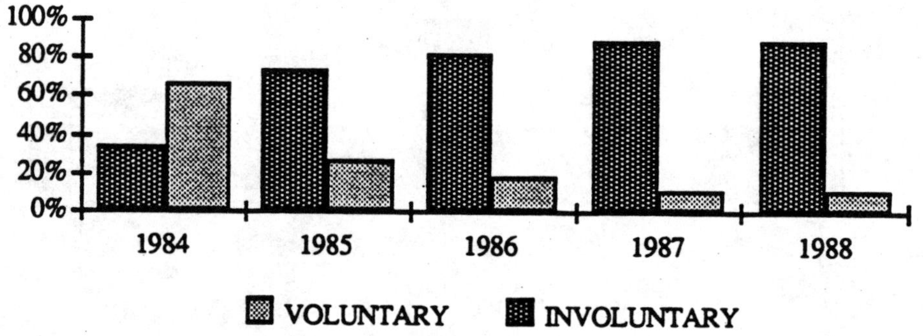

Admissions from Maverick County

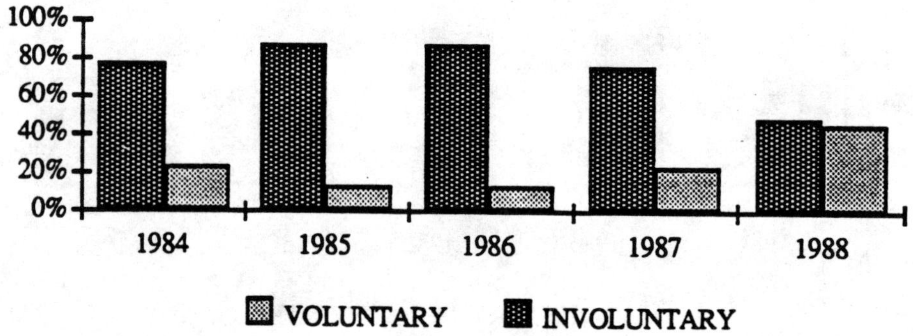

Figure 5.4 cont.

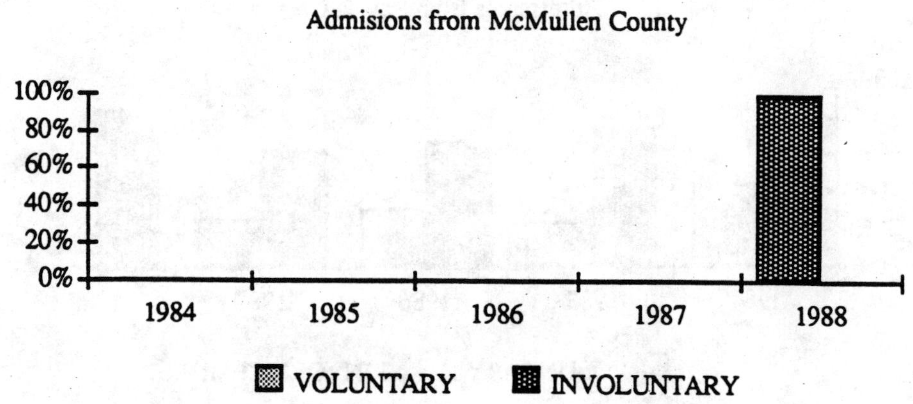

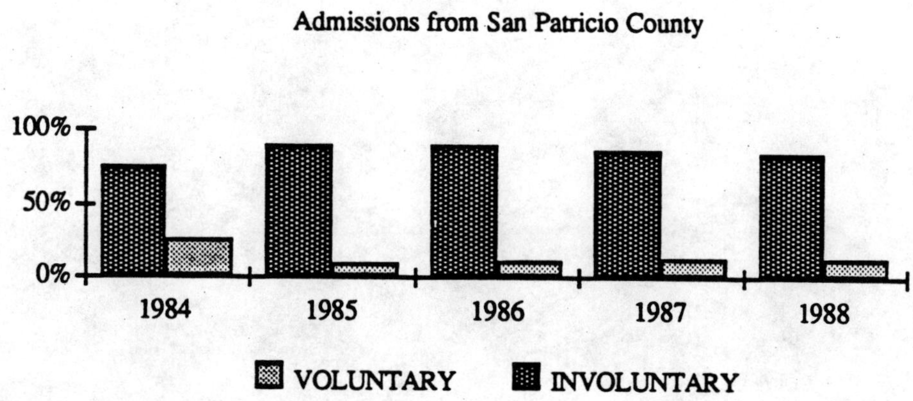

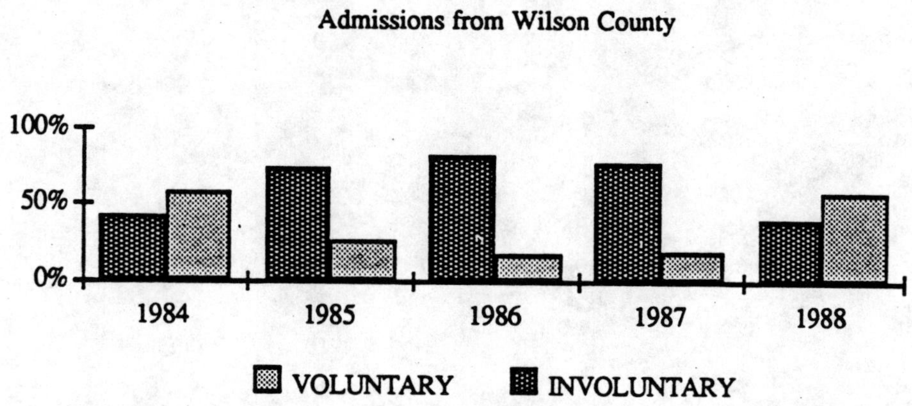

Figure 5.4 cont.

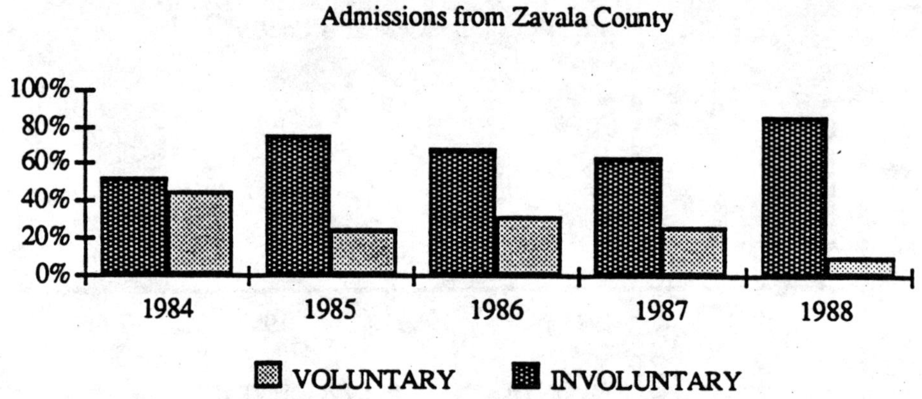

Source: TDMHMR, 1988

Figure 5.5 shows the percentage of total admissions that were first-time admissions for each of the counties in the outreach area. This is further broken down by the percentage of first admissions that were voluntary and involuntary. First admissions represent, in a limited way, the incidence of mental illness in a community which is severe enough to require hospitalization. Increasing rates of first admissions to the state hospital can be indicative of several underlying dynamics. Increasing rates can result from not only an increased community awareness of available services at the state hospital, but also lack of services within the community. In many cases, it may be some combination of the two. Generally, the actual incidence of serious mental illness in the population is fairly stable over time; therefore, local variations are generally indicative of local differences.

Atascosa and Live Oak counties showed a consistent upward trend in their first admissions over the five-year period. During 1988 and 1987, the first admissions from Atascosa County were almost evenly split between voluntary and involuntary. LaSalle and Wilson counties had an even split between voluntary and involuntary first admissions in 1988; however, from 1985 to 1987 they had more involuntary admissions. The opposite pattern held in 1984. The following counties have always had more voluntary first admissions than involuntary: Frio, Comal, Bee, Maverick, Aransas, Zavala, San Patricio, and Gonzales.

Several of these counties, along with LaSalle and Wilson, showed slight peaks in first-time admissions during 1986. Karnes and Guadalupe counties, prior to 1988, had more involuntary first admissions. Overall, their rate of first admissions has remained fairly constant; however, in 1988 the ratio shifted toward more voluntary than involuntary first admissions. When all of the counties are considered together, there is a slight increase in the percentage of first admissions from 38 percent in 1984 to 52 percent in 1988.

Figure 5.6 shows the five-year history for short-term versus long-term stays in inpatient facilities from the counties in the outreach area. For purposes of this case study, short-term is defined as 7 days or less and long-term is defined as 60 days or more. The levels of short-term stays in the state hospital may relate to the type of emergency care available in the community, while the level of long-term stays may be an indication of the needs of individual clients for extensive rehabilitation not available in the community.

Several counties have shown consistently more long-term stays in the inpatient facilities: Zavala, Wilson, San Patricio, and Gonzales. Of these counties, Zavala and Wilson have also shown increases in both short-term and long-term admissions during the past two years.

Dimmit and Maverick counties have consistently had more short-term than long-term admissions, and Atascosa and Frio had the opposite pattern until 1988, when they too had more short-term than long-term admissions. LaSalle, Karnes, and Aransas counties have recently shifted to having more long-term admissions.

In Live Oak, Guadalupe, Comal, and Bee counties there are about equal numbers of short-term and long-term admissions. Overall, short-term admissions account for between 16 percent to 20 percent of the total admissions over the past five years, with a slight increase in 1988. Long-term stays account for 21 percent to 26 percent of the admissions and peaked in 1985.

The overall impression that one derives from examining the above utilization patterns is one of wide diversity. No one trend can be seen to unify these impressions. All of the counties seem to use the state hospital facility for some of their short-term admissions; but at the same time, they send their longer-term clients to the state hospital facility as well. The differences in voluntary and involuntary commitment patterns may represent disparate and differing attitudes among county judges. In sum, there are many potential

Figure 5.5. Percentages of Admissions to SASH and Other Inpatient Facilities that Are First Admissions

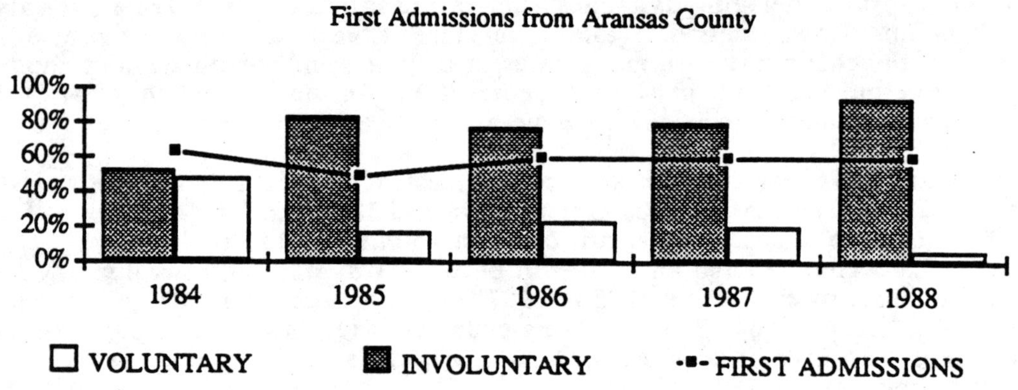

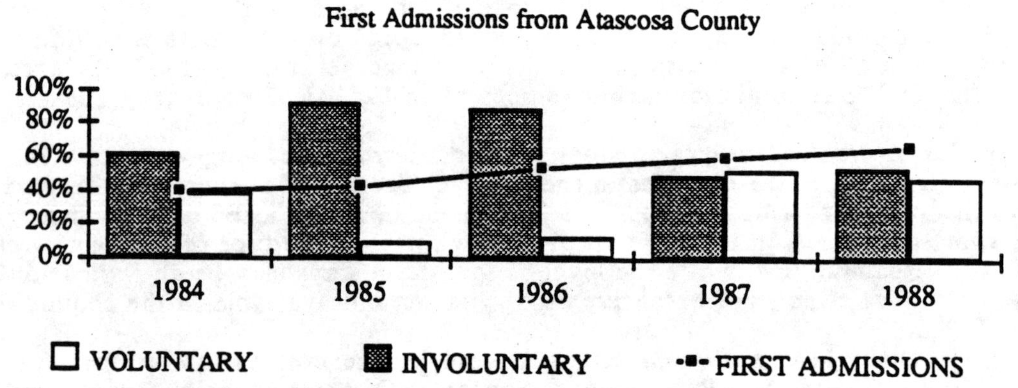

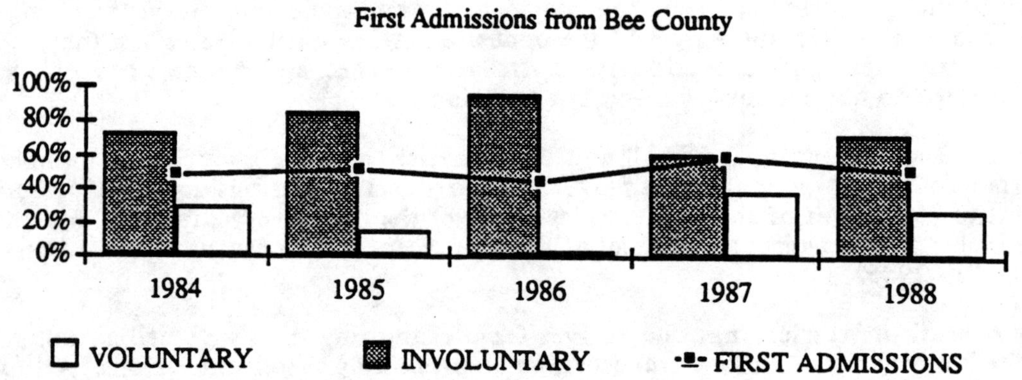

Figure 5.5 cont.

First Admissions from Comal County

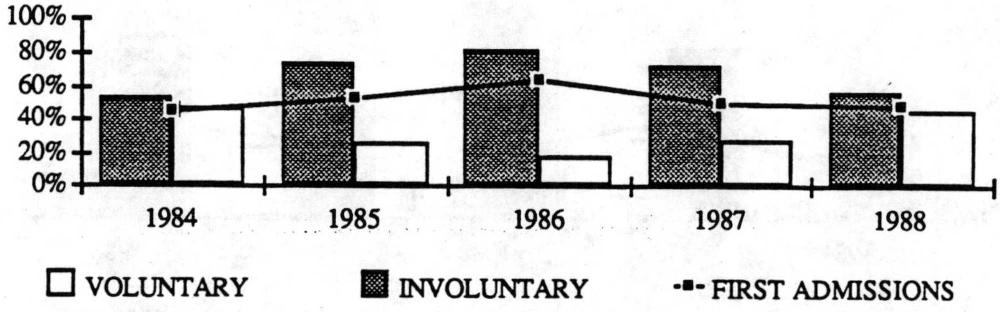

First Admissions from Dimmit County

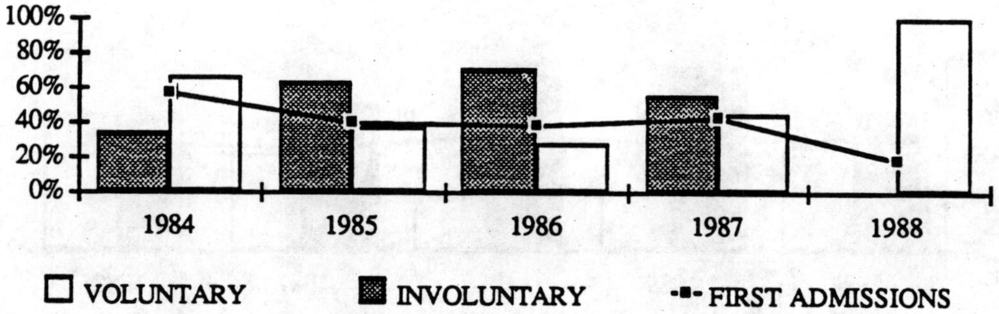

First Admissions from Frio County

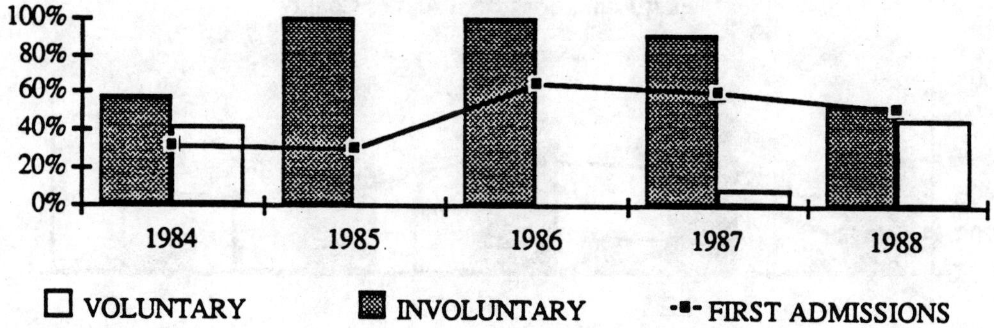

Figure 5.5 cont.

First Admissions from Gonzales County

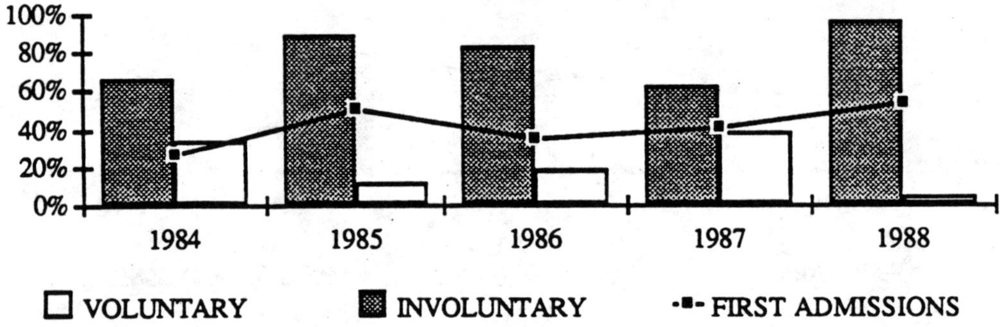

First Admissions from Guadalupe County

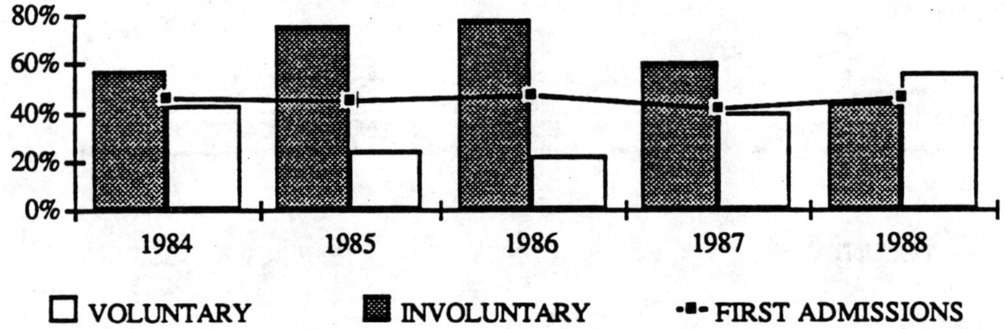

First Admissions from Karnes County

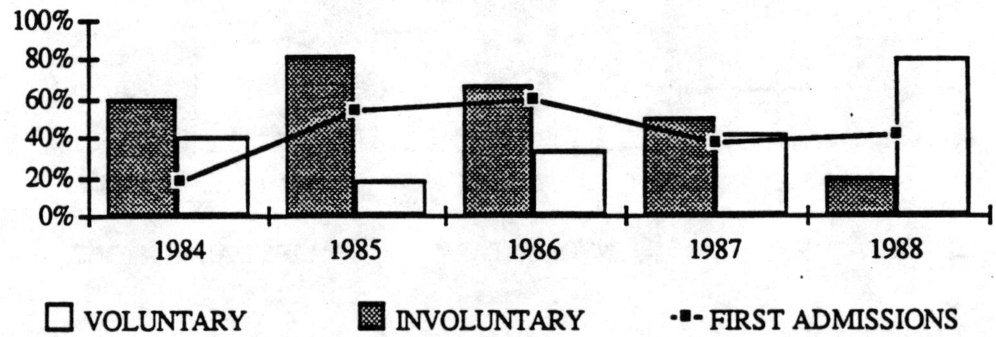

Figure 5.5 cont.

First Admissions from LaSalle County

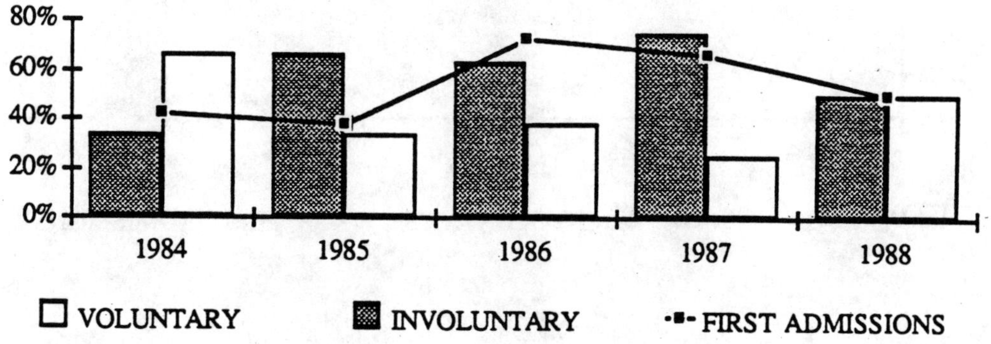

First Admissions from Live Oak County

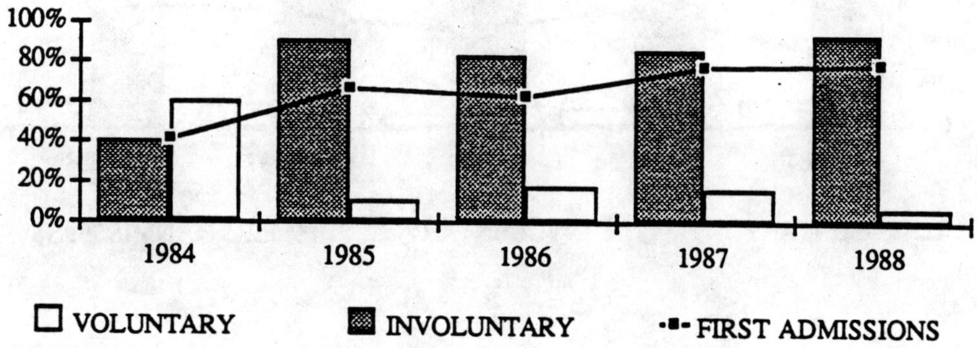

First Admissions from Maverick County

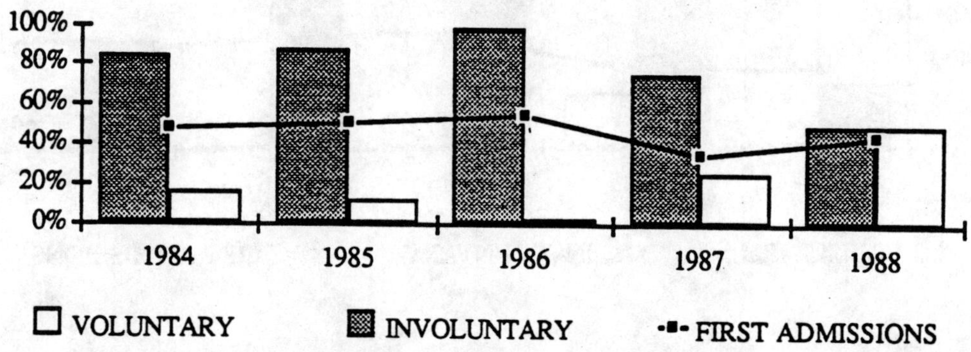

Figure 5.5 cont.

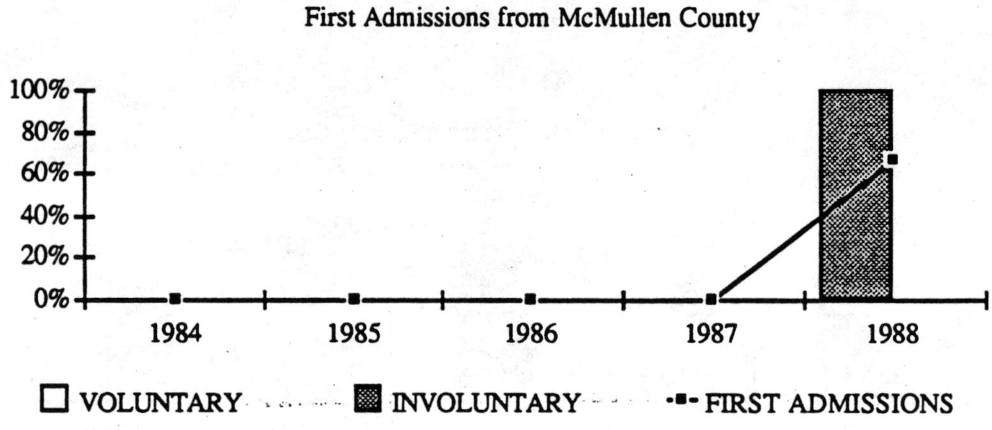

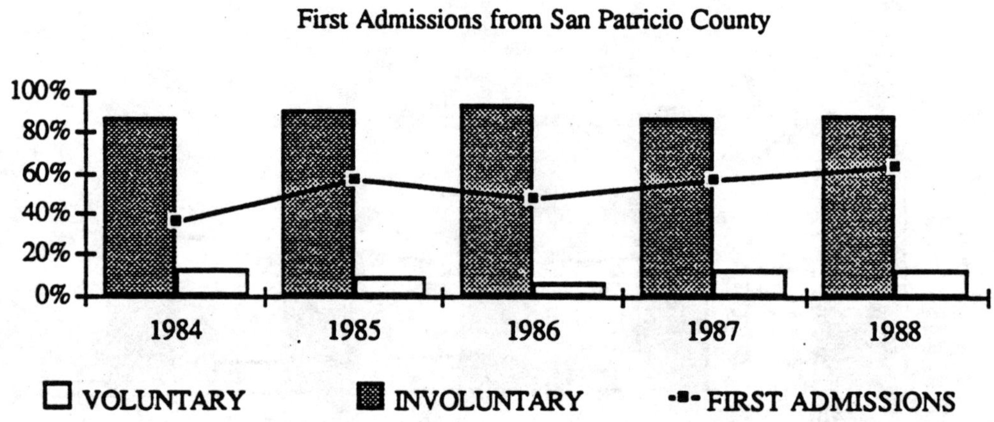

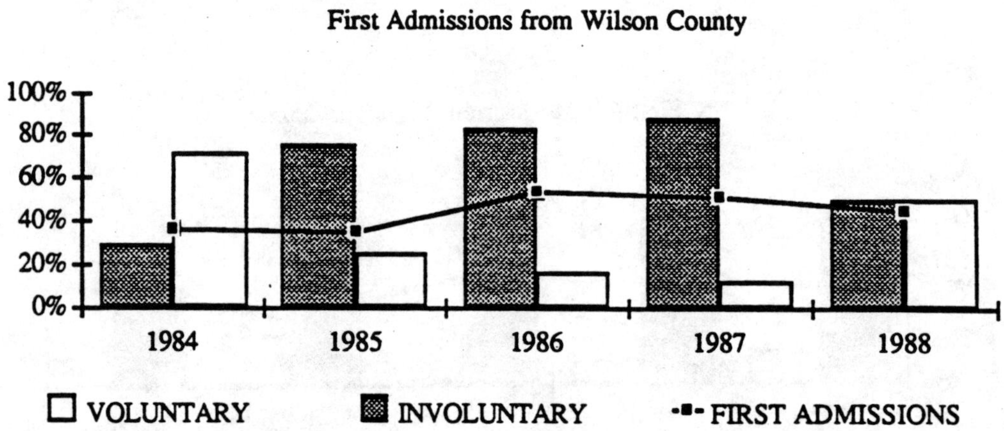

Figure 5.5 cont.

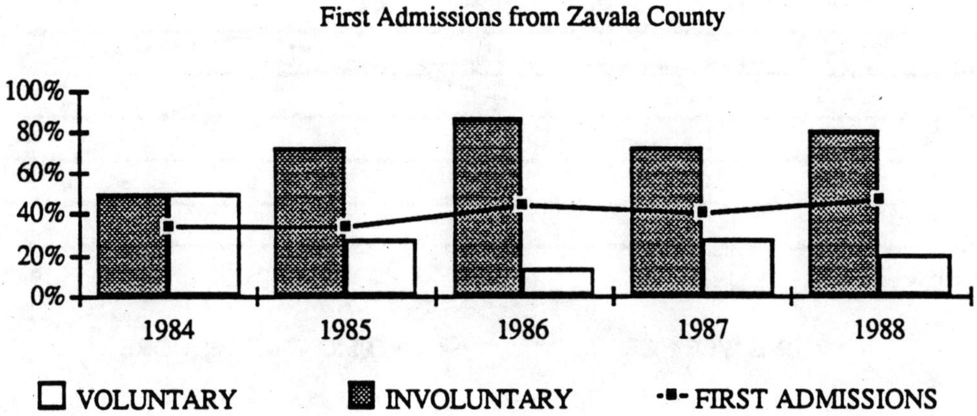

Source: TDMHMR, 1988.

Figure 5.6. A Comparison of Short-Term and Long-Term Admissions to Inpatient Facilities by County

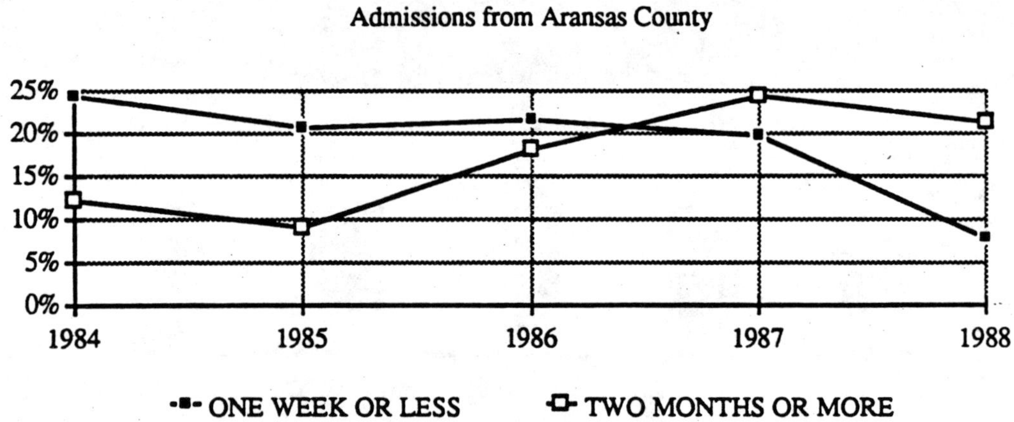

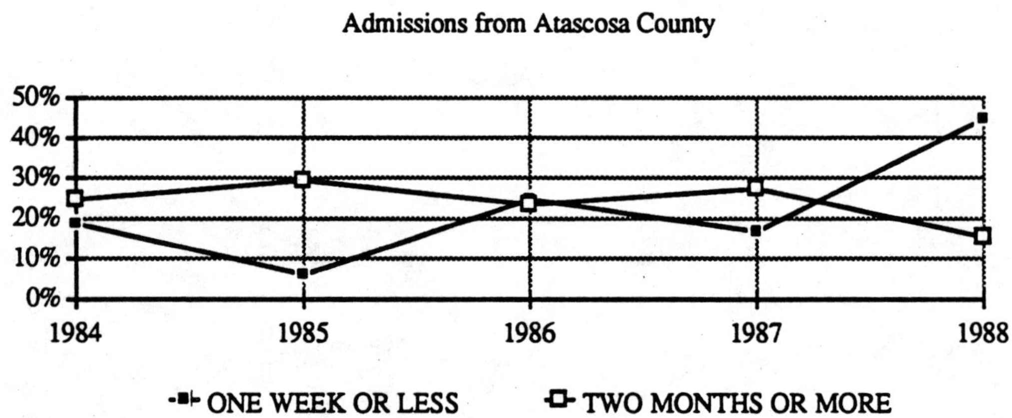

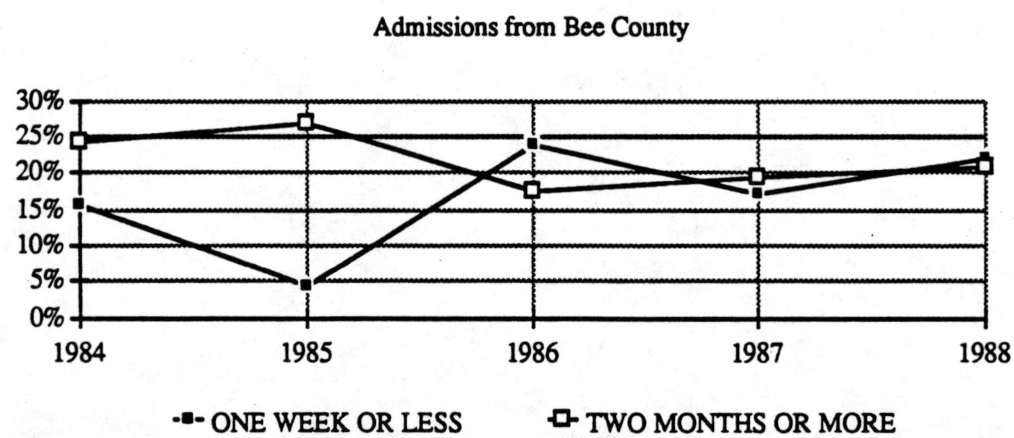

Figure 5.6 cont.

Admissions from Comal County

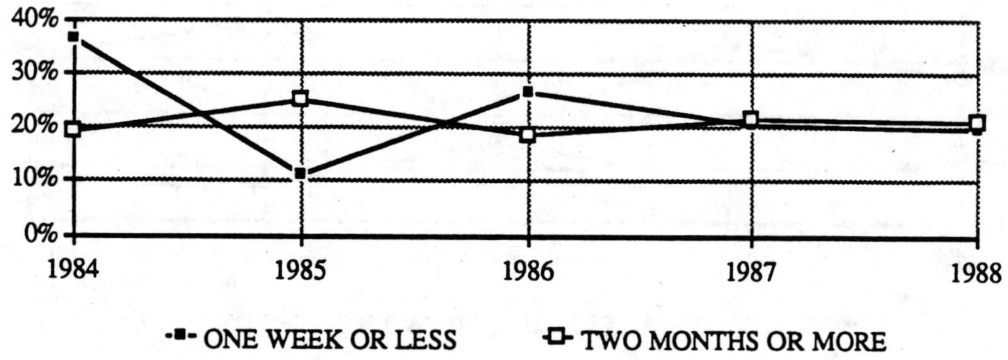

Admissions from Dimmit County

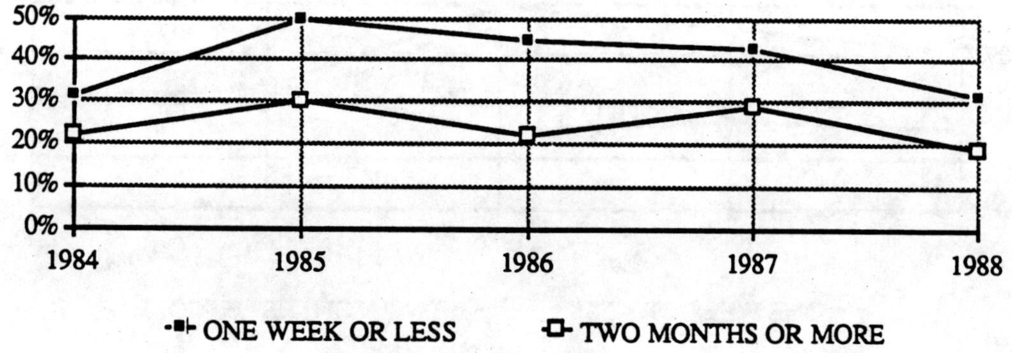

Admissions from Frio County

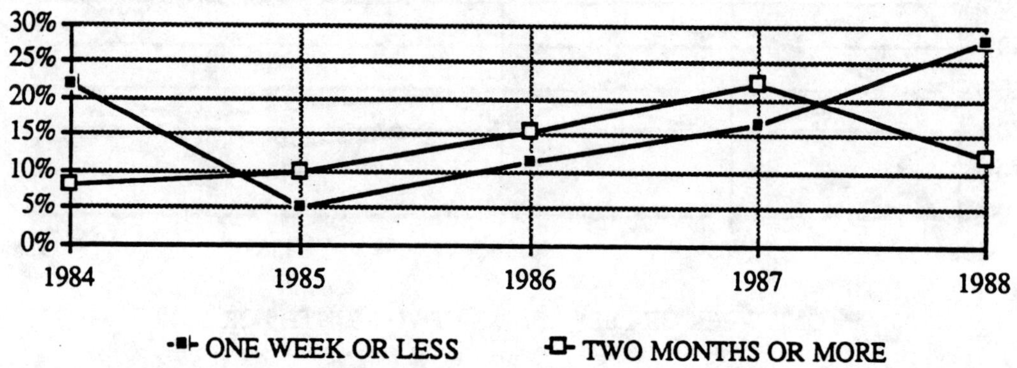

Figure 5.6 cont.

Admissions from Gonzales County

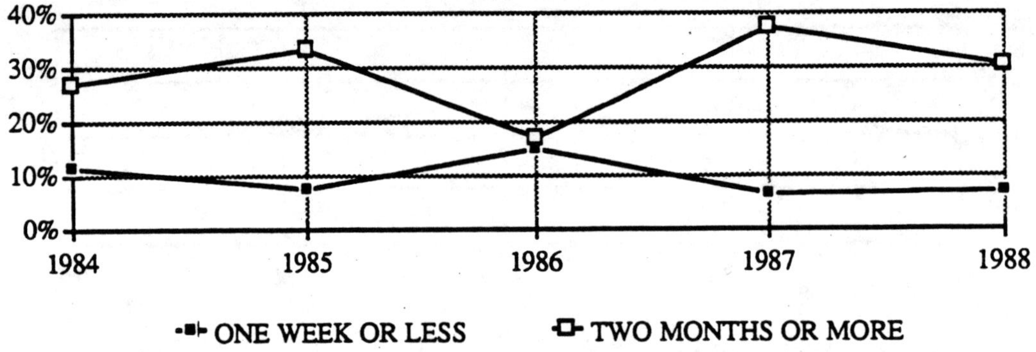

Admissions from Guadalupe County

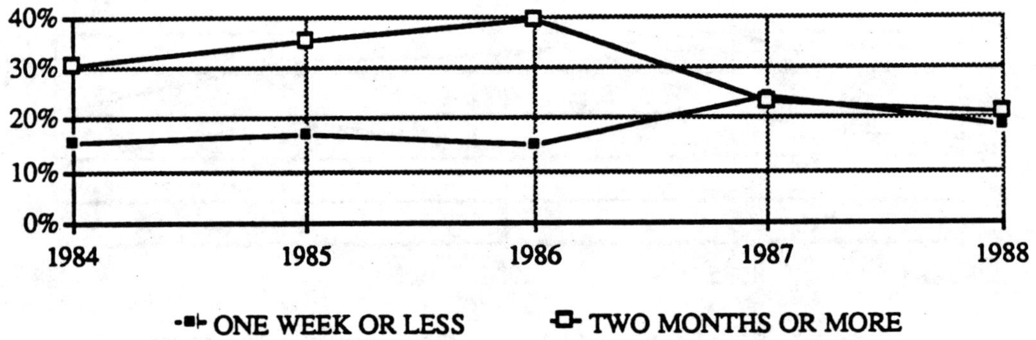

Admissions from Karnes County

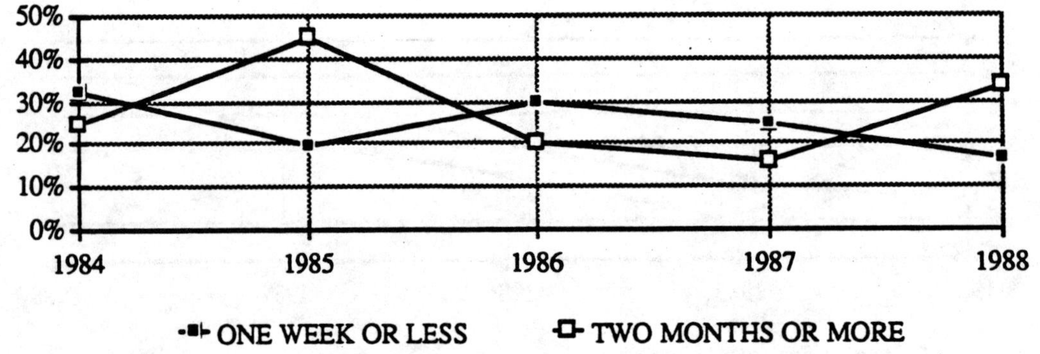

Figure 5.6 cont.

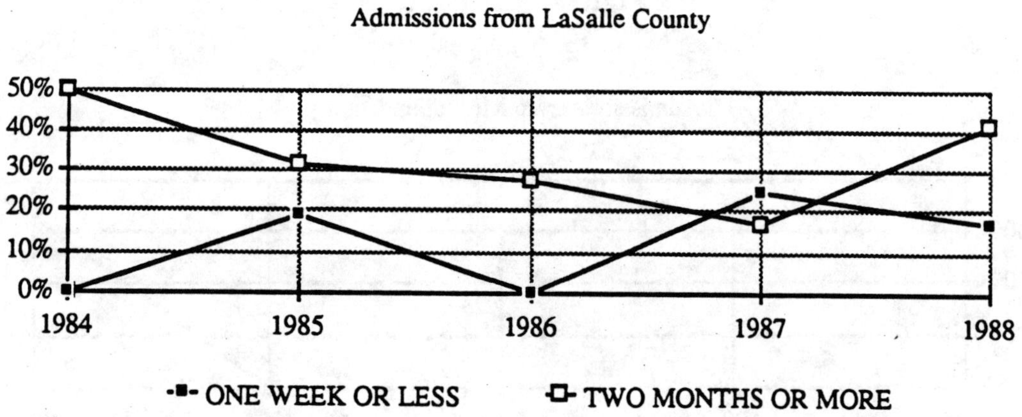

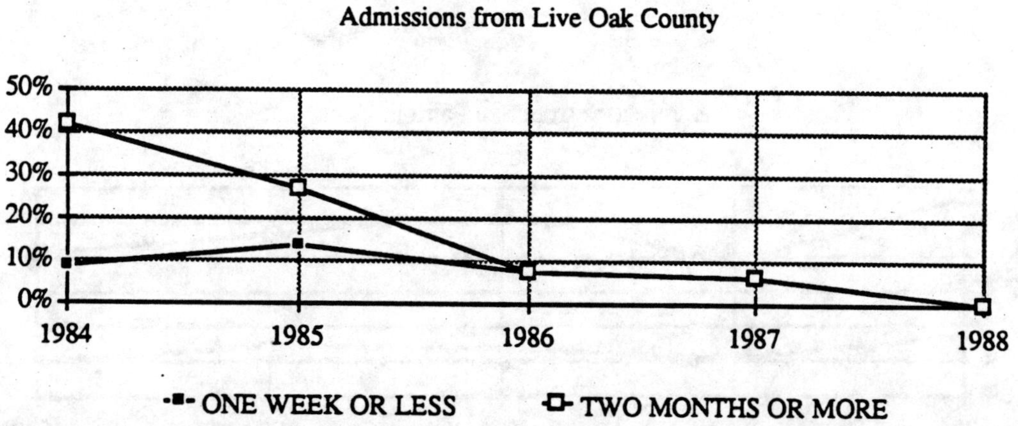

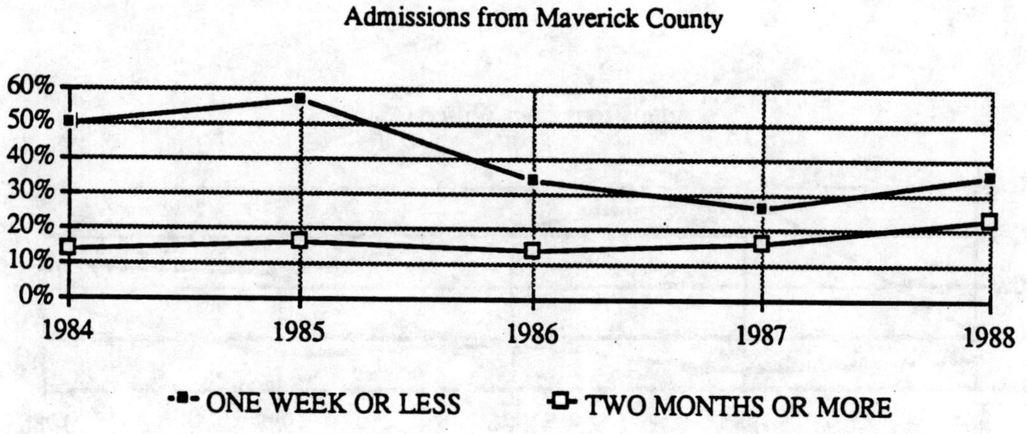

Figure 5.6 cont.

Admissions from McMullen County

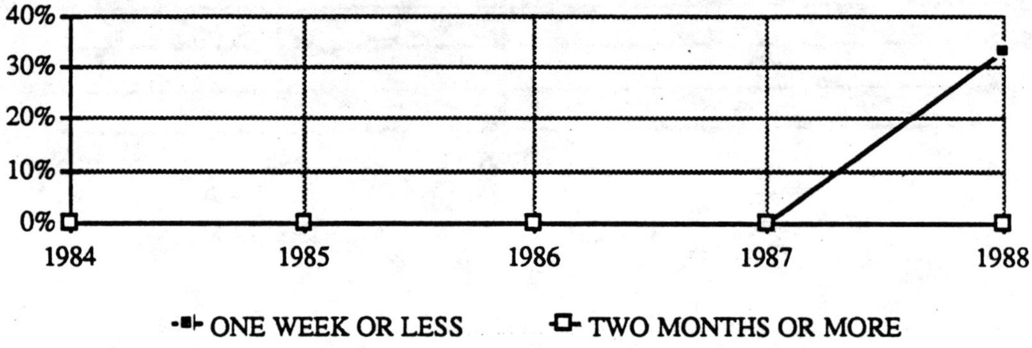

Admissions from San Patricio County

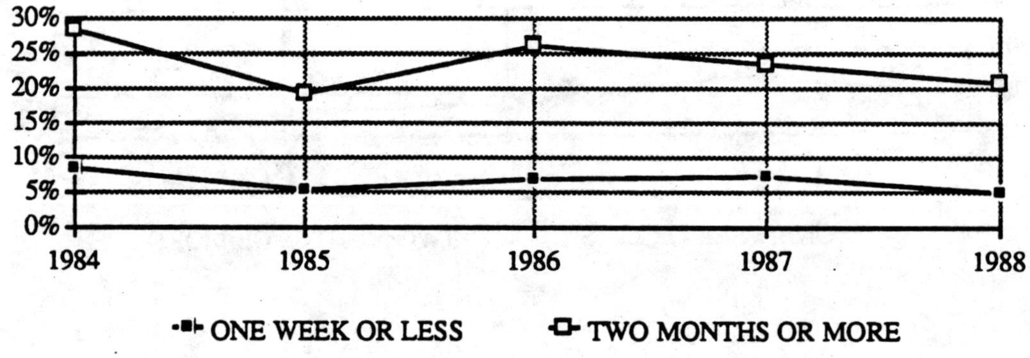

Admissions from Wilson County

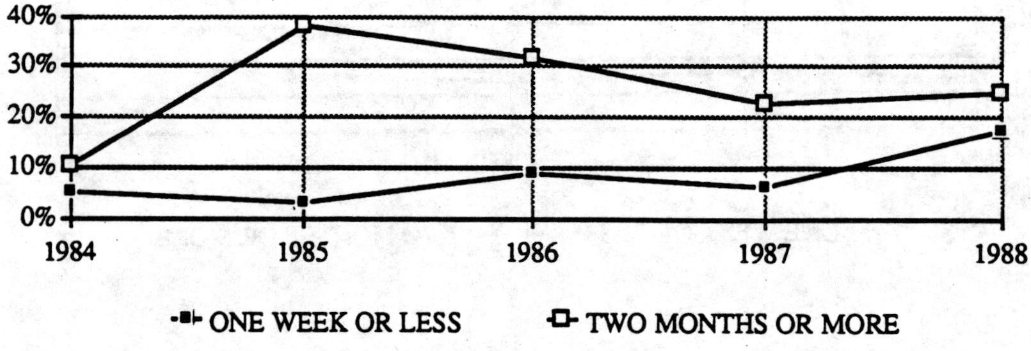

Figure 5.6 cont.

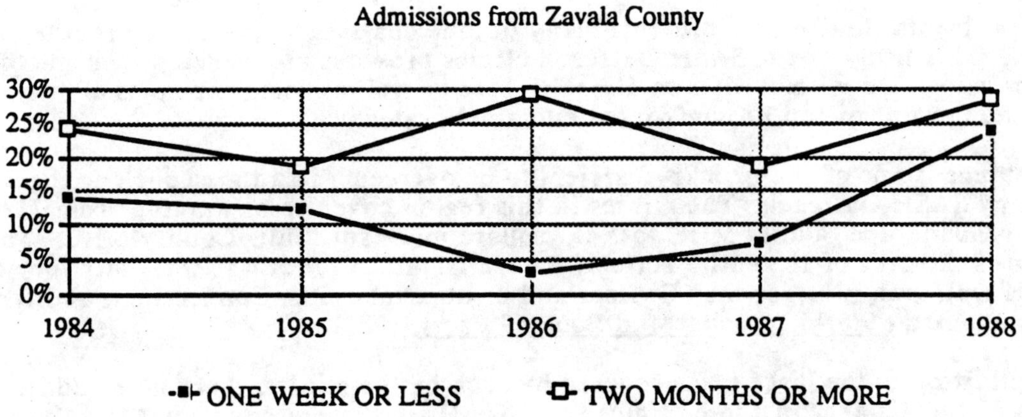

Source: TDMHMR , 1988.

factors concerning commitment to state hospital facilities impacting the utilization patterns seen among these different counties. In fact, the only thing which these counties may have in common is that they all receive mental health care through SASH.

CONCLUSIONS AND RECOMMENDATIONS

Rural mental health care presents many unique challenges to service providers and planners. This study of the SASH Outreach clinics provides an overview of some of the problems associated with rural mental health care as well as some examples of ways in which these problems can be confronted and ameliorated.

Distance is one of the primary barriers to be overcome in an area such as the one covered by SASH Outreach. The clinics in this region cover areas ranging from 713 square miles for Guadalupe County MHC to 3,457 square miles for Multi-County MHC. That is three times the area of the entire state of Rhode Island. In fact, the total territory covered by SASH Outreach is larger than Switzerland or Massachusetts, Connecticut, and Rhode Island combined (World Almanac and Book of Facts, 1987).

In addition to the large areas covered by each of the clinics, there is the additional problem of the distance of those clinics from SASH itself. Not counting Multi-County MHC, which has its home base at SASH and its community elsewhere, the nearest clinic is about 30 miles from SASH and the farthest is 140 miles away. The state hospital must often be relied upon for vital services not available in the smaller communities. It is also the home base for the professional mental health consultants who circulate from clinic to clinic providing psychiatric and psychological services not available full-time in the small clinics. In addition to these routine services, clients must often be transported to and from SASH for hospitalization when their needs cannot be met in the community. Because of the time involved in transit and the small staff at most of the clinics, this must often be done by law enforcement officials or families, rather than by staff who are familiar with the clients' problems and are trained to handle any unforeseen complications along the way.

Inadequate funding interacts with the problem of distance and isolation to create staffing shortages at most of the clinics. Recruiting and retaining well-trained staff in the rural community is a challenge at best. As noted in the introduction, there are few mental health professionals in rural communities across the state of Texas, and this area is no exception. Several of the clinics reported difficulty in recruiting master's-level staff even when they had openings. Paraprofessional staff must therefore be relied upon heavily in these areas to provide basic care to those in need. Although paraprofessionals can and do provide many valuable services in the community, this can seriously limit the range of services offered in a clinic. Psychological testing, medication evaluation, and professional counseling are available in most of the clinics only on a part-time basis, when the consultants visit from SASH. The need for these services in the community may not be part-time, however.

The rural counties with their respective small towns covered by SASH Outreach suffer from a paucity of many of the essential resources thought to be necessary for community care of the mentally ill. Hospitals in the rural area, when they exist, are often small and unequipped to provide the types of specialized care required by psychiatric emergencies. Five of the counties in the SASH Outreach area do not even have a hospital (Walker, Mountain, Barry, & Mayo, 1986).

Communities, therefore, often use the state facility as their psychiatric inpatient unit, for both long-term and short-term care. Alternative forms of housing for the mentally ill are more or less nonexistent in this rural community. Even nursing homes are scarce. Three of the SASH Outreach counties do not have even one nursing facility.

Vocational training and rehabilitation is difficult in an area in which jobs are not available for many of the general citizenry, much less for those with mental illness. The unemployment rate in the SASH Outreach area ranges from about 6 percent in Wilson County to 30 percent in Maverick County (Suniga, 1989).

The overall low level of funding available for mental health care in Texas interacts with the problems idiosyncratic to rural mental health care. Recruiting staff may be especially difficult in rural areas, but it is much harder when adequate salaries and incentives cannot be offered. The large distances that must be traveled by any one staff person could be shortened if there were more staff available to cover those distances. And community resources can often be developed through education and consultation. Additional funds would help in all of these situations.

There are several recommendations that can be made based on this study of the SASH Outreach. Some require additional funding for adequate implementation; others do not. Most build upon efforts already in place at this time.

An area that the SASH Outreach clinic staff has emphasized as being extremely important in the provision of mental health care in their communities is that of community involvement. All of the clinics rely heavily on local physicians, law enforcement officers, and others in the community for a variety of services. They provide a network of knowledgeable individuals who can refer clients in need, help clients obtain public assistance when eligible, transport them to the hospital, and aid in the evaluation of emergency situations. A more formalized emphasis on community education might do much to improve services in these areas. The SASH psychiatrists who currently visit the clinics to see clients might be able to serve more actively as consultants to the local physicians in emergency situations and to conduct short seminars for local physicians. This type of backup, combined with some formal training for those physicians in up-to-date use of psychotropic medications might permit many more emergencies to be handled locally by the family physicians rather than requiring transport to SASH for evaluation and treatment. Local hospital staff, with some additional training, might be able to handle more varied psychiatric emergencies in their own facility. Education of law enforcement officers in the handling of psychiatric emergencies might allow them to defuse many situations before they result in incarceration and/or commitment. Expansion of the family education groups might allow many crises to be averted in the home itself. None of these suggestions require extensive funds, just knowledgeable staff, working in concert with families, and in most cases the groundwork is already in place. In some of the counties, there is already an informal network which provides similar services. Community education at many levels can go far to develop community resources.

Recruiting and retaining staff in rural communities requires incentives over and above salary level. The professional isolation associated with rural areas must be addressed as well. In some ways, SASH is in a good position to solve this problem. The state hospital, as home base for the Outreach operations, could serve a dual purpose for training and staff enrichment opportunities. For example, if staff from the Outreach clinics came together with their co-professionals at the hospital regularly for meetings and training, several benefits would ensue. Isolation would be reduced, information would be shared, and morale might benefit. In addition, this would encourage the development of the kind of ongoing professional relationships among the inpatient and outpatient staff that would help to ensure continuity of care when clients from the Outreach clinics are hospitalized at SASH. One of the limitations of this type of plan is that currently, with the small staff available at the Outreach clinics, it would be difficult to spare key personnel for meetings in San Antonio very often. With increased staffing, however, this may become more feasible. It would also be a good idea for some training to be done in the home community.

Linkages with community agencies, such as the local Texas Rural Health Initiative Clinics, and community colleges might be initiated. There might be multiple benefits for all concerned if such alliances could be made.

Education of another type might also bolster the Outreach clinic's staffs. If relationships could be developed with colleges and universities for the placement of interns from various mental health disciplines at rural centers for their supervised practica, all concerned might benefit. The clinics would gain trained staff, and the interns would gain invaluable experience in rural mental health care. Many might even decide to continue to work with mental health programs (i.e., early childhood development, mental health clinics, etc.) in rural communities after finishing their education.

Cultural relevance is another important issue in the recruitment of staff for the SASH Outreach area, since 10 of the counties in this area are over 50 percent Hispanic. It is very important to recruit staff that are bilingual and familiar with the Hispanic culture to work in this area. Training in bi-cultural issues should also be provided for the current staff when needed. This training should not be limited to the staff at the clinic sites, but also be offered to those professionals who provide consultant services in this area. The resulting knowledge of relevant cultural issues may lead to more appropriate care.

There are some specific problems that relate more to the structure of the Outreach system than to rural mental health per se. Outreach, being funded through the state hospital, has been particularly vulnerable to the funding priorities set by the superintendent of the hospital. The current requirement that outreach budgets conform to a specific community-based funding formula should eliminate much of this vulnerability.

Another area of concern is with the structure of the case management system for outreach. Since case management services are housed at the state hospital administratively, there is the potential for less than perfect coordination with the clinics themselves. This type of administrative structure makes it essential that good communication be developed between case management and clinic staffs in order that there be less overlap of services, quicker response to emergencies, and better linkages with clinic staff and some system for follow-up care. It should also be recognized that in rural areas caseloads cannot be as large as they can be in more urban areas where less travel is required. At SASH, in particular, the case manager often has to cover an extremely large area. For example, there is one case manager for all of Dimmit and Zavala counties. This represents over 2,500 square miles that must be covered by one person (Brechtel, 1989).

The problems in rural mental health care are numerous but not insurmountable. From this case study, it can be seen that SASH Outreach clinics are not able, under the current funding levels and organizational structure, to fulfill all of the requirements of SB 633 and SB 257. Officials of TDMHMR, aware of funding and other related problems, have in some ways added to the problem. By trying to cope with the problems experienced by the outreach clinics, there has been a tendency to "cut them some slack" (Collier, 1989) when it comes to fulfilling the TDMHMR requirements for core services. But, by not holding outreach clinics to the same standard as the CMHCs, it follows that the people of rural Texas are not always receiving adequate mental health care. From the information presented in the previous sections it seems reasonable to assume that the greater rate of admissions to the state hospital from these outreach counties is related to and associated with the lack of adequate community services in these outreach areas. This situation forces the outreach clinics to use the state hospital more than CMHCs for basic mental health care.

In spite of these problems, however, there is a sense of dedication and competence at the SASH Outreach clinics that has allowed them to do much with what little they have to work with in rural, sparsely populated areas. Perhaps with some additional funding, which has been granted for FY 1990-1991, continued support from the SASH administration, and the continued creativity and enthusiasm witnessed among the Outreach clinic staff, the mental health services to this area will continue to improve and to grow.

Appendix 5.A. Mental Health Services Questionnaire

«Clinic» LSA «lsa»

«phone» «contact»

Contact Person :

______________________________Position____________________

How many clients are on your active caseload?

What is the cost of providing an hour of service?

What percent of your clients are unable to pay for services?

How many of your clients are on SSI? SSDI? Food Stamps?

What is the most frequent diagnosis?

How many people are on your staff currently?

What are their educational backgrounds?

Do you have any open staff positions to be filled?

<u>Crisis Stabilization Services</u>

24 hour crisis stabilization service is one of the core services which is supposed to be available to clients from each of the local service areas. How are these services provided by your center?

Do you contract with a local hospital for emergency beds?

How do you typically handle an emergency situation in which a client requires immediate hospitalization?

Is the state hospital typically used for crisis stabilization?

Is law enforcement generally cooperative in situations where commitment may be necessary?

What about the client who requires some additional supervision, but may not need hospitalization? Do you offer any supervised family living programs in which a client can be stabilized within a home situation where there is 24 hour supervision and on-call medical backup?

Emergency Screening

Do you have a 24 hour crisis hot line?

If not, how do clients in crisis access the mental health center after hours and on weekends?

Is there a crisis intervention team in your service area which provides emergency screening for clients who need to be seen by a professional because of their problems in order to determine if hospitalization is necessary?

Where is this team based?

How is it staffed?

This service may be provided through the emergency room of a hospital? If it is, are center staff involved, or is the crisis handled by whatever physician is on duty at the time?

Is the state hospital often used as an emergency screening facility?

If so, how are clients transported to and from the hospital for assessment?

Multidisciplinary Assessment

If a client is seen in crisis either in a hospital or in his home by a crisis team, his situation is supposed to be assessed within 24 hours by mental health professionals representing more than one discipline - specifically a physician (preferably a psychiatrist) and one or more representatives of nursing, psychology or social work. How is this service typically handled in your center's area?

Is this service typically handled at the state hospital?

Family Support Including Respite

What services do you offer to the families of your clients? Do you have support groups, provide education on the nature of mental illness and medications, etc?

Is there any provision in your area for respite care for the families of your clients? This can include homemaker services, visiting nurses, etc?

Case Management

How many of your clients are receiving case management services?

Where is the case management service based in your area?

Do you find that this arrangement allows for close enough supervision of the clients under case management?

What problems have you experienced with the case management system as it stands in your area/

Medication Related Services

Do you operate a medication clinic at your center?

How do you do the laboratory screening that is required for some medications?

Do you provide medication education / how / how often ?

Do you provide education on basic mental health issues and coping stategies for your clients?

Do you provide medications at your center?

Are clients charged for their medications?

Psychosocial Rehabilitation

What kinds of social support activities are provided through your center?

Are their social clubs for clients?

What about weekend outings, or other social gatherings?

Is their a day treatment program? If so, what is typically done in the program, and who attends?

Do you offer vocational or pre-vocational training training through your center?

Is there any opportunity for sheltered employment?

This service may be provided through collaboration with TRC or local Community Colleges, etc. If they don't mention either of these, ask if they work with these agencies to provide this service.

<u>Housing Services</u>

What kinds of residential services are available for your clients who need this kind of help?

Nursing Home Placement?

Board and Care Homes?

Half Way Houses?

Personal Care Home?

Group Homes?

Supervised Apartments?

Fairweather Lodges?

Other?

How many of your clients receive some kind of residential services?

References

Battle-Ledford, Susie. 1989. Director, Comal County Mental Health Clinic, New Braunfels, Texas. Telephone interview by Minh Ly Griffin, March 9.

Bayne, Calvin. 1989a. Business Manager, San Antonio State Hospital, San Antonio, Texas. Letter to Nicholas Hoover, July 13.

_________. 1989b. Business Manager, San Antonio State Hospital, San Antonio, Texas. Telephone Interview with Nicholas Hoover, July 26.

Brechtel, Joann. 1989. Chief of Case Management, San Antonio State Hospital, San Antonio, Texas. Telephone interview by Pam M. Diamond, June 1.

Bruce, Vivian. 1989. Director, Atascosa County Mental Health Clinic, Jourdanton, Texas. Telephone interview by Minh Ly Griffin, March 14.

Burk, Frances. 1989. LVN and Acting Director, San Patricio County Mental Health Clinic, Sinton, Texas. Telephone interview by Minh Ly Griffin, March 6.

Collier, Cathy. 1989. Assistant Deputy Commissioner of Region III, Texas Department of Mental Health and Mental Retardation. In-class presentation to Policy Research Project, April 4.

Crabtree, Shirley. 1989. Director, Gonzales County Mental Health Clinic, Gonzales, Texas. Telephone interview by Minh Ly Griffin, March 1.

Esparza, Profirio. 1989a. Director, SASH Outreach Services, San Antonio, Texas. Interview by Pamela Diamond, Minh Ly Griffin, and Nicholas Hoover, February 11.

_________. 1989b. Director, SASH Outreach Services, San Antonio, Texas. Telephone interview by Nicholas Hoover, March 28.

Flores, Raymond. 1989. Director, Dimmit County Mental Health Clinic, Carrizo Springs, Texas. Telephone interview by Minh Ly Griffin, March 1.

Gonzalez, Rigoberto, Regional Support Specialist TDMHMR. 1989. "Region III Mental Health Quarterly Report: FY 1989."

Parsons, Ann. 1989. Director, Multi-County Mental Health Clinic, San Antonio, Texas. Telephone interview by Minh Ly Griffin, March 6.

Rossett, Allen Ray. 1989a. Director and LVN, Karnes County Mental Health Clinic, Kenedy, Texas. Interview by Pamela Diamond, Minh Ly Griffin, and Nicholas Hoover, February 11.

_________. 1989b. Director and LVN, Karnes County Mental Health Clinic, Kenedy, Texas. Telephone interview by Minh Ly Griffin, March 7.

San Antonio State Hospital. 1989a. "San Antonio State Hospital Monthly Operating Report by Fund and Department"; Run Date 1/17/89 as of 12/31/88. Fund 05: Community Services.

_________. 1989b, "San Antonio State Hospital Outreach Services," San Antonio, Texas, January 4.

Schnee, Steven B. 1989. Superintendent, San Antonio State Hospital, San Antonio, Texas. Telephone interview by Pamela Diamond, June 21.

Smith, Jerry. 1989. Budget Director, Texas Department of Mental Health and Mental Retardation, Austin, Texas. Telephone interview by Nicholas Hoover, June 6.

Smith, Jim. 1989. Budget Analyst, Texas Department of Mental Health and Mental Retardation, Austin, Texas. Telephone interview by Nicholas Hoover, July 18.

Stockley, John. 1989. Director, Maverick County Mental Health Clinic, Eagle Pass, Texas. Telephone interview by Minh Ly Griffin, March 13.

Texas Department of Health. 1988. "State Health Planning and Resource Development," Austin, Texas.

Texas Department of Mental Health and Mental Retardation (TDMHMR). 1989a. "Future Directions." (June 23). (Working Draft).

_________. 1989b. "Strategic Planning." (February 13).

_________. 1989c. "Characteristics of SASH MH Clients with Open Community Assignments." (February 8). (Computer printout).

_________. 1988. "CARE system database; records for all inpatient clients with admissions from 9/1/83 to 10/1/88." Austin, Texas.

_________. 1987. "CARE: Reference Manual." Austin, Texas.

World Almanac and Book of Facts. 1987. Pharos Books.

Ward, Mike. 1989. "MHMR Settlement Opposed: Court Appointed Monitor Faults State Appropriations." Austin American Statesman, June 30.

Zuniga, Rosemary. 1989. Information Specialist, Texas Department of Commerce, Austin, Texas. Telephone interview by Pam Diamond, June 2.

Chapter 6. Summary and Conclusions

When community mental health centers were created by the federal Community Mental Health Center Act of 1963, their mission was not entirely clear. Between that time and the early 1980s, a dual system for treatment of the mentally ill evolved. The community mental health and mental retardation centers, which during their early years were primarily funded through local and federal monies, were attempting to meet the mental health needs of their communities under general federal guidelines as they saw fit. TDMHMR primarily concentrated on the state hospitals and state centers, although its hold over the state hospitals was tenuous because the hospitals were line items in the TDMHMR budget, and essentially received funds directly from the legislature. What developed was one ideology emphasizing community-based care, with little or no money, and another ideology emphasizing institutionalization, which was underfunded but still received most of the state's monetary attention.

With the advent of psychotropic drugs and new psychotherapies, the emphasis on state institutions has become somewhat anachronistic. Two other events had a significant effect on the financial relationship between TDMHMR and CMHMRCs. The first was the shift from categorical grants, which went directly to the centers from the federal government, to block grants in 1981. This move reduced the federal financial commitment to mental health care and also made TDMHMR the primary conduit of federal funds to the CMHMRCs. The second major financial change came about because of the <u>R. A. J v. Jones</u> settlement agreement. This forced the state legislature to invest more money into mental health care delivery. One irony of this increased financial attention is that the level of funding for state hospitals has increased while the average daily census has decreased.

Even with the court suit, Texas has lagged in allocating funds for the chronically mentally ill. In FY 1988, Texas allocated approximately $500 million for the chronically mentally ill, of which about $90 million was for community care (Warner, Crumpton, and Watts, forthcoming, p. 185). In 1985 the national average for per capita mental health expenditures was $38.40, compared with only $18.70 per capita in Texas. Not only is the level of state support for community-based care quite limited, it also is quite variable between the different community centers, especially with regard to state hospital outreach areas. Now that 60 percent of the total funds being received by the community centers for mental health services are state monies, there is a greater demand by the state for accountability, uniformity of services, and availability of care to persons across the state. These centers still continue to have an ambivalent role since as 501-C3 entities they are independent of the state and accountable to their boards and local funding sources. On the other hand, since most of their funding comes from the state to take care of persons who are at least in one sense partially wards of the state, they are extensions of the state mental health system.

By examining these four community-based mental health delivery systems, it can be seen that accessibility, continuity, and level of funding vary greatly. The Legislative Budget Board's report to the 71st Legislature points out, "The cost per services vary greatly between mental health service areas for reasons not totally explained by geographical or other economic circumstances" (LBB, 1989, p. 145).

To illustrate this point, Table 6.1 shows the characteristics, revenue sources, expenditures, and service provision for the three CMHCs and one state hospital outreach that we analyzed.

The first notable variation in service is in the number of clients served within the service area. The highest level in this category, as in almost all categories, is Tri County MHMRC, which has 694 clients per 100,000. Dallas County MHMR and Concho Valley are

Table 6.1. Variation in Fiscal Year 1988 Characteristics, Revenue, Expenditure, and Services Provision Among the Mental Health Services Providers in Case Studies

	Provider			
	Concho Valley	Dallas	Tri County	SASH Outreach
PROVIDER CHARACTERISTICS				
Square Miles	9,369	880	3,007	15,031
Area Population	117,700	1,810,294	325,852	363,600
Per Square Mile	12.56	2,057.15	108.36	24.19
Total MH Clients	611	8,751	2,262	1,406
Clients Served per 100K	519.12	483.40	694.18	386.69
PROVIDER REVENUE SOURCES				
Total MH				
Revenues FY 1988	$1,114,640	$19,956,391	$4,112,153	$1,127,278
Per Capita	$9.47	$11.02	$12.62	$3.10
Local	$322,252	$4,606,909	$1,959,004	N/A
Per Capita	$2.74	$2.54	$6.01	
Local Tax Revenue	* $119,657	$3,963,138	* $135,848	N/A
Per Capita	$1.02	$2.19	$0.42	
Percent of Local Funds				
as Local Taxes	37.13%	86.03%	6.93%	
State	$736,470	$10,935,953	$2,015,567	$1,127,278
Per Capita	$6.26	$6.04	$6.19	$3.10
Federal	$55,918	$450,379	$137,582	N/A
Per Capita	$0.48	$0.25	$0.42	
PROVIDER EXPENDITURE CHARACTERISTICS				
MH Expenditures by Program				
Residential Services	$240,428	$6,743,068	$1,216,803	N/A
Percent of Budget	21.57%	42.13%	25.16%	
Expenditure per client	$393.50	$770.55	$537.93	
Client and Family				
Support Services	$675,191	$7,188,189	$2,929,886	N/A
Percent of Budget	60.57%	44.91%	60.58%	
Client to Expenditure	$1,105.06	$821.41	$1,295.26	
Case Management	$74,121	$522,499	$167,295	N/A
Percent of Budget	6.65%	3.26%	3.46%	
Client to Expenditure	$121.31	$59.71	$73.96	
Management & Support	$124,900	$1,550,444	$522,027	
Percent of Budget	11.21%	9.69%	10.79%	N/A
Client to Expenditure	$204.42	$177.17	$230.78	
PROVIDER SERVICE PROVISION				
State Hospital Admissions	142	1400	41	842
Per 100K population	120.65	77.34	12.58	231.57
Number of Case Managers	3	10	7	6
Case Managers Per Client	204	875	323	234
Total Residential Beds	15	417	66	0
Per 100K population	12.74	23.03	20.25	0.00
Crisis Stabilization Beds	1	80	18	0
Per 100K population	0.85	4.42	5.52	0.00

* Local tax revenue for mental health for Concho Valley and Tri County MHMRC were calculated by multiplying the percentage of the total budget allocated for mental health by the total local tax revenue.

roughly comparable with about 500 per 100,000 population. SASH Outreach is lowest, with a rate of 387 per 100,000 population. The reasons for this become clearer when the revenue sources of the CMHCs are examined.

The category with the most dramatic variation is total per capita funding, ranging from $12.62 at Tri County to $3.10 at SASH Outreach. Tri County spends four times per capita more than SASH and roughly 40 percent more than Dallas County or Concho Valley. In FY 1988, while the three community centers all received direct state aid from TDMHMR amounting to between $6.00 and $6.26 per capita, San Antonio State Hospital Outreach, whose only source of revenue was TDMHMR, only received $3.10 per capita in state funding. This low figure is somewhat deceiving since outreach services does receive off-budget aid from the state hospital, such as for crisis stabilization beds. But even with all support from SASH taken into account, this is still a very low figure considering the needs of the population.

A major difference between the three CMHMRCs (keeping in mind that SASH Outreach is not a CMHMRC) is the level of local funding per capita. The category of local funds includes local taxes, combined with funds from other sources generated by local efforts including contracts with other state agencies and Medicaid/Medicare funds. In terms of total local funds, Tri County received $6.01 per capita compared with $2.75 for Concho Valley and $2.54 for Dallas County. When local tax effort only is examined, the range was from a low of $0.42 per capita for Tri County to a high of $2.19 for Dallas County. As a percentage of total local funds, the figures are even more telling. For Dallas County MHMRC, local taxes made up 86 percent of the total local funds, for Concho Valley they made up 37 percent, but for Tri County they made up only 7 percent of the total local effort. This very low percentage is primarily the result of Tri County's aggressiveness in obtaining funds from other state agencies, in spite of limited funding from local counties.

The most significant difference between these centers is in service provision. The number of case managers does not seem to significantly correlate with the number of state hospital admissions, nor does residential beds per 100,000 in the service area. However, the number of crisis stabilization beds per 100,000 seems to be related to the reduction in hospital admissions. The availability of crisis beds within the service area seems to provide an avenue for the centers to stabilize those who might otherwise be in the state hospital. SASH Outreach is a very good example of this, with 232 admissions per 100,000 and no crisis stabilization beds. There are crisis stabilization beds for SASH Outreach, but they happen to be at the San Antonio State Hospital and therefore not part of the outreach budget. However, since the point of crisis stabilization beds is to keep people out of the state hospitals, and since these beds are at times 200 miles from the patients, the result is that the SASH Outreach area uses the hospital much more than other areas. At Concho Valley, with only one crisis bed, the rate was reduced to 120 admissions per 100,000. Since only 365 days at a local private hospital are budgeted, Concho Valley must be quite restrictive as to how many patients it puts in the crisis unit and thus how quickly it runs out of funds before the end of the year. Concho Valley must refer a number of clients to Big Spring State Hospital who would probably be assigned to crisis residential beds if they were available.

Dallas County, with 80 crisis residential beds, had a rate of 77 admissions per 100,000. This admission rate compares favorably with that of Concho Valley but is significantly above the reported rates of 23 admissions in Harris County and 50 per 100,000 in Tarrant County. In these cases, both Harris County and Tarrant County benefit from state-funded hospitals in their counties to which admissions are not counted as state hospital admissions.

Finally, Tri County's state hospital admissions are an order of magnitude below that of the other centers. In 1988, its rate of 12.58 admissions per 100,000 was the lowest of all the community centers in the state. In part this is due to the availability of 25 structured crisis residential beds and a higher ratio of such beds per capita than are available at the other three centers. It is also no doubt due to a quite aggressive treatment approach to clients who live in the Tri County area. A final consideration may be, ironically, the lack of availability of housing in the Tri County area. There are no board and care facilities in the three counties, and local law enforcement does not permit persons to sleep on the street. These factors might mean that some of the chronically mentally ill, without stable housing arrangements from family or the few apartments available through the community center, emigrate to Houston, Dallas, or Austin where either board and care homes are available or sleeping outside is permitted. The subsequent hospital admissions of such persons would not generally be counted against the Tri County hospitalization rate.

This variation in service provision is not only evident with these four case studies, but also throughout the 63 local Mental Health Authorities within the state. This points to a need to rethink the funding relationship between the CMHMRCs and TDMHMR. The legislature recognizes the need for appropriating increased funds for care at the community mental health centers. The accountability system with regard to monitoring care is quite limited. Equitable treatment of centers is difficult when some centers have much more serious problems with homeless persons and unsupervised board and care homes. This is even further complicated by the presence in some areas of Texas of state-funded state centers, or in Harris and Tarrant counties of psychiatric hospitals, which exist in parallel to local community centers and are not counted in the local budgets or the local hospital rates.

One method of having better accountability, and a more efficient use of state funds, is to move away from contracted services to a purchased services approach to funding CMHMRCs. The TDMHMR board has been given the authority to cancel or modify contracts, or to recoup payment from contracting CMHMRCs that do not meet specified criteria. However, it is hesitant to do so unless the circumstances are extreme. The result of this practice is that services may be purchased from the CMHMRCs by TDMHMR with state funds but never received (LBB, 1989, p. 154). During FY 1988, the LBB found that the contracts of the various CMHMRCs fell short of their goals. As an example of this shortfall, Table 6.2 shows the number of structured bed days and semi-independent bed days that were contracted for by TDMHMR and how many days were actually used by the CMHMRCs.

Table 6.2. Mental Health Services--Contracted vs. Actual FY 1988

	Contracted	Actual	Variation
Structured Bed Days	208,946	182,818	26,146
Semi-Independent Bed Days	318,434	275,489	42,854
Totals	527,308	458,307	69,000

Source: Legislative Budget Board, Performance Report to the 71st Legislature (Austin, January 1989), p. 154.

According to the LBB, a total of 69,000 mental health bed days were purchased but not received. The LBB estimates that this amounted to a loss of service valued at $1.8 million in state funds (LBB, 1989, p. 154).

One funding mechanism that, in theory, would avoid this inefficient use of state funds would be for TDMHMR to purchase these services from the CMHMRCs after they have been delivered rather than before. Clients would use the core services at the CMHMRCs, which would then bill TDMHMR for the services actually used. This could provide the centers with an added incentive to find clients who have been released from state hospitals or are at risk of being admitted. The state could set minimum levels of service that the centers must provide, but would give them extra funds to bring in those who need service. This method could be an effective application of the concept of funds following the client. Further, it would help the centers develop the level of documentation necessary in the future to bill Medicaid for some services.

The concept that funds follow the client is quite sound, but it falls apart if no one is following the client and making sure that appropriate services are being provided. Between 1983 and 1988, there were 61,599 individuals admitted to the state hospitals in Texas. Of that number, 43.7 percent have never been registered at a CMHMRC (TDMHMR, 1988). The CMHMRCs need to be given the funds and incentives to give these clients care after they have been released from the state hospital.

Alternative approaches to funding community-based care include arrangements such as those in Wisconsin, where the county is the funding authority; if the patient needs care at the county hospital, the care is purchased by the mental health authority. Different approaches to capitation of the chronically mentally ill are being developed whereby the responsible local authority receives a capitation payment for each mentally ill client assigned to it and in return must provide full services to all such clients assigned. In either case, the responsibility is firmly in the hands of the local mental health authority.

One of the major obstacles for the CMHMRCs in treating the chronically mentally ill in the community is lack of affordable housing. In some areas, such as the SASH Outreach services area, the problem of housing is acute. The chronically mentally ill who live in the major urban areas have been served by the registered and unregistered board and care homes. But for those in local MHAs with few housing alternatives, the chances of returning to the state hospitals are greater. Funds need to be made available for housing clients. Needed housing ranges from contracting with board and care homes to the purchase of houses and apartment complexes so that centers can offer alternatives to meet the diverse needs of their clients.

In most MHAs, the shortage of funds is particularly reflected in limitations on psychosocial programs. In the SASH Outreach area there is a minimum of such services. At Dallas County MHMR in particular, there is exemplary psychosocial programming, but service availability falls far short of demand. Staff at Dallas County estimated that Independence House could be replicated in another part of the county and effectively treat another 250 clients.

One of the important shortcomings that these case studies point out is the failing of Texas to provide adequate mental health care in the rural areas of the state. These neglected areas are forced to use the state hospitals at a higher rate, as illustrated by the figures for SASH Outreach in Table 6.1. Steps should be taken to provide the funding and personnel needed to provide these areas with adequate mental health clinics.

It is hoped that this volume of case studies illuminates the problems and potentials of community-based mental health care delivery throughout Texas. The variation in care shown by these four delivery systems indicates the need for changes in how TDMHMR manages and funds the CMHMRCs and state hospital outreach services. Development of new funding approaches and more comprehensive services may lead to more adequate care of this most dependent and fragile population in Texas.

References

Crumpton, Laurie, Chandler Stolp, and David Warner. 1989. Hospital Care for Schizophrenia in California in 1984. Working Paper Series No. 54. Austin: Lyndon B. Johnson School of Public Affairs, University of Texas at Austin.

Legislative Budget Board (LBB). 1989. Performance Report to the 71st Legislature. Austin, January 10.

Texas Department of Mental Health and Mental Retardation (TDMHMR). 1988. "Care System" Data.

Torrey, E. Fuller, et al. 1988. Care of the Seriously Mentally Ill: A Rating of State Programs. 2nd ed. Washington D.C./Arlington Va.: Public Citizen Health Research Group/National Alliance for the Mentally Ill.

Warner, David C., Laurie Crumpton, and Gary Watts. Forthcoming. "Financial Costs of Caring for the Chronically Mentally Ill in Texas." In Community Care of the Chronically Mentally Ill. ed. Charles Bonjean, Marion Coleman, and Ira Iscoe. Austin: Hogg Foundation for Mental Health.